THE NEUROSCIENCE
OF CLINICAL
PSYCHIATRY

THE PATHOPHYSIOLOGY OF BEHAVIOR
AND MENTAL ILLNESS

THE NEUROSCIENCE OF CLINICAL PSYCHIATRY

THE PATHOPHYSIOLOGY OF BEHAVIOR AND MENTAL ILLNESS

Edmund S. Higgins, MD

Clinical Associate Professor of Family Medicine and Psychiatry
Medical University of South Carolina
Charleston, South Carolina

Mark S. George, MD

Distinguished Professor of Psychiatry, Radiology, and Neurosciences
Medical University of South Carolina
Charleston, South Carolina

Director, MUSC Center for Advanced Imaging Research
Medical University of South Carolina
Charleston, South Carolina

Illustrations by Edmund S. Higgins, MD

Wolters Kluwer | Lippincott Williams & Wilkins
Health
Philadelphia · Baltimore · New York · London
Buenos Aires · Hong Kong · Sydney · Tokyo

Acquisitions Editor: Charles W. Mitchell
Managing Editor: Sirkka Howes Bertling
Project Manager: Rosanne Hallowell
Manufacturing Manager: Kathleen Brown
Marketing Manager: Adam Glazer
Design Coordinator: Teresa Mallon
Cover Designer: Karen Klinedinst
Production Services: Laserwords Private Limited, Chennai, India
Printer: R. R. Donnelley

Library of Congress Cataloging-in-Publication Data

Higgins, Edmund S.
  The neuroscience of clinical psychiatry : the pathophysiology of behavior and mental illness / Edmund S. Higgins, Mark S. George ; illustrations by Edmund S. Higgins.
     p. ; cm.
  Includes bibliographical references and index.
  ISBN-13: 978-0-7817-6655-5
  ISBN-10: 0-7817-6655-9
  1. Mental illness—Pathophysiology. 2. Psychiatry. I. George, M. S. (Mark S.), 1958- II. Title.
  [DNLM: 1. Mental Disorders—physiopathology. 2. Nervous System—physiopathology.
3. Neuropsychology—methods. WM 140 H636n 2007]
  RC483.H54 2007
  616.89—dc22

                                                                    2007004849

Care has been taken to confirm the accuracy of the information presented and to describe generally accepted practices. However, the authors, editors, and publisher are not responsible for errors or omissions or for any consequences from application of the information in this book and make no warranty, expressed or implied, with respect to the currency, completeness, or accuracy of the contents of the publication. Application of this information in a particular situation remains the professional responsibility of the practitioner.

The authors, editors, and publisher have exerted every effort to ensure that drug selection and dosage set forth in this text are in accordance with current recommendations and practice at the time of publication. However, in view of ongoing research, changes in government regulations, and the constant flow of information relating to drug therapy and drug reactions, the reader is urged to check the package insert for each drug for any change in indications and dosage and for added warnings and precautions. This is particularly important when the recommended agent is a new or infrequently employed drug.

Some drugs and medical devices presented in this publication have Food and Drug Administration (FDA) clearance for limited use in restricted research settings. It is the responsibility of health care providers to ascertain the FDA status of each drug or device planned for use in their clinical practice.

The publishers have made every effort to trace copyright holders for borrowed material. If they have inadvertently overlooked any, they will be pleased to make the necessary arrangements at the first opportunity.

To purchase additional copies of this book, call our customer service department at (800) 639-3030 or fax orders to (301) 824-7390. International customers should call (301) 714-2324. Lippincott Williams & Wilkins customer service representatives are available from 8:30 am to 6:00 pm, EST, Monday through Friday, for telephone access. Visit Lippincott Williams & Wilkins on the Internet: http://www.lww.com.

10 9 8 7 6 5 4 3 2

To my eldest son Fess, for his assistance with the artwork on Tuesday mornings at local coffee shops while waiting for school to open.

—ESH

To Eloise, my dance partner for 27 years now, who has acetylated large portions of my DNA through wonderful shared life experiences.

—MSG

Contents

SECTION III
Disorders

Preface

Neuroscience is the basic science of psychiatry. Neuroscience describes the brain mechanisms that

- gather information from the external and internal world,
- analyze the information, and
- execute the best response.

Psychiatric disorders are the result of problems with these mechanisms.

The increased accessibility to the workings of the brain in the last 25 years has resulted in an explosion of information about neuroscience. Different lines of research such as brain imaging and animal studies along with more traditional postmortem analysis, medication effects, and genetic studies have transformed the way we conceptualize normal and abnormal behavior.

Bits and pieces of the neuroscience literature have filtered up to the practicing clinician, but a comprehensive understanding of the field is almost inaccessible to all but the most dedicated self-educators. The jargon is foreign and difficult to navigate. The standard textbooks are thick with multiple authors and almost impossible to read cover to cover. The relevance to the practice of psychiatry can sometimes be hard to appreciate.

We hope this book will provide a way for residents and practicing clinicians to gain a thorough appreciation for the mechanisms within the brain that are stimulating (or failing to stimulate) their patients. We also hope that the reader will have more accurate answers for the patient who asks, "What's causing my problem?" Likewise, we hope the reader will be better prepared for the increasingly difficult neuroscience questions that are appearing on board certification tests.

If we've learned anything from our studies of the brain, it is that LEARNING IS WORK! The brain increases its metabolism when conducting academic assignments. The process of focusing one's attention, understanding the concepts, and storing the new information requires energy. There is no passive learning.

Consequently, when learning is interesting and relevant it requires less energy. We have made every effort to make this material appealing and easy to consume. Pictures, drawings, and graphs have been liberally incorporated to allow the reader to learn the concepts quickly and efficiently. Every effort has been made to keep the material short and concise, but not too simple. Finally, we think information that is relevant to the reader is easier to retain, so we have tried to keep bringing the focus back to the practice of psychiatry.

We intend our book to be for three populations. First, it is for those in training: psychiatrists, psychologists, counselors and allied physicians. Second, it is for psychiatric residents seeking to review the topics in preparation for their board examinations. And last, it is for the practicing clinician who was trained before the revolution in neuroscience who would like to become more up-to-date and familiar with the field.

We hope that the reader will have a thorough—soup to nuts—understanding of the important topics in neuroscience and henceforth, be able to read and comprehend the future research in this field.

Edmund S. Higgins, MD
Mark S. George, MD

Acknowledgments

The authors wish to thank the following people for their assistance with this manuscript: Sherri A. Brown for her assistance with the artwork; Pamela J. Wright-Etter, MD, and Robert J. Malcolm Jr., MD, who reviewed individual chapters; and Laura G. Hancock, DO, and L. William Mulbry, MD, residents, who reviewed the entire book.

Figures 3.6, 3.7, 3.8, 12.5, and 19.1 were drawn by Fess Higgins.

About the Authors

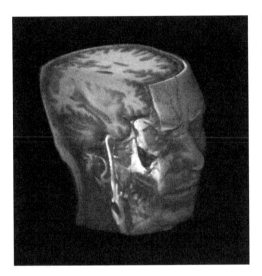 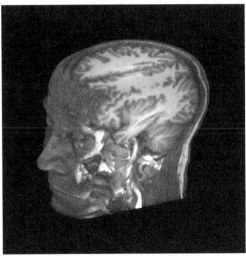

Edmund S. Higgins, MD   Mark S. George, MD

Edmund S. Higgins, MD, is a Clinical Associate Professor of Family Medicine and Psychiatry at the Medical University of South Carolina (MUSC). He received his medical degree from Case Western Reserve University School of Medicine. He completed residencies in Family Practice and Psychiatry at MUSC. He is currently the Department Editor for Neuroscience News in *Current Psychiatry*. He is also the Medical Director for Psychiatric Services at the Charleston County Detention Center and has a private psychiatric practice. He lives on Sullivan's Island, South Carolina.

Mark S. George, MD, is a Distinguished Professor of Psychiatry, Radiology, and Neurosciences as well as Director of the Center for Advanced Imaging Research and the Brain Stimulation Laboratory, Psychiatry, at the Medical University of South Carolina, Charleston. He received his medical degree and completed dual residencies at MUSC in both neurology and psychiatry and is board certified in both areas. After a fellowship in London and four years at NIMH, he returned to Charleston where he has conducted pioneering work with functional imaging of the brain, transcranial magnetic stimulation, and vagus nerve stimulation. He is on several editorial review boards, has published over 300 scientific articles or book chapters, has eight patents, and has written or edited four books. He too resides on Sullivan's Island, South Carolina.

The Basic Structures

Historical Perspective

One of the most remarkable paradigm shifts that has occurred during our lives has been the recognition that most of our behavior is inherited. Eccentric, compassionate, outgoing, irritable, and so on: Traits such as these travel in families from generation to generation. And as we all know, inheritance equals biology. Figure 1.1 shows the relationship between shared genes and the likelihood of developing schizophrenia if a relative has the disease.

Perhaps even more remarkable is the power of inheritance to interact with the environment to dictate our personality. Bouchard and others have studied this eloquently by looking at personality characteristics in monozygotic (identical) and dizygotic (fraternal) twins reared together and apart. Using personality tests to assess five major personality traits, they found more correlations for monozygotic twins compared with dizygotic twins regardless of whether they were raised together or apart (see Table 1.1). In other words, the monozygotic twins reared apart shared more personality characteristics than dizygotic twins reared in the same household. Their overall conclusion was that these personality traits are strongly influenced by inheritance and only modesty affected by environment. (The lay press unfortunately summarized this research as "Parents Don't Matter.")

Figure 1.2 shows a remarkable example of identical twins separated when 5 days old, raised in different households—one in Brooklyn, the other in New Jersey—who met for the first time at the age of 31. Both are firemen, bachelors, with mustaches and metal frame glasses. Not only do they have the same mannerisms but they also laugh at the same jokes and enjoy the same hobbies. Yet, they were exposed to entirely different environmental influences throughout their lives.

Our individuality—who we are, how we socialize, what we like, even our religious beliefs—may be influenced more by the brain we are born with and its predetermined development than by the experiences we have along the way. We are not excluding the importance of environment in molding our character, particularly the negative influence of trauma. It is just that our brains are more programmed than we previously believed.

The brain has not always been of interest to humankind. Most ancient cultures did not consider the brain to be an important organ. Both the Bible and Talmud fail to mention diseases related to the brain. Egyptians carefully embalmed the liver and the heart but had no use for the brain; they scooped it out and threw it away. (If there really is an Egyptian afterlife—those poor pharaohs are spending eternity without a brain.)

But, first, how did we go from ignoring the brain to where we are now?

BRIEF HISTORY OF NEUROSCIENCE

Thomas Willis—after whom the Circle of Willis at the base of the brain was named—was the first neurologist. In the 17th century, he moved us into what one author has called the *Neurocentric Age*. Before Willis—and actually for a considerable time after him—physicians based their understandings of illness on the writings of the great physicians from antiquity. Willis took the unusual approach of describing a patient's behavior,

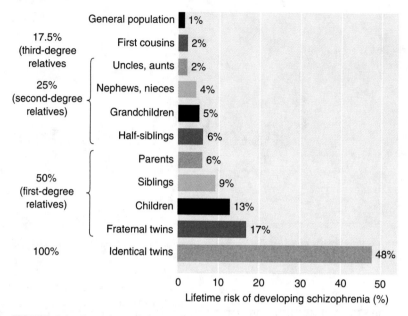

FIGURE 1.1 ● As the shared genetic profile with someone having schizophrenia increases, the risk of developing schizophrenia also increases. (Adapted from Gottesman II. *Schizophrenia genesis.* New York: WH Freeman; 1991.)

then examining the brain after death and making correlations.

He was the first to coin terms such as *lobe, hemisphere*, and *corpus striatum*—terms that we still use. Comparing the human central nervous system (CNS) anatomy with that of animals and conducting postmortem dissection of interesting

cases, he made surprisingly accurate conclusions about higher brain functions versus lower brain functions. For example, he deduced that human functions such as memory were likely to reside in the "outmost banks" (gray matter) of the cerebral hemispheres because these areas were smaller in animals and damaged in individuals with severe

TABLE 1.1

The Correlations for Five Personality Traits in Monozygotic Twins Reared Apart and Together, and Dizygotic Twins Reared Apart and Together

Personality Trait	Monozygotic, Apart	Monozygotic, Together	Dizygotic, Apart	Dizygotic, Together
Extraversion	0.41	0.54	0	0.19
Neuroticism	0.49	0.48	0.44	0.19
Conscientiousness	0.54	0.54	0.07	0.29
Agreeableness	0.24	0.39	0.09	0.11
Openness	0.57	0.43	0.09	0.11
Mean	**0.45**	**0.48**	**0.17**	**0.18**

The mean correlations are surprisingly similar to the lifetime risk of developing schizophrenia for identical (monozygotic) and fraternal (dizygotic) twins shown in Figure 1.1.

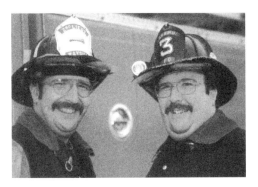

FIGURE 1.2 ● Gerald Levy (left) and Mark Newman are identical twins who were separated at birth, yet have made many of the same choices in life. (From The Image Works, Woodstock, New York.)

Central sulcus

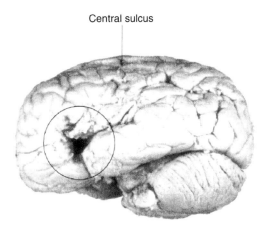

FIGURE 1.3 ● The preserved brain of the patient who helped Broca convince physicians that some functions—in this case the ability to speak—were localized in the cerebrum. (Adapted from Bear MF, Connors BW, Paradiso MA, eds. *Neuroscience: Exploring the Brain,* 3rd ed. Baltimore: Lippincott Williams & Wilkins; 2007.)

head injuries who had lost memory. He believed that the brainstem likely controlled basic functions such as breathing and heart rate. However, he also thought that the white matter was the seat of imagination—so he was not entirely on target, but he started the process of matching structures with behaviors.

At the start of the 18th century, it was still not clear how nerves worked. *Luigi Galvani*, an Italian physician (memorialized by the term *galvanic skin response*), demonstrated through extensive experimentation that a frog muscle will twitch when stimulated with electricity. This demonstrated that the substance flowing through the nerves was not air, fluid, or spirits, but electricity. Galvani proposed that the brain secretes electricity, which is then distributed to the muscles by the nerves. He also believed that the electricity did not leak into the surrounding tissue because the nerves were covered with a fatty insulation, which we now know is myelin. Not all his beliefs were accurate, but he made the big leap to recognizing that mammals have intrinsic electrical activity that coordinates movement.

Before the 1860s the brain was seen as a single multipurpose organ, much the way we currently view the liver or pancreas. The French physician *Paul Broca* with his famous case in 1861 confirmed for the first time that certain functions were localized to specific regions of the brain (see Figure 1.3). The patient in this case exhibited a loss of articulate speech, although he retained oral dexterity, and he could understand and hear. All he could utter was one syllable: "tan." His speech could have great emotional tone, but the syllable never changed. After his death, an autopsy revealed a lesion of his left frontal lobe—what is now called *Broca's aphasia*. The fact that almost

all similar cases were on the left hemisphere and that similar right hemispheric lesions did not affect speech also led Broca to identify cerebral dominance for some functions.

David Ferrier of Scotland and *Eduard Hitzig* of Germany independently identified the specialized cortical areas controlling motor function. Using the techniques of stimulation and ablation in experimental animals, they localized and mapped out what we now call the motor cortex. This new understanding of the brain provided the first examples of useful neurosurgical treatment given on the basis of the patient's motor symptoms. There is a case report from 1879 of a teenage girl with seizures of the right face and arm who had a left meningioma accurately diagnosed and removed. With the development of antiseptic techniques and effective anesthesia, surgeons could successfully localize and remove some tumors using Ferrier's map of the motor cortex.

It is noteworthy that both men speculated about higher brain functions and the lobes in front of the motor cortex—the prefrontal cortex. Ferrier noted problems with attention in monkeys with damaged frontal lobes. Experimenting with dogs, Hitzig came to believe that the frontal cortex played an important role in abstract thought.

The discovery of individual neurons was a major step in the development of neuroscience. In order to be able to see nerve cells, it was necessary to be able to fix the brain (which can have the consistency of gelatin) and to cut thin slices; in addition, microscopes of sufficient power

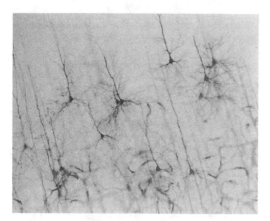

FIGURE 1.4 ● Individual pyramidal nerve cells can be identified after incubation with Golgi's silver stain. (Adapted from Bear MF, Connors BW, Paradiso MA, eds. *Neuroscience: Exploring the Brain,* 3rd ed. Baltimore: Lippincott Williams & Wilkins; 2007.)

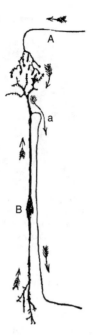

FIGURE 1.5 ● Drawing of neurons by Cajal showing the unidirectional nature of impulses in the communication between neurons A and B. (From Ramon y Cajal S. *Recollections on my life. Transactions of the American Philosophical Society,* Vol. 8, Part 2. Philadelphia: The American Philosophical Society; 1937.)

were needed. An Italian physician, *Camillo Golgi,* discovered a selective silver stain that allowed researchers to visualize the individual nerve cells in what was otherwise a uniform blob of color. For the first time, researchers could see sharp black images of the nerve cells and identify specific parts such as the cell body and the dendritic branches (see Figure 1.4). Termed the *Golgi stain,* this technique is still used today.

Santiago Ramón Cajal, a Spanish physician, used Golgi's stain, a Zeiss light microscope, and 25 years of patient observation to become perhaps the first modern neuroscientist. He proposed that individual nerve cells are the singular unit of the brain—a new concept at that time, which has since been called the *neuron doctrine.* By tracing neurons from sensory organs such as the eye back to the cortex and from the motor cortex to the muscles, he concluded that the dendrites are receptive, the cell body is executive, and the axon transmits the information over a long distance.

Cajal went on to show that nerve impulses flow only in one direction—what he called his *law of dynamic polarization.* Figure 1.5 is one of his drawings, with little arrows showing the direction of the impulses between two communicating neurons. Additionally, Cajal observed and meticulously drew the embryonic development of neurons. He was the first to document the growth of an axon that ultimately branches with dendrites and collateral axons. In 1894, Cajal stated in a lecture to the Royal Society of London, "the ability of neurons to grow in an adult and their power to create new connections can explain learning."

This is often cited as the origin of the synaptic theory of memory. Both Golgi and Cajal received the Nobel Prize for Physiology and Medicine in 1906.

Charles Sherrington, an English neurophysiologist, did extensive studies of animal nerves. Focussing mostly on the spinal and peripheral nerves, he advanced the understanding of sensory dermatomes and reflexes. He is best known for giving us the term *synapse.* Although he never actually saw one—and they wouldn't be seen until the development of the electron microscope— Sherrington theorized that a physical junction existed between nerves to pass along an impulse.

Another English neurophysiologist (who shared the 1932 Nobel Prize with Sherrington), *Edgar Adrian* is best known for recognizing the "all-or-nothing" properties of the action potentials. With regard to behavior and the brain, his major discoveries dealt with habituation and the sensory cortex. Adrian found that a stimulus to a nerve cell is followed by a burst of action potentials coursing down the axon. However, the quantity of action potentials decreases over time even if the stimulus remains unchanged. This explains at the level of the neuron the basis for a well-known treatment for anxiety: exposure therapy.

In the beginning of the 20th century, it was not known how neurons communicate with each other or how a neuron can make a muscle contract. Some believed the communication was electrical—as though a spark jumped from one neuron to another. Others believed a chemical process transmitted the signal. No one had evidence establishing one system or another. *Henry Dale* and *Otto Loewi*, an Englishman and a German, shared the Nobel Prize in 1936 for their work in establishing the chemical transmission of nerve impulses. Dale was working with the autonomic nervous system and established that an epinephrine-like compound had activating effects on the sympathetic nervous system, and that acetylcholine could activate the parasympathetic nervous system as well as skeletal muscles. Unfortunately, Dale was unable to show that epinephrine (or really norepinephrine) and acetylcholine were excreted by the neurons to elicit these effects.

It was Otto Loewi who in 1921 performed the elegant little experiment that proved the neurochemical transmission of nerve impulses. Legend has it that Loewi dreamed the experiment and, upon awaking early in the morning, rushed down to the laboratory and performed it. The experiment is depicted in Figure 1.6. Loewi's clever experiment showed that stimulating the vagus nerve slowed down the beating of the frog heart bathed in Ringer's solution. He then transferred some of that solution to another isolated frog heart and, without electrical stimulation, its rhythm also slowed down—as though its vagus nerve had been stimulated. He concluded that a chemical was excreted from the synapses of the first heart when the vagal nerve was stimulated. This chemical then

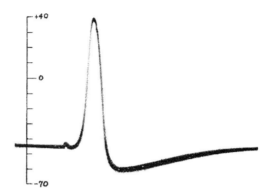

FIGURE 1.7 ● First-published intracellular recording of an action potential. (From Hodgkin AL, Huxley AF. Action potentials recorded from inside a nerve fibre. *Nature*. 1939;144:710–711.)

flowed into the container holding the second heart and induced bradycardia.

In 1939, *Hodgkin* and *Huxley* published the first intracellular recording of an action potential (see Figure 1.7). Before this time, no one had directly measured the electrical charge in an axon as an action potential passed. Hodgkin and Huxley were able to accomplish this by inserting microelectrodes into the giant axons of squids.

One of the more amazing accomplishments of a developing neuron is the ability to accurately make the correct connection between the brain and the motor neuron—which in the case of a whale may be 60 feet. *Robert Sperry*, in the 1940s, utilized the amphibian capacity to regenerate axons and established that the connections are determined precisely. He cut the optic nerve of a newt and rotated the eye 180 degrees. With the eye back in the socket, axons regenerated, taking a convoluted path to the original locations in the vision center of the amphibian brain. However, because the eye was upside down, the poor newt had his ups and downs crossed—for example, he would lift his head to bite a bug on the ground. Sperry speculated that growing nerves recognized their appropriate location through a mechanism of chemical guidance, although he did not find a specific messenger. It has been the work of many others in the intervening years that has identified the multitude of molecules that attract, inhibit, and repulse the growing neuron.

Sperry is best known in psychology circles for his work with "split-brain" individuals. Some patients with intractable seizures have had their corpus callosum cut to prevent the seizures from spreading from one side of the brain to the other (see Figure 1.8). The procedure often produced remarkable improvements without appearing to

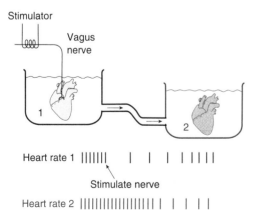

FIGURE 1.6 ● Otto Loewi's famous experiment establishing that a chemical from the vagus nerve of one heart can induce bradycardia in a second unstimulated heart.

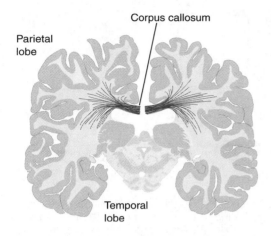

Parietal lobe

Corpus callosum

Temporal lobe

FIGURE 1.8 ● The corpus callosum contains millions of axons crossing between the two hemispheres. Sperry established that surgical resection of this structure interrupts the passage of information from one hemisphere to another.

affect the individual's personality or intellectual functioning. Sperry, with careful experimentation, was able to show that the left and right hemispheres no longer share information in such individuals. With further experimentation, he established that the left hemisphere has superior language and arithmetic skills whereas the right hemisphere has better spatial skills.

The discovery of trophic factors that promote the development and survival of nerve cells was the result of *Rita Levi-Montalcini* et al. recognizing the significance of an accidental finding. They discovered that sensory nerves grew unusually large when cultured next to a specific mouse sarcoma. With some effort they isolated the protein that they called *nerve growth factor* (NGF). Figure 1.9 shows the profound impact NGF has on the growth of sensory neurons. Since this landmark discovery, many other growth factors have been isolated. Some of these growth factors may play important roles in the development of psychiatric disease and will be discussed in subsequent chapters.

MODERN RESEARCH
Imaging

Researchers such as Willis and Broca were forced to wait for a patient to die before they could examine the brain. These scientists were studying patients with damaged brains using what some have called the *lesion method*. Although this remains an important tool for the modern neuroscientist (now there are large "brain banks" preserving brains of patients with similar illnesses), the noninvasive analysis of the CNS has transformed the way we study behavior and mental disorders.

Early attempts to image the brain were unhelpful, painful, and even dangerous. An ordinary x-ray provides little information because the brain is soft tissue and not radiopaque. Searching for displacement of calcified structures could provide indirect evidence of a mass. Pneumoencephalography, in which cerebrospinal fluid (CSF) is removed and replaced with air to enhance visualization of the CNS, is an example of the painful and dangerous extremes that were foisted on patients in earlier times.

The development of noninvasive imaging techniques (see Table 1.2) has led to another small revolution in neuroscience. Although the functional studies (positron emission tomography [PET], single photon emission computerized tomography

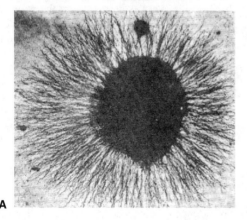

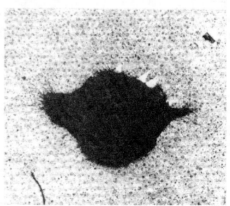

A

B

FIGURE 1.9 ● The sensory nerves in (**A**) show robust growth when exposed to nerve growth factor. (From Levi-Montalcini R. The nerve growth factor. *Ann NY Acad Sci.* 1964;118:149–170.)

POINT OF INTEREST

The Figure shows a method of using imaging studies frequently found in the literature. That is, one functional study is subtracted from another and the result is superimposed on a structural image. In this case the subject is performing a finger opposition task with his right fingers while in a SPECT scanner (A). The white arrow shows the activation of the left motor cortex. (B) A SPECT scan in the controlled state is also produced. (C) The control image is substrated from the task image. (D) The results are superimposed on an MRI of the same location and drawings of the human homunculus along the motor cortex are added for further understandina.

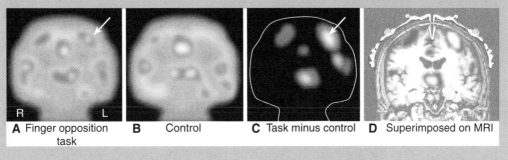

| A Finger opposition task | B Control | C Task minus control | D Superimposed on MRI |

Functional imaging substraction study superimposed on structural image.

[SPECT], and functional magnetic resonance imaging [fMRI]) remain largely limited to research, the noninvasive structural analyses (computed tomography [CT] and magnetic resonance imaging [MRI]) have transformed the practice of neurology.

Animal Studies

Animal studies provide the second major technique for understanding the workings of the brain. Some clinicians unfairly discount the significance of "rat studies." Clearly, animals do not possess a similarly developed human cerebral cortex, nor can we ever be sure they actually have psychiatric symptoms. However, they can provide sophisticated analyses that are beyond the scope of human studies. Besides the well-known microelectrode stimulation or ablation studies that we will mention throughout this book, there are several new techniques that seem almost unbelievable and are worth explaining.

Microdialysis

While we speculate that psychiatric medications increase the neurotransmitters at the synapse, it is difficult to prove this. Microdialysis involves a small, permanently implanted micropipette that allows continuous sampling of the neurochemistry at specific locations in the CNS in active animals. This technique was used to show that cocaine will increase the excursion of dopamine at the nucleus accumbens (see Chapter 9, Pleasure).

Markers of Gene Activation

Neurochemical transmission between two neurons in some situations can have more lasting effects than just depolarization of the membrane. The transmission of the signal ultimately leads to activation of the DNA or what is frequently called *gene expression*. Researchers can measure mRNA or proteins that are a result of this "gene expression" as a way of determining where a specific neurotransmitter operates. Cyclic adenosine monophosphate responsive element-binding protein (CREB) and proteins in the Fos family are two transcription factors that are frequently used as markers of gene expression. Identifying CREB or FOS in a postmortem brain slice helps pinpoint the areas in the brain that were active in the animal during the experimental manipulation.

Knockout Mice

Animals (typically mice) can be bred to establish a population that does not have a particular receptor—or has the receptor in markedly reduced numbers. The mice can be observed for certain behaviors or how they respond to established interventions. For example, mice bred deficient in the corticotrophin-releasing hormone receptor 1 (Crhr-1) showed a reduction in anxiety-related

TABLE 1.2

A Brief History of Imaging Methods Used to Analyze the Central Nervous System

Date	Initials	Name	Method	Specifics
1918	X-ray	Pneumoencephalography	Replacing CSF with air	Painful and dangerous
1927	X-ray	Cerebral angiography	Injecting contrast into circulation	Visualizes the cerebral vasculature
1970s	CT	Computed tomography	Ionizing radiation	Changed the way we practice medicine
	PET	Positron emission tomography	Decay of positron-emitting radionuclides	Measures activity of brain by analyzing blood flow
	SPECT	Single photon emission computed tomography	Single photon emission	More widely available than PET; lower resolution
1980s	MRI	Magnetic resonance imaging	Magnetic changes induced in molecules	No radiation; noninvasive; high resolution
	fMRI	Functional magnetic resonance imaging	Measures changes in blood oxygen used by brain regions	Has allowed extensive explorations of brain localization of function

CSF, cerebrospinal fluid.

behaviors, suggesting neuroendocrine involvement in fear and anxiety (see Chapter 19, Anxiety).

However, there are limits to the assumptions we can make about the brain and behavior from knockout mice. We never know what profound effect the absence of that receptor may have had on normal development. Likewise, we do not know what unintended downstream effects are caused by the missing receptor.

DNA Microarrays—Also Called Gene Chips

DNA microarrays enable researchers to compare the mRNA (and therefore gene activity) from tissue sample to DNA with known activity. The microarray is a chip no bigger than a postage stamp with thousands of different DNA molecules, multiplied, segregated, and attached in separate tiny locations (see Figure 1.10).

The mRNA from the tissue being studied is transcribed to DNA, labeled with fluorescent markers, and dropped onto the microarray chip. The single-stranded DNA from the tissue sample will bind with similar single-stranded DNA on the microarray. The chip is then read in a scanner that calculates the amount of binding between the tissue DNA and the chip DNA in each discrete spot, giving an estimate of that specific gene activity in the tissue. As an example, this procedure was done with small samples from

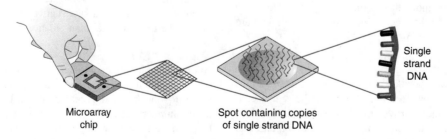

Microarray chip

Spot containing copies of single strand DNA

Single strand DNA

FIGURE 1.10 ● The microarray chip contains multiple copies of many different genes so that a broad spectrum of gene activity can be analyzed quickly in a scanner.

the prefrontal cortex of schizophrenic and control postmortem brain. Remarkably, the schizophrenic brains showed reduced expression of myelination-related genes, suggesting a disruption in the myelin as part of the pathogenesis of schizophrenia (see Chapter 20, Schizophrenia).

Viral-Mediated Gene Transfer

Researchers can use viruses to introduce a sequence of DNA into the neurons at specific locations in the brain of laboratory animals. For example, using a virus to implant the DNA for the vasopressin receptor in the ventral pallidum of promiscuous voles, researchers were able to create monogamous voles (see Chapter 14, Social Attachment).

The Controlled Trial

It is discouraging to realize that the brain is so resistant to change. It is more discouraging to read about eccentric clinicians, parents, teachers, and other meddlers expounding the effectiveness of their unproven interventions to reduce symptoms or improve behavior. Sugar and hyperactivity are "known" to have a cause and effect relationship that has unfortunately failed to materialize in controlled trials.

We tend to conceptualize the pathogenesis of psychiatric disorders as the absence of what we are replacing with our treatment (neurotransmitters, a superego, the corrective emotional experience, etc.). It is important to prove that these interventions are actually working. Perhaps the greatest research tool in health care has been the controlled trial. With this technique we can determine with some confidence how effective interventions might be, which then gives us some insight into the working of the brain.

QUESTIONS

Part 1: Match the names in the right column with the events in the left column.

L 1. Started the Neurocentric Age

E 2. The brain has intrinsic electric activity.

B 3. Localization of function

D 4. The motor cortex

F 5. Silver stain

C 6. Individual nerve cells are the singular unit of the CNS.

J 7. Coined the term *synapse*

A 8. "All-or-nothing"

H 9. Neurochemical transmission of nerve impulses

G 10. First action potential

K 11. Chemical guidance of regenerating nerves

I 12. Nerve growth factors

A. Edgar Adrian

B. Paul Broca

C. Santiago Ramón Cajal

D. David Ferrier

E. Luigi Galvani

F. Camillo Golgi

G. Hodgkin and Huxley

H. Otto Loewi

I. Rita Levi-Montalcini

J. Charles Sherrington

K. Robert Sperry

L. Thomas Willis

Part 2: Match the columns.

13. Implanted micropipette   P

14. Activation of DNA   N

15. Missing receptors   O

16. Single-stranded DNA   M

17. Implanting specific traits   Q

M. DNA microarray

N. Gene expression

O. Knockout mice

P. Microdialysis

Q. Viral-mediated gene transfer

See Answers section at end of book.

Neuroanatomy

CEREBRAL CORTEX

There are many large textbooks with extensive writings and illustrations providing all the known specifics about the anatomy of the nervous system. If you are looking for that sort of detail, then you are reading the wrong book. We—on the other hand—have tried to limit our discussion of neuroanatomy to those structures that are frequently identified in the scientific articles that are relevant to the clinician treating mental illness.

The cerebral cortex is made up of white matter and gray matter. The white matter is primarily myelinated axons transporting impulses between the gray matter and lower brain structures. The gray matter is where the nerve cells and synapses reside, that we so often discuss in mental health treatment. The architectural order of cells and fibers in the gray matter conforms to a basic structural plan with subtle differences.

Brodmann's Areas

In the early part of the 20th century many neuroanatomists were struggling to divide the neocortex into structurally distinct regions. Korbinian Brodmann, a German neurologist, was working in a psychiatric clinic where he was influenced by Alois Alzheimer to pursue a career in neuroscience basic research. After extensive analysis of the human and monkey neocortex, he published in 1909 his classic work *Comparative Localization Studies in the Brain Cortex, its Fundamentals Represented on the Basis of its Cellular Architecture.* He had divided the neocortex into 52 regions based on the size, number, and density of the cells

as well as the local connections and long tract projects to and from the subcortical regions (see Figure 2.1).

Brodmann's scheme is still widely used and often mentioned in the scientific literature. For example, in the studies using microarrays to analyze schizophrenia mentioned in Chapter 1, Historical Perspective, the researchers removed tissue from region 46 in the postmortem brains. Another group that replicated the study sampled tissue from region 9.

The neocortex that Brodmann examined and categorized is made up of six layers, with few exceptions (see Figure 2.2). The pyramidal neurons with their triangular-shaped cell bodies make up approximately 75% of the cortical neurons. They have a single apical dendrite pointed toward the pial surface and a number of basilar dendrite branches projecting horizontally. The axons project to other cortical regions or the subcortex. Likewise, excitatory projections come in from the other brain regions. The local connections or interneurons are typically inhibitory γ-aminobutyric acid (GABA) neurons.

The neuroanatomy most commonly cited in neuroscience literature, discussing behavior and mental disorders, is shown in Figure 2.3 and reviewed in the subsequent text.

Prefrontal Cortex

The prefrontal cortex (PFC) is in front of the motor cortex. This is one of the anatomic structures that distinguishes humans from other mammals. Brodmann calculated that the PFC as a percentage of the total cortex is 3.5% in the cat, 7% in the dog, 8.5%

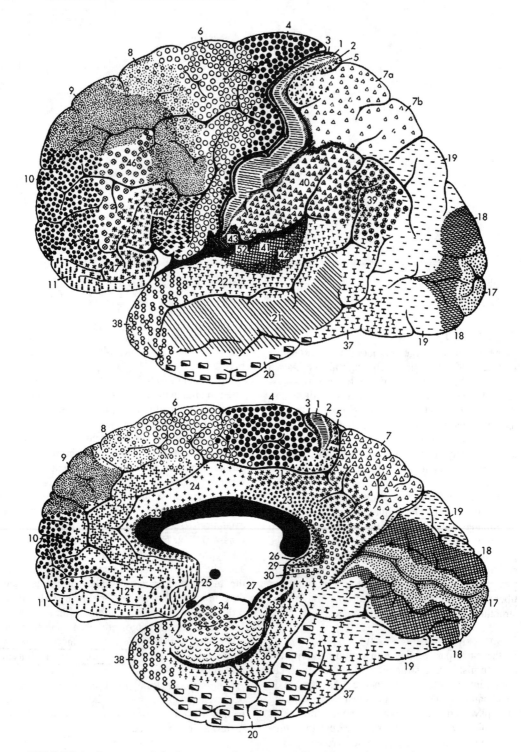

FIGURE 2.1 ● Areas of the human cerebral cortex defined by Brodmann in his 1909 publication.

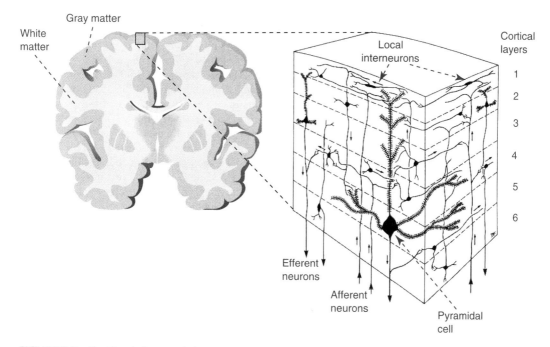

FIGURE 2.2 ● The six layers of the neocortex, from the pial surface above layer 1 to the white matter below layer 6. (Adapted from Bear MF, Connors BW, Paradiso MA, eds. *Neuroscience: exploring the brain,* 3rd ed. Baltimore: Lippincott Williams & Wilkins; 2007; and Snell RS. *Clinical neuroanatomy: a illustrated review with questions and explanations,* 3rd ed. Philadelphia: Lippincott Williams & Wilkins; 2001.)

in the lemur, 11.5% in the macaque, 17% in the chimpanzee, and 29% in humans. Dysfunction in the PFC is implicated as a possible source of pathology in many psychiatric disorders—depression, schizophrenia, anxiety, and attention deficit hyperactivity disorder (ADHD) as well as anger and violence.

There are four regions of the PFC that are mentioned frequently in the scientific literature and are shown in Figure 2.4. Unfortunately, there is no consensus on the wording of the general regions.

Different terms are combined frequently to describe a specific region, for example, ventrolateral or medial orbital. The astute clinician needs to have an understanding of the general regions and be ready to adapt.

Neurologists, assessing and following up patients with injuries (e.g., Phineas Gage—see Chapter 11, Anger and Aggression), have identified three different syndromes associated with frontal lobe damage. The location, core characteristics, and common symptoms are briefly outlined

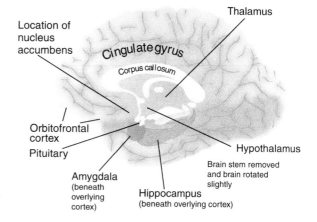

FIGURE 2.3 ● Several of the important brain structures involved in behavior. (Adapted from Bear MF, Connors BW, Paradiso MA, eds. *Neuroscience: exploring the brain,* 3rd ed. Baltimore: Lippincott Williams & Wilkins; 2007.)

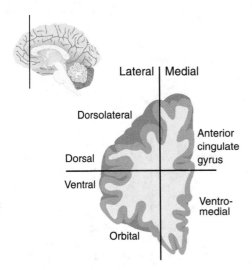

Lateral | Medial

Dorsolateral

Dorsal

Ventral

Anterior
cingulate
gyrus

Ventro-
medial

Orbital

FIGURE 2.4 ● A section of the prefrontal cortex cut just anterior to the genu of the corpus callosum. (Adapted from Lewis DA. Structure of the human prefrontal cortex. *Am J Psychiatry.* 2004;161[8]:1366.)

in Table 2.1. The three syndromes roughly correlate with the three regions of the PFC. Although it is appealing to associate a location with specific behavioral pattern, it is not that simple. Most patients have clinical features of more than one of the syndromes because few lesions are confined to one region. Furthermore, recent imaging studies do not always find correlation between the anatomy and the traditional syndromes.

Hippocampus

The hippocampus and the amygdala are the essential structures of what is commonly called the *limbic lobe*—although there is no specific lobe. The hippocampus is a folded structure incorporated within the temporal lobe and dorsal to other important cortical structures of the rhinal sulcus (or primitive smell brain). The hippocampus is made up of two thin sets of neurons that look like facing "C"s—the dentate gyrus and the Ammon's horn. Ammon's horn has four regions of which only CA3 and CA1 are shown in Figure 2.5.

The hippocampus plays an essential role in the development of memories (see Chapter 15, Memory) and is one of the few locations in the brain where we know that stem cells reside (see Chapter 7, Adult Development and Plasticity). Additionally, the volume of the hippocampus is decreased in various psychiatric disorders (e.g., post-traumatic stress disorder [PTSD] and major depression), suggesting that these regions may play a role in the pathogenesis of these disorders.

Amygdala

The amygdala lies within the temporal lobe just anterior to the hippocampus (see Figure 2.6). Using the anatomy and connections, the amygdala can be divided into three regions: the medial group, the central group, and the basolateral group. The basolateral group, which is particularly large in humans, receives input from all the major sensory systems. The central nucleus sends output to the hypothalamus and brain stem regions. Therefore, the amygdala links sensory input from

TABLE 2.1

The Three Traditional Frontal Lobe Syndromes and the Associated Regions and Symptoms

Location	Syndrome	Symptoms
Orbital (orbitofrontal)	Disinhibited	Poor impulse control
		Explosive outburst,
		Inappropriate behavior
Dorsolateral (dorsal convexity)	Disorganized	Cognitive dysfunction
		Diminished judgment, planning, and insight
		Concrete and inflexible
		Decreased spontaneous behavior
Medial (ventromedial)	Apathetic	Paucity of spontaneous behavior
		Sparse verbal output

TREATMENT: PREFRONTAL LOBOTOMY

The infamous prefrontal lobotomy was developed in Portugal in 1935 by the neurologist Egas Moniz. He coined the term *psychosurgery* and later even won the Nobel Prize for Medicine for his work. The procedure was intended to sever the afferent and efferent fibers of the prefrontal lobe and produce a calming effect in patients with severe psychiatric disease.

Walter Freeman popularized and simplified the procedure in the United States. He developed a minimally invasive technique, shown in the figure, called the *transorbital lobotomy*. An instrument resembling an ice pick was inserted under the eyelid through the orbital roof and blindly swept left and right. It is hard to believe what Freeman reported in 1950—that out of 711 lobotomies 45% yielded good results, 33% produced fair results, and 19% left the patient unimproved or worse.

Although initially received with enthusiasm, in part due to the unavailability of other effective treatments, the development of unacceptable personality changes (unresponsiveness, decreased attention span, disinhibition, etc.) led to a decline in the procedure. Ultimately, the development of effective pharmacologic treatments brought an end to this drastic intervention.

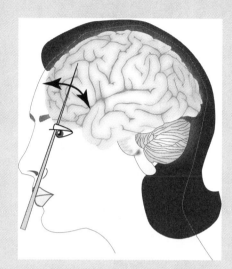

Transorbital frontal lobotomy. (Adapted from Bear MF, Connors BW, Paradiso MA, eds. *Neuroscience: exploring the brain,* 3rd ed. Baltimore: Lippincott Williams & Wilkins; 2007.)

DISORDER: LIMBIC LOBE

The limbic lobe concept is a term that occasionally appears in psychiatric literature, but not one that we will use. It was originally introduced in 1878 by Broca, who noted that the cingulate gyrus, hippocampus, and their connecting bridges formed a circle on the medial side of the hemispheres. He called the structure *le grand lobe limbique*. Paul MacLean in the mid-1950s popularized the concept by linking the structure to emotional functions. Historically, this was a big step in associating emotions with neuroanatomy and has had a large impact on biologic psychiatry.

Exactly what constitutes the limbic system has never been well defined nor is it clear that the structures involved (amygdala, hippocampus, cingulate gyrus) have unique connections that process emotions. The problem originates from the attempt to impose emotional functions on to a number of closely related structures, rather than trying to find which structures are responsible for particular emotions. We prefer to identify the neuroanatomy involved with a specific emotion instead of using the more ambiguous limbic system concept.

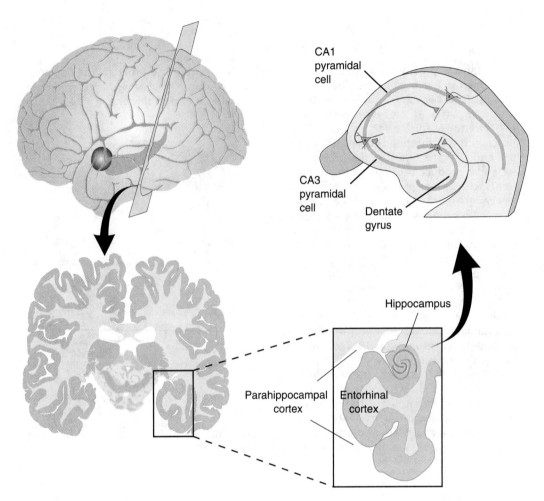

FIGURE 2.5 ● Different views of the hippocampus. (Adapted from Bear MF, Connors BW, Paradiso MA, eds. *Neuroscience: exploring the brain,* 3rd ed. Baltimore: Lippincott Williams & Wilkins; 2007. and Kandel ER, Schwartz JH, Jessell TM, eds. *Principles of neural science,* 4th ed. New York: McGraw-Hill; 2000.)

cortical regions with hypothalamic and brain stem effectors. The amygdala is active when people are anxious and/or angry, which will be discussed further in subsequent chapters. Likewise, when the organ is removed these emotions are impaired.

Hypothalamus

If there were little tiny persons that sit inside our head (which there are not), watching the "control panel" from our body and making decisions about internal settings, they would sit at the hypothalamus. This small cluster of nuclei makes up less then 1% of the brain mass yet has powerful effects on the body's homeostasis. The hypothalamus controls such basic functions as eating, drinking, sleeping, and temperature regulation, to name a few. A small lesion in the hypothalamus has devastating effects on the body's basic functions.

The suprachiasmatic nucleus is an example of a small cluster of cells within the hypothalamus that has a profound impact on our daily lives (see Chapter 12, Sleep).

The hypothalamus sits in a commanding position within the central nervous system (CNS), between the cortex and brain stem (see Figure 2.7). It receives input from four sources: the higher cortex, the brain stem, internal chemoreceptors, and hormonal feedback. The cortex relays filtered cognitive and emotional information about the external environment. The sensory neurons in the body send signals about the internal milieu up through the brain stem. The hypothalamus has its own chemoreceptors that measure glucose, osmolarity, temperature, and so on, in the blood. Finally, the hypothalamus receives feedback from the steroid hormones and neuropeptides.

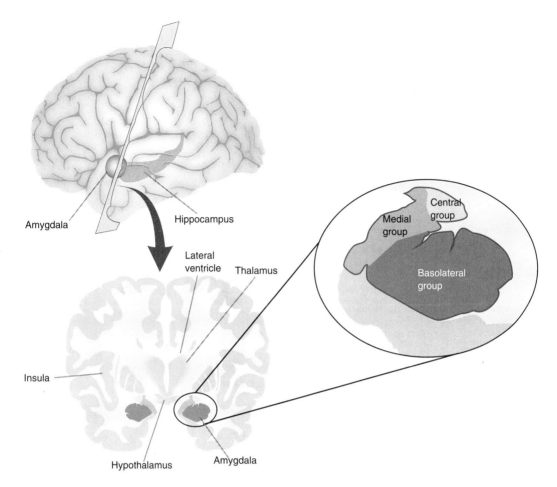

FIGURE 2.6 ● The location and groups (often called *nuclei*) of the amygdala.

The hypothalamus lies on either side of the third ventricle and is divided into three zones. The lateral zone controls arousal and motivated behavior. The medial zone is more involved with homeostasis and reproduction. The periventricular zone is of most interest to us. It includes the suprachiasmatic nucleus, cells that control the autonomic nervous system (ANS) (discussed in the subsequent text), and the neurosecretory neurons that extend into the pituitary (see Chapter 6, Hormones and the Brain).

AUTONOMIC NERVOUS SYSTEM

The ANS can be thought of as the brain's extensions to the vital organs of the body (see Figure 2.8.) There are two branches. There is the sympathetic division, which originates in the posterolateral region of the periventricular zone of the hypothalamus. The other branch is the parasympathetic division, which originates in the anterior cells of the same zone in the hypothalamus. The sympathetic and parasympathetic divisions appear to operate in parallel but with opposite effects and use different neurotransmitters.

The sympathetic division, in a simplified sense, controls the fight–flight response and plays a prominent role in the physical symptoms of anxiety, for example, racing heart. These neurons send out their axons from the thoracic and lumbar regions to preganglionic neurons, which primarily reside in the sympathetic chain on either side of the spinal cord. The postganglionic sympathetic neurons innervate the smooth muscles of the vital organs as well as the walls of blood vessels. The preganglionic neurons are cholinergic, whereas the postganglionic neurons use norepinephrine. The postganglionic norepinephrine receptors likely explain why β-blockers can be used to quell the physical symptoms of anxiety, for example, performance anxiety.

The parasympathetic neurons mediate functions that the body performs in times of calm, for

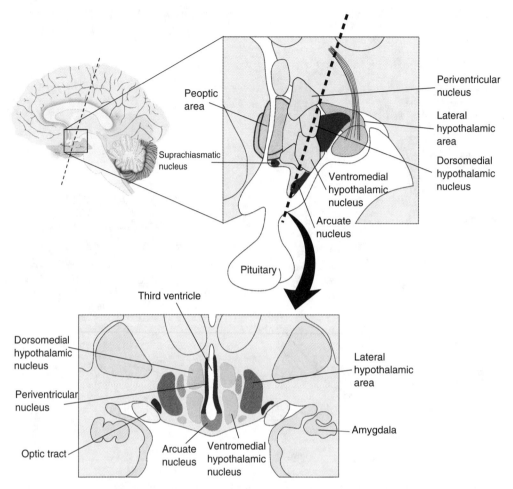

FIGURE 2.7 ● The hypothalamus lies on either side of the third ventricle in close proximity to the pituitary gland. The hypothalamus can be subdivided into multiple nuclei, many of which are not shown. (Adapted from Kandel ER, Schwartz JH, Jessell TM, eds. *Principles of neural science*, 4th ed. New York: McGraw-Hill; 2000.)

example, digest food. These neurons emerge from the brain stem and sacral region of the spinal cord. The axons travel longer distances and innervate ganglia typically located at the end organ. Unlike the sympathetic neurons, the parasympathetic neurons are exclusively cholinergic.

For the psychiatrist, the ANS occasionally complicates the treatment of mental disorders—particularly when using the tricyclic antidepressants. Side effects such as dry mouth, tachycardia, and constipation can be seen as an imbalance between the sympathetic and parasympathetic divisions. These symptoms are not so much the result of sympathetic stimulation as they are the result of parasympathetic blockade. The likely culprit is blockade of the muscarinic receptor in the cholinergic neurons of the parasympathetic division (see Chapter 4, Neurotransmitters).

CEREBELLUM

The cerebellum sits on top of the brain stem, at the back of the skull, below the cerebral cortex. Once considered the "lesser brain" and only involved with the coordination of movement, more recent functional imaging studies have shown that the cerebellum "lights up" in a wide variety of behaviors. Not only is it active in sensation, cognition, memory, and impulse control but it has also been implicated to be playing a role in the pathophysiology of autism, ADHD, and schizophrenia.

Fossil records document that the cerebellum has grown throughout human evolution and actually contains more neurons than any other part of the brain. Yet, its function is not clearly understood. Of particular interest, if the cerebellum is totally removed, especially in young persons, they can with time regain almost normal function.

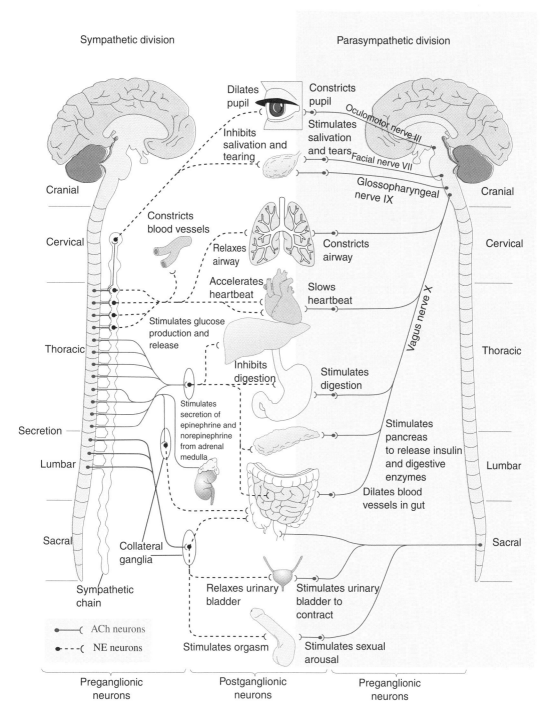

FIGURE 2.8 ● The two divisions of the autonomic nervous system and the end organs they inner-vate. (Adapted from Bear MF, Connors BW, Paradiso MA, eds. *Neuroscience: exploring the brain,* 3rd ed. Baltimore: Lippincott Williams & Wilkins; 2007.)

This does not happen with similar removal of the motor or sensory cortex, in which case the person remains impaired.

It appears that the cerebellum is a supportive structure for the cerebral cortex. Some have speculated that it grew throughout evolution to provide extra computational support for an overburdened cortex. This reasoning proposes that the cerebellum is not responsible for any one particular task, but rather functions as an auxiliary structure for the entire cerebral cortex—not just movement. We anticipate increased reports of the important role of the cerebellum in mental illness, in the future.

BLOOD–BRAIN BARRIER

The brain needs to be bathed in a pristine extracellular environment. If the brain is exposed to the fluctuations in hormones, amino acids, or ions that occur in the rest of the body, unexpected neuronal activity could result. The *blood–brain*

barrier (BBB) is one mechanism the brain uses to maintain a controlled environment, isolated from the rest of the body.

Historically, it was thought that the barrier was produced by the astrocytes that hold the capillaries with their foot processes. Later it became clear that it is the tight junctions between the endothelial capillary cells that form the continuous wall preventing many substances from entering the CNS (see Figure 2.9). There are a few areas of the brain that have gaps in the BBB. The pituitary gland and some parts of the hypothalamus are two examples of these BBB gap regions. This is logical because these areas need to receive unfiltered feedback regarding the status of the endocrine system by way of the circulating blood.

The BBB is not an impenetrable wall, as the brain needs constant supplies to perform its functions. Lipid-soluble substances can readily diffuse through the lipophilic cell walls. Conversely,

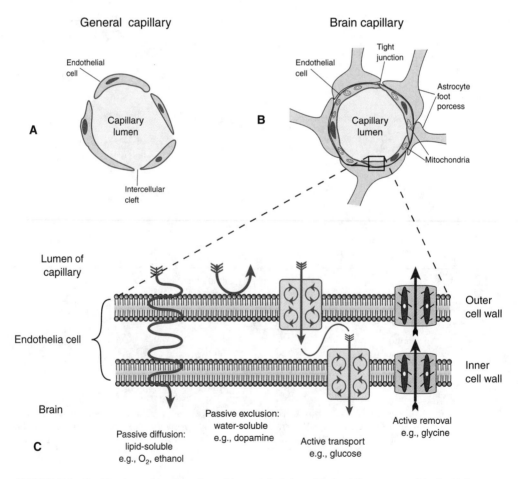

FIGURE 2.9 ● The loose junctions found in peripheral capillaries (**A**) contrast with the tight junctions formed in the brain endothelial cells (**B**). Passive and active transport mechanisms allow the movement of substances between the brain and blood stream (**C**).

TREATMENT: NERVE GROWTH FACTORS

An ongoing struggle for the pharmaceutical industry is how to get potential therapeutic molecules across the BBB. It is estimated that 70% of drugs are excluded from the brain. Of particular interest are the nerve growth factors that have exceptional potential to heal, but cannot cross the BBB. Recent work has focused on alternative methods to circumvent the BBB. Researchers at the University of Wisconsin have used stem cells to deliver glial cell line–derived neurotrophic factor (GDNF) to primates with Parkinson's disease. The stem cells were engineered to produce GDNF, a growth factor known to affect the growth and survival of dopamine neurons. When injected into the striatum of the animals, GDNF was delivered to the substantia nigra and parkinsonian symptoms were decreased. This remarkable intervention has potential for other treatment-resistant neurologic diseases such as multiple sclerosis (MS) and amyotrophic lateral sclerosis (ALS).

water-soluble substances are deflected by the endothelial cell wall. Yet, the brain needs some water-soluble substances, such as glucose, and indeed there are active transport mechanisms within the endothelial cell wall to bring these essential substances into the brain.

The endothelial cells also actively transport offensive substances out of the brain's extracellular environment. The P-glycoprotein is such a transporter. Found in the gut as well as the brain, this protein actively removes a wide variety of drugs and deposits them in the capillary lumen. For example, the nonsedating antihistamines are excluded from the CNS by this protein whereas the older antihistamines such as diphenhydramine are not—hence their different effects on fatigue.

QUESTIONS

1. Brodmann's areas are differentiated by the
   a. Cortical morphology.
   b. Cellular architecture.
   c. Afferent connections.
   d. Predominant neurotransmitter.

2. The orbitofrontal aspect of the PFC describes the area
   a. Above the corpus callosum.
   b. Posterior to the amygdala.
   c. At the base of the PFC.
   d. Anterior to the cingulate gyrus.

3. Lesions of the medial (also ventromedial) PFC are associated with
   a. Paucity of spontaneous behavior—apathetic.
   b. Disorganized cognitive function.
   c. Concrete thinking.
   d. Poor impulse control.

4. All of the following are true about the hippocampus except that it
   a. Is smaller in some psychiatric disorders.
   b. Is involved with memory.
   c. Is disrupted by frontal lobotomy.
   d. Contains undifferentiated stem cells.

5. The "command center" of the brain is the
   a. Hippocampus.
   b. Amygdala.
   c. ANS.
   d. Hypothalamus.

6. All of the following are true about the sympathetic nervous system except that it
   a. Stimulates digestion.
   b. Is associated with anxiety.
   c. Stimulates secretions from the adrenal medulla.
   d. Relaxes the airways.

7. The cerebellum
   a. Solely functions to support movement.
   b. Has been implicated with autism.
   c. Is similar to the motor cortex.
   d. Is relatively small in humans.

8. The BBB can be crossed by all of the following except
   a. Lipid-soluble molecules.
   b. Active transport across the cell wall.
   c. Breaches in the tight junctions.
   d. Most medications.

See Answers section at end of book.

Cells of the Nervous System

THE NEURONAL CELL

The human brain is the most complex organ known to exist in the universe. The workhorse of the brain is the neuron. It is estimated that we have 100 billion neurons with 100 trillion connections. The most prominent neuron in the cerebral cortex is the pyramidal cell. These neurons have a diamond-shaped cell body and usually reside in layers III or V of the gray matter (see Figure 3.1).

The cell body of the neuron is full of the usual assortment of organelles, although not in the same proportions as seen in nonneural cells. Structures such as the *endoplasmic reticulum* and *mitochondria* are found more frequently in neurons than in other brain cells, presumably because of the increased need for protein synthesis and energy. The instructions for the functioning of the cell are contained in the DNA, which resides in the nucleus. The instructions are enacted when the DNA is *transcribed* into messenger ribonucleic acid (mRNA) which is *translated* into proteins in the cytoplasm (see Figure 3.2). As mentioned in Chapter 1, Historical Perspective, this process is often called *gene expression*.

The *ribosome* is the organelle in which mRNA is translated into proteins (see Figure 3.3). The ribosomes are usually attached to the *endoplasmic reticulum* (rough ER), but can also be floating freely in the cytoplasm. The proteins, once they are refined, are used by the cell for structural (e.g., receptors), functional (e.g., enzymes), or communication (e.g., neuropeptides) purposes, to name a few.

The *Golgi apparatus*, which looks like endoplasmic reticulum without the ribosomes, is where much of the "posttranslation" refinement, sorting, and storage of proteins occurs (see Figure 3.4). This apparatus enables proteins to be appropriately transported to distant sites within the cell such as the dendrites.

The *mitochondria* are the energy generators of the neuron and are abundant in these cells, which reflects the active nature of the brain. The mitochondria convert adenosine diphosphate (ADP) into adenosine triphosphate (ATP) and it is ATP that the cell uses to perform its functions.

The *dendrites* are the part of the neuron that sprout off the cell body and look like tree branches. They have been called the *ears* of the neuron for they receive input from other neurons and relay it to the cell body. Most dendrites have little knobs along their stalks that are called *dendritic spines*. Each spine is the postsynaptic receptor for an incoming signal. The morphology and quantity of the branches and spines of the dendrites have been a focus of considerable interest. Dendritic abnormalities are the most consistent anatomic finding of mental retardation. Although the exact morphology varies depending on the cause of retardation, a typical finding is a reduction in the number and length of dendritic branches along with sparse and thin spines.

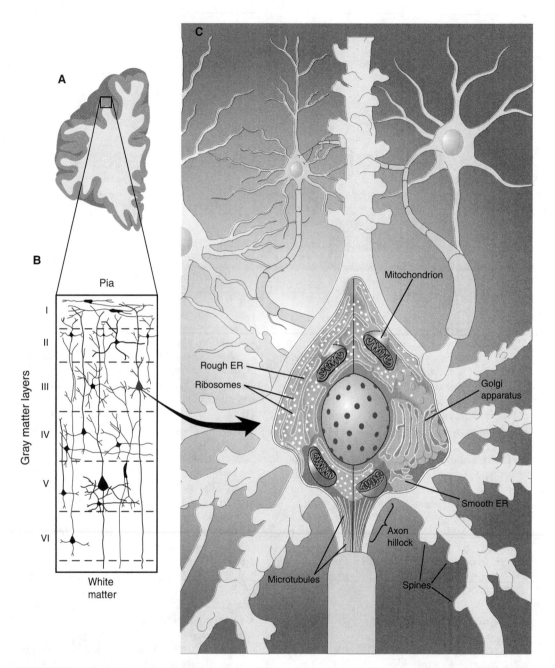

FIGURE 3.1 ● **A:** Cross section of the right prefrontal cortex (PFC). **B:** The six layers of neurons in the gray matter of the PFC. **C:** A stereotypical pyramidal neuron found in layer three of the cerebral cortex. ER, endoplasmic reticulum. (Adapted from Bear MF, Connors BW, Paradiso MA, eds. *Neuroscience: Exploring the Brain,* 3rd ed. Baltimore: Lippincott Williams & Wilkins; 2007.)

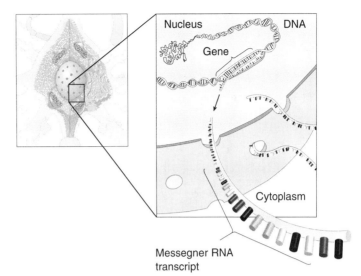

FIGURE 3.2 ● Messenger ribonucleic acid (mRNA) carries the genetic instructions from the nucleus to the cytoplasm where translation into proteins occurs. (Adapted from Bear MF, Connors BW, Paradiso MA, eds. *Neuroscience: Exploring the Brain,* 3rd ed. Baltimore: Lippincott Williams & Wilkins; 2007.)

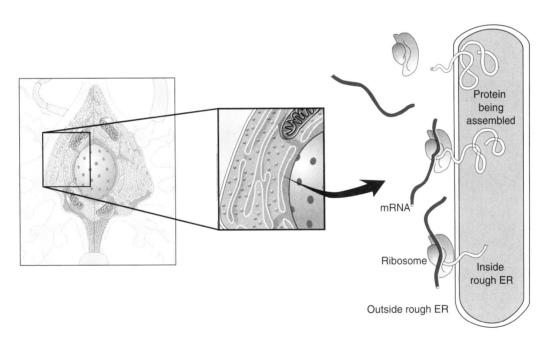

FIGURE 3.3 ● Messenger ribonucleic acid (mRNA) binds to a ribosome, initiating protein synthesis. Proteins synthesized on the rough endoplasmic reticulum (ER) as shown are eventually inserted into the membrane. Proteins synthesized on free ribosomes (not shown) are utilized in the cytosol. (Adapted from Bear MF, Connors BW, Paradiso MA, eds. *Neuroscience: Exploring the Brain*, 3rd ed. Baltimore: Lippincott Williams & Wilkins; 2007.)

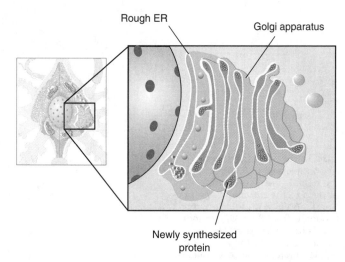

Rough ER

Golgi apparatus

Newly synthesized
protein

FIGURE 3.4 ● The Golgi apparatus where proteins are refined
and stored. ER, endoplasmic reticulum. (Adapted from Bear MF,
Connors BW, Paradiso MA, eds. *Neuroscience: Exploring the Brain,* 3rd
ed. Baltimore: Lippincott Williams &
Wilkins; 2007.)

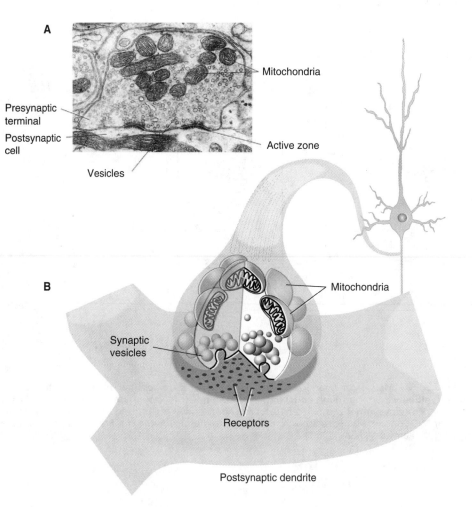

A

Mitochondria

Presynaptic
terminal

Postsynaptic
cell

Active zone

Vesicles

B

Mitochondria

Synaptic
vesicles

Receptors

Postsynaptic dendrite

FIGURE 3.5 ● A synapse as seen with an electron microscope (**A**) and in a schematic
drawing (**B**). Note the high concentration of vesicles filled with neurotransmitter and mitochondria to power the rapid processing. (Adapted from Bear MF, Connors BW, Paradiso
MA, eds. *Neuroscience: Exploring the Brain,* 3rd ed. Baltimore: Lippincott Williams &
Wilkins; 2007.)

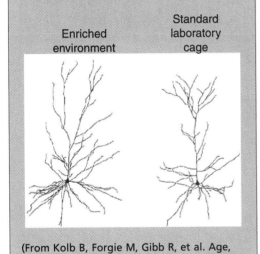
The *axon* is perhaps the most unique struc-
ture of the neuron. Starting at the *axon hillock*
and running either only a few micrometers or the
length of the spinal cord, the axon can transmit a
signal quickly without degradation to other neurons or end organs. For this reason the axon is
often conceptualized as the telephone wire of the
brain. Because the axon is devoid of ribosomes
and incapable of protein synthesis, a process called
axoplasmic transport enables the neuron to send
material down the microtubules to the distal ends
of the cell.

The terminal end of the axon forms the synapse
(see Figure 3.5). Here the electrical signal sent
down the axon is converted into a chemical signal, so that the neuron can communicate with its
neighbor. The neurotransmitters that form the basis of the chemical signal are stored in vesicles
and diffuse across the synaptic cleft to the receptors on the postsynaptic dendrite when the vesicles
open (this is discussed in more detail later in the
chapter).

ELECTRICAL SIGNALING

All living cells maintain a negative internal elec-
tronic charge relative to the fluid outside of the
cell—roughly −60 mV in a neuron. Nerve cells
use the depolarization of this charge to signal other
nerves or end organs. There are two basic steps
in this process. The neuron first receives signals
through the dendrites—what are called *postsynaptic potentials.* Second, the cell sums the incoming
impulses and if high enough sends an impulse
down the axon—an *action potential.*

Postsynaptic Potentials

A single pyramidal cell will receive input from
1 to 100,000 neurons through the postsynaptic
synapses on the dendrites and cell body. When
the neurotransmitters bind with the receptor at the
postsynaptic synapse, ions flow into the neuron
and generate a potential or in other words a signal,
but not an action potential. An action potential is
generated only in the axon.

There are two ways to change the potential of
the dendrite:

depolarize (excite) with an influx of positive ions
    such as Na^+ and
hyperpolarize (inhibit) with an influx of negative
    ions such as Cl^-.

These are appropriately called *excitatory postsynaptic potentials* (*EPSPs*) and *inhibitory postsynaptic potentials* (*IPSPs*) (see Figures 3.6 and 3.7).
The EPSP and IPSP are, the accelerator and brake,
respectively, for the brain. The goal for a healthy
brain is to maintain the correct balance—too much
excitation and one can have a seizure, too much
inhibition and the brain can be sluggish, even
comatose.

The Action Potential

The most important words in regard to the action potential are *threshold* and *all-or-none.* The
neuron will sum up all the incoming EPSPs and
IPSPs at the axon hillock. If the potential has de-
polarized to the threshold then an action potential
is generated. This occurs by the opening of the
voltage-gated sodium channels and the rapid influx of positive ions. Like other ion channels, the
voltage-gated sodium channel is a protein embedded in the lipid member of the cell. The "gated"
nature of the channel means that this type of

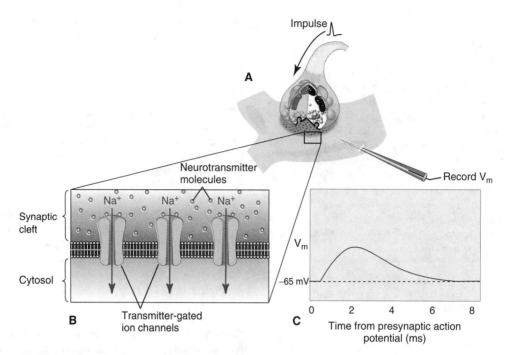

FIGURE 3.6 ● Excitatory postsynaptic potential (EPSP). When an impulse arrives at the dendrite from an excitatory neuron (**A**), the neurotransmitter binds with the receptor and allows the entry of positively charged sodium ions (**B**). The resulting depolarization generates an EPSP (**C**). (Adapted from Bear MF, Connors BW, Paradiso MA, eds. *Neuroscience: Exploring the Brain*, 3rd ed. Baltimore: Lippincott Williams & Wilkins; 2007.)

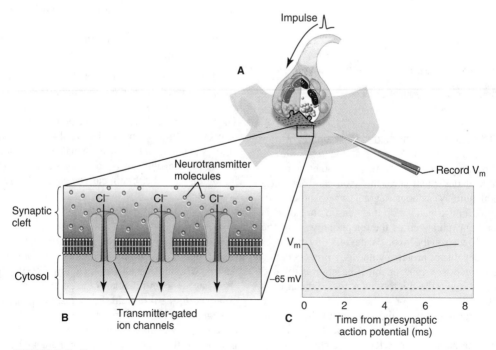

FIGURE 3.7 ● Inhibitory postsynaptic potential (IPSP). When an impulse arrives at the dendrite from an inhibitory neuron (**A**), the neurotransmitter binds with the receptor and allows the entry of negatively charged chloride ions (**B**). The resulting hyperpolarization generates an IPSP (**C**). (Adapted from Bear MF, Connors BW, Paradiso MA, eds. *Neuroscience: Exploring the Brain*, 3rd ed. Baltimore: Lippincott Williams & Wilkins; 2007.)

TREATMENT: CALM DOWN

As clinicians, we are often treating patients who have too much cerebral excitation. Anxiety, attention deficit hyperactivity disorder (ADHD), insomnia, and mania are four conditions in which the brain is going too fast and the goal of treatment is to calm down the brain. We can conceptualize that, for whatever reason, such patients do not have enough inhibition. It is encouraging that more research is being directed toward treatments that increase inhibitory potentials (e.g., γ-aminobutyric acid [GABA]). The challenge is to selectively inhibit the offending trait either for the whole brain or, even better, in the disordered region.

pore allows a large and fast influx of the particular ions once the threshold has been crossed. Figures 3.8 through 3.10 show how the neuron requires enough depolarization (excitation) and not too much hyperpolarization (inhibition) to generate an action potential.

If the threshold (−40 mV) has been reached at the axon hillock, the neuron "pulls the trigger" and shoots an action potential down the axon. Because of the unique feature of the voltage-gated sodium channels, the action potential maintains its integrity as it proceeds along the axon—there is no diminution in voltage. Axons wrapped with myelin can speed along an action potential at up to 15 times faster than those without myelin.

Electrochemical Signaling

As Otto Loewi demonstrated in 1921, the communication within the nervous system is *both* electrical and chemical. Figure 3.11 shows a representation of the arrival of the action potential at the synaptic terminal, the release of the neurotransmitters, and the generation of an excitatory or inhibitor postsynaptic potential in the dendrite

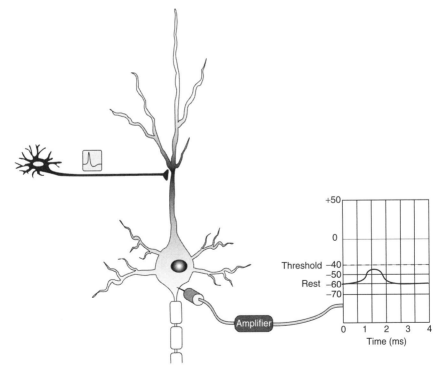

FIGURE 3.8 ● The black neuron on the left sends an excitatory impulse to the central neuron. The impulse generates an excitatory postsynaptic potential, but it is not strong enough to reach the threshold and start an action potential.

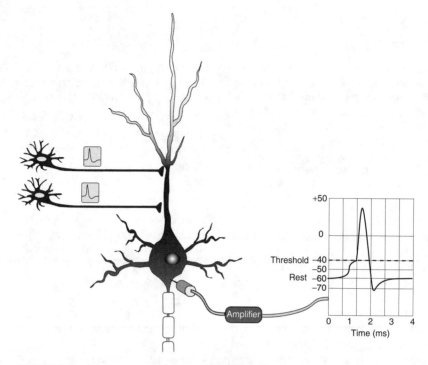

FIGURE 3.9 ● In this case, two excitatory neurons are simultaneously sending impulses to the central neuron. This generates an excitatory postsynaptic potential that is strong enough to cross the threshold and start an action potential down the axon.

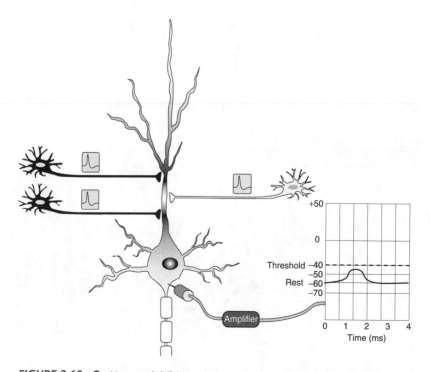

FIGURE 3.10 ● Here an inhibitory neuron sends an impulse that hyperpolarizes the central neuron (inhibitory postsynaptic potential). This has the effect of diminishing the excitatory potential, which is now no longer able to reach the threshold. So no action potential is generated.

Electrical

1. The action potential arrives at the presynaptic terminal

2. Depolarization causes voltage-gated calcium channesl to open and results in a large influx of Ca^{2+}

3. Exocytosis: Ca^{2+} causes the vesicles to fuse with the membrane and release the neurotransmitter

4. Excitatory postsynaptic potentials (EPSP) spread out over the dendrite

Chemical

A. Precursor molecules and enzymes are transported down the axon from the cell body along the microtubules

B. Enzymes in the synaptic terminal convert the precursor molecules into active neurotransmitter

C. The neurotransmitter is stored in the vesicles until released by the influx of Ca^{2+}

D. The released neurotransmitter binds with the receptors on the postsynaptic terminal and generates an EPSP

E. Reuptake of the neurotransmitter limits the duration of the signal and allows the cell to recycle the neurotransmitter

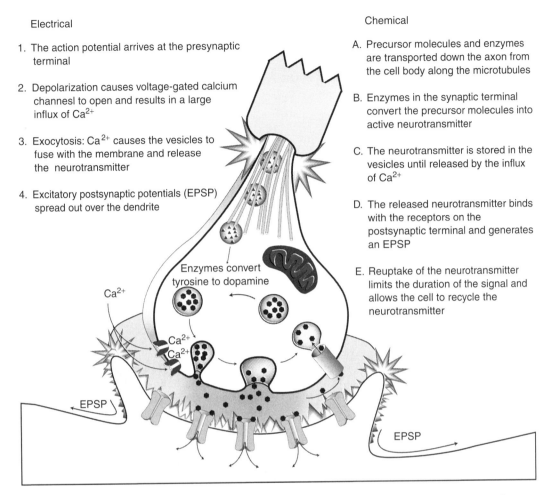

Enzymes convert tyrosine to dopamine

Ca^{2+}

Ca^{2+}
Ca^{2+}

EPSP

EPSP

FIGURE 3.11 ● This is an example of the electrochemical signaling from a dopamine neuron. If this were an inhibitory neuron, γ-aminobutyric acid or glycine for example, the postsynaptic potential would be an inhibitory postsynaptic potential (IPSP) and not an excitatory postsynaptic potential (EPSP). (Adapted from Rosenzweig MR, Breedlove SM, Watson NV. *Biological Psychology,* 4th ed. Sunderland, MA: Sinauer; 2005.)

of the neighboring neuron. This example is of a dopamine neuron that is an excitatory neuron, but the same principles apply to all the neurons and neurotransmitters.

The arrival of the action potential at the terminal depolarizes the membrane, which opens the *voltage-gated calcium channels*. The voltage-gated calcium channels are similar to the voltage-gated sodium channels except they are permeable to Ca^{2+}. Consequently, there is a large and rapid influx of Ca^{2+}, which is required for *exocytosis* and the release of the neurotransmitter.

NON-NEURONAL CELLS

The glial cells that make up the rest of the cells in the central nervous system (CNS) actually outnumber the neurons by 9:1. Traditionally seen as supportive cells with no roll in communication, recent research has shown that glial cells modulate the synaptic activity. There are three kinds of glial cells: astrocyte, oligodendrocyte, and microglia. The microglia are similar to macrophages found in the peripheral tissue. They respond to injury with a dramatic increase in their numbers and remove cellular debris from the damaged area.

The oligodendrocyte is considered the CNS equivalent of the Schwann cell in the peripheral nervous system (see Figure 3.12). They are the cells that wrap myelin around the axons of the neurons and by acting as an electrical insulator greatly increase the speed of the transmission of the action potential. This process of myelinization is not complete at birth and proceeds rapidly in

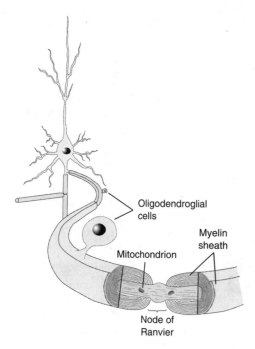

Oligodendroglial cells

Myelin sheath

Mitochondrion

Node of Ranvier

FIGURE 3.12 ● Oligodendroglial cells wrap a myelin sheath around the axon, providing electrical insulation and greatly enhancing the speed of the action potential and hence the efficiency of the brain. (Adapted from Bear MF, Connors BW, Paradiso MA, eds. *Neuroscience: Exploring the Brain*, 3rd ed. Baltimore: Lippincott Williams & Wilkins; 2007.)

the first years of life, which has a dramatic effect on behavior. In children, this process results in improved motor skills as they mature. Complete myelinization of the prefrontal cortex is delayed until the second and even third decade of life. With our teenagers, we hope they will stay out of trouble until this process is complete.

Alternatively, demyelinating disorders such as multiple sclerosis and Guillain-Barré have devastating effects on patients. Clearly, a neuron without its myelin is not as effective. Regarding mental illness, recent research suggests that some failure in myelination may play a role in schizophrenia (see Chapter 20, Schizophrenia).

The astrocyte is the star-shaped cell that fills the spaces between the neurons (see Figure 3.13). We have already seen that the astrocyte plays a role in maintaining the blood–brain barrier, but other functions include regulating the chemistry of the extracellular fluid, providing structural support, and bringing nutrients to the neurons. Even more interesting is the role the astrocyte plays in modulating the electrical activity at the synapse. Research has shown that astrocytes encircle the

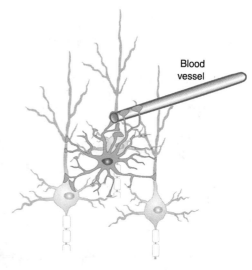

Blood vessel

FIGURE 3.13 ● The astrocyte not only supports the neurons and blood vessels but also has some role in modulating the transmission of information.

synapse and have receptors that respond to the neurotransmitters released by the neuron. The astrocyte may in turn release its own neurotransmitter, which has the effect of enhancing the transmission of the signal. This may facilitate learning and memory. Additionally, there is evidence that the presence of astrocytes or the proteins they excrete increases the number of synapses a neuron will form. Clearly, the glial cells are more involved in the communication within the brain than previously thought.

DISORDER: EPILEPSY

Increasing evidence is pointing to the astrocyte as playing an instigating role in epilepsy—a problem historically assigned to dysfunctional neurons. Analysis of specimens after surgical resection for epilepsy often shows prominent gliosis. Glutamate released from astrocytes can trigger experimental models of seizures. Finally, several effective antiepileptic drugs (valproate, gabapentin, and phenytoin) potently reduce astrocytic Ca^{2+} signaling—an event believed to precede seizure activity. If aberrant astrocytes are the nidus for seizures, then new treatments could be created that calm the astrocyte without dulling the neurons.

QUESTIONS

1. The pyramidal cells in the gray matter reside predominantly in which layers?
   a. I and III.
   b. II and IV.
   c. III and V.
   d. IV and VI.

2. Protein synthesis requires all of the following except
   a. Rough endoplasmic reticulum.
   b. Gene expression.
   c. Transcription and translation.
   d. mRNA.

3. Enhanced arborization of the dendrites is found with
   a. Mental retardation.
   b. Stimulating environments.
   c. Usual laboratory environments.
   d. Schizophrenia.

4. An inhibitory postsynaptic potential
   a. Results from the influx of sodium ions.
   b. Depolarizes the cell.
   c. Can induce seizures.
   d. Hyperpolarizes the cell.

5. The neuron generates an action potential based on the postsynaptic potential at the
   a. Axon hillock.
   b. Synapse.
   c. Nucleus.
   d. Node of Ranvier.

6. Exocytosis of the neurotransmitters at the synapse requires opening of the
   a. Voltage-gated sodium channels.
   b. Voltage-gated calcium channels.
   c. Excitatory postsynaptic channels.
   d. Inhibitory postsynaptic channels.

7. The cell responsible for myelin in the CNS is
   a. Astrocyte.
   b. Microglia.
   c. Schwann cell.
   d. Oligodendrocyte.

8. Modulates electrochemical activity at the synapse.
   a. Astrocyte.
   b. Microglia.
   c. Schwann cell.
   d. Oligodendrocyte.

See Answers section at end of book.

Neurotransmitters

POINT OF INTEREST

It is not uncommon in our practices for patients to announce at the initial evaluation, "Doc, I have a chemical imbalance" as though it is some sort of Diagnostic and Statistical Manual of Mental Disorders (DSM) diagnosis. Whether a "chemical imbalance" is the source of mental illness remains to be determined, but most assuredly the manipulation of these chemicals are the bread and butter of psychiatry. They are the chemical part of the "electrochemical" communication and the focus of this chapter.

A "neurotransmitter" is technically defined by meeting three criteria.

1. The substance must be stored in the presynaptic neuron.
2. It must be released with depolarization of the presynaptic neuron induced by the influx of Ca^{2+}.
3. The substance must bind with a specific receptor on the postsynaptic neuron.

Neurotransmitters differ from hormones by their close physical proximity of the release to the receptor—although this turns out to be less straightforward than one might imagine, as we will see in Chapter 6, Hormones and the Brain.

The classic neurotransmitters—the ones we frequently discuss—are small molecules designed for ease of use. For neurotransmitters, the body needs a substrate that can be produced quickly, with ease, and be recycled—much like the daily newspaper. Figure 4.1 shows some representative neurotransmitters compared to a neuropeptide substance P. The common neurotransmitters such as γ-aminobutyric acid (GABA) and norepinephrine (NE) are small and constructed with elements that are easy for the body to find. This facilitates the rapid creation and deployment of information that is so important for the functioning of the brain.

POINT OF INTEREST

The body—in all its wisdom—has developed a small number of neurotransmitters. Rather than having a billion separate molecules that each transmits a specific message, the body has a limited number of neurotransmitters that mean different things in different places. Much like the alphabets where 26 letters can create innumerable words, the body uses only a few hundred neurotransmitters to coordinate the most complex organ in the universe. In addition to these limited set of neurotransmitters performing many different functions in the brain, they are also used in other organs.

An extensive review of all known neurotransmitters is beyond the scope of this book. We will

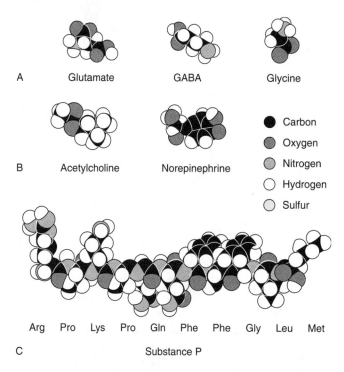

A   Glutamate   GABA   Glycine

B   Acetylcholine   Norepinephrine

● Carbon
● Oxygen
● Nitrogen
○ Hydrogen
● Sulfur

Arg Pro Lys Pro Gln Phe Phe Gly Leu Met

C   Substance P

FIGURE 4.1 ● A sample of neuro-transmitters showing the relative size of the amino acids (**A**), two of the amines (**B**) and a neuropeptide (**C**). GABA, γ-aminobutyric acid. (Adapted from Bear MF, Connors BW, Paradiso MA, eds. *Neuroscience: exploring the brain*, 3rd ed. Baltimore: Lippincott Williams & Wilkins; 2007.)

focus on the relevant molecules in the following three basic categories:

1. The classic neurotransmitters.
2. Neuropeptides.
3. Unconventional neurotransmitters.

CLASSIC NEUROTRANSMITTERS
Amino Acids

Glutamate. This is the major workhorse of the brain, with glutamate neurons making up more than half of the *excitatory* neurons. Without glutamate the brain does not get started or

POINT OF INTEREST

Of the classic neurotransmitters, the monoamines are the ones we typically talk about, for example, dopamine (DA), serotonin, and NE. Hanging around psychiatrists, one might imagine that the brain is predominately made up of these neurons and neurotransmitters. Amazingly, these agents are in minority in the brain. The largest number of neurons and the ones that do the heavy lifting in the brain come from the amino acid group, of which glutamate and GABA are the most prominent. The pie chart gives a very rough estimate of the relative proportion of several important neurotransmitters. The neuropeptides (discussed later) would only be a line on this chart.

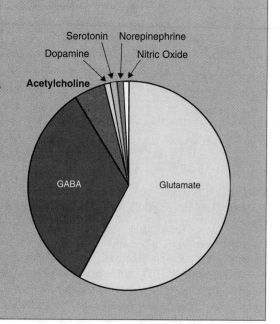

keep running. Glutamate and another excitatory transmitter *aspartate* are nonessential amino acids that do not cross the blood–brain barrier. Consequently, glutamate must be synthesized in the brain from glucose and other precursors. Glial cells assist in the reuptake, degradation, and resupply of glutamate for neurons.

DISORDERS

Glutamate neurons are believed to be involved in the formation and storage of memories. Changes in the receptors—termed *synaptic plasticity*—are well documented and seem to be involved in the physical manifestation of learning (see Chapter 15, Memory). Too much glutamate, as occurs with a stroke, is toxic to the nerve cells. Not only is the cell deprived of oxygen but also the glutamate that is released by the dying cell results in further damage. Efforts are underway to find an agent that will block the toxic effects of glutamate during ischemic events to limit the secondary damage. More recently, glutamate has been implicated as a possible culprit in the pathophysiology of schizophrenia. Postmortem studies and therapeutic trials suggest that glutamatergic dysregulation may be present in patients with schizophrenia (see Chapter 20, Schizophrenia).

GABA and Glycine. GABA is the major inhibitory transmitter in the brain and is used by approximately 25% of the cortical neurons. Glycine is the other inhibitory amino acid, but is less common. GABA puts the brakes on the brain: not enough GABA and one can have seizures. The GABA neurons are primarily the interneurons in the gray matter providing local constraint over cortical circuitry. Figure 3.11 in the previous chapter shows an example of a GABA neuron hyperpolarizing the pyramidal neuron such that it no longer generates an action potential.

Similarly, Figure 4.2 shows how input from a GABA interneuron quiets an overactive neuron. One can see how increasing GABAergic activity can be an effective treatment for epilepsy. More recently, increasing GABAergic activity has been used to treat insomnia, pain, and anxiety, and to

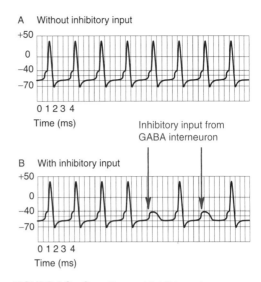

FIGURE 4.2 ● Effects of inhibitory input. **A:** Without GABA inhibition (or any other inhibition) the neuron fires regularly. **B:** With input from a GABA interneuron (in brown), some action potentials are inhibited. GABA, γ-aminobutyric acid.

assist in the management of mania—all situations where too much central nervous system (CNS) activity is a component of the disorder.

Monoamines

Catecholamines. There are two principle classes of monoamines: *catecholamines* (DA, NE, and epinephrine) and *indoleamines* (serotonin and melatonin). All the monoamines are inactivated and degraded when taken back by the neuron. (Clinicians often refer to this as the reuptake pump, but neuroscientists call this the *transporter*, e.g., the DA transporter.) The class of enzymes in the terminal that degrades the neurotransmitters is the monoamine oxidases (MAOs). Consequently, MAO inhibitors cause an increase in catecholamines (e.g., DA, NE, and serotonin), by limiting the degradation process, with well-known benefits for depression and anxiety.

Unfortunately, some food products and medications can cause an increased release of NE. When the MAOs are inhibited, an excessive amount of NE is released. This can result in dangerous elevations in blood pressure, which has resulted in stroke and even death in some cases.

Starting with the catecholamines, we see in Figure 4.3 that the transmitters are synthesized from the essential amino acid tyrosine that must be obtained from the diet. Note that L-dopa is synthesized into DA. This shows why L-dopa can be given as a treatment for Parkinson's disease. The trick is to allow the synthesis in the CNS,

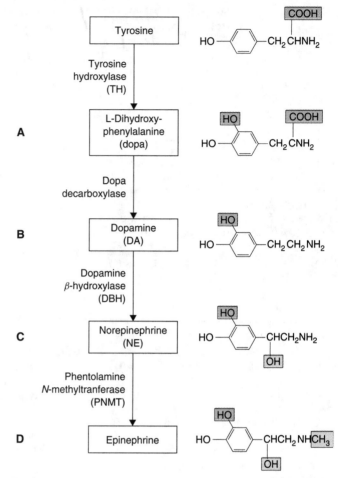

FIGURE 4.3 ● The synthesis of catecholamines from tyrosine. (Adapted from Bear MF, Connors BW, Paradiso MA, eds. *Neuroscience: exploring the brain*, 3rd ed. Baltimore: Lippincott Williams & Wilkins; 2007.)

but inhibit the enzyme dopa decarboxylase in the periphery so that the patient is not too nauseated.

Dopamine. DA neurons constitute approximately half a million of the cells in the brain—a tiny percentage out of the 100 billion total cells—from three primary nuclei (see Figure 4.4). The *substantia nigra* located in the ventral midbrain has primary projections to the caudate and putamen (collectively called the *striatum*). This pathway is called the *nigrostriatal system* or *mesostriatal system*. As part of the basal ganglia this pathway is integral to voluntary movement. Parkinson's disease is the result of a loss of DA neurons in the substantia nigra. The extrapyramidal side effects due to antipsychotic medications can induce parkinsonian symptoms by blockade of these neurons.

The cells of the *ventral tegmental area,* also in the ventral midbrain, project to the nucleus accumbens, prefrontal cortex, amygdala, and hippocampus. These innervations, called the *mesolimbocortical DA system*, are particularly dense in primates. Some writers subdivide these branches into the *mesolimbic* (nucleus accumbens, amygdala, and hippocampus) and *mesocortical* (prefrontal cortex), which seems artificial as they originate from the same cell bodies.

DISORDERS

The branches to the nucleus accumbens are involved with reward and substance abuse. The branches to the prefrontal cortex are involved with attention and cognition, and seem to be impaired in patients with attention deficit hyperactivity disorder (ADHD). Some speculate that problems with the mesolimbic system cause the positive symptoms of schizophrenia whereas negative symptoms are caused by impairment in the mesocortical system.

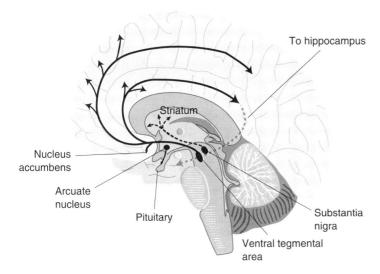

FIGURE 4.4 ● The dopaminergic system. The substantia nigra forms the nigrostriatal pathways to the caudate and putamen. The ventral tegmental area projects to the nucleus accumbens and cortex. The arcuate nucleus of the hypothalamus projects to the tuberoinfundibular area of the hypothalamus.

The short tracts in the *arcuate nucleus* of the hypothalamus—called the *tuberoinfundibular DA system*—release DA into the portal veins of the pituitary gland. The synthesis and release of prolactin in the anterior pituitary is inhibited by this DA. Any process that interrupts the action of DA on the prolactin-producing cells will lead to hyperprolactinemia. Hence, antipsychotic medications that block the DA receptor can cause an increase in prolactin, although it appears to be less with the newer antipsychotic agents for unclear reasons.

Norepinephrine. Called *noradrenaline* in the UK and hence noradrenergic neurons, these neurons contain an additional enzyme in their terminals that converts DA to NE. Approximately 50% of the NE neurons are located in the locus coeruleus. We have two in each side of our

brain stem with approximately 12,000 neurons in each nucleus. The remainder of the NE neurons is found in loose clusters in the medullary reticular formation (see Figure 4.5).

Although small in number, these noradrenergic neurons are very important. They project to virtually every area of the brain and spinal cord. For example, knockout mice that are deficient in NE cannot survive. The NE neurons play an important role in alertness. The firing of the locus coeruleus increases along a spectrum from drowsy to alert, with the lowest found when we sleep and the highest when we are hypervigilant. Clearly, the noradrenergic neurons are important in handling danger. In a threatening situation, the locus coeruleus is active as are the sympathetic neurons of the autonomic nervous system (ANS) where the peripheral noradrenergic neurons are found.

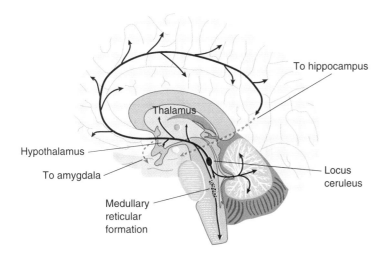

FIGURE 4.5 ● The noradrenergic system. With projections to almost every area of the brain and spinal cord, the NE system plays an important role in alertness and anxiety. NE, norepinephrine.

TREATMENT

Inappropriate noradrenergic activity, both centrally and peripherally, plays an important role in anxiety and depression. Not only is a rapid heart rate a symptom of anxiety but also a high resting heart rate after a motor vehicle accident is a predictor of later post-traumatic stress disorder (PTSD). Reducing the activity of these neurons is one goal of pharmacological treatment.

Recently, the Food and Drug Administration (FDA) approved vagus nerve stimulation (VNS) as a treatment for medication resistant depression. Incoming signals to the brain from the vagus nerve provide the locus ceruleus with information about the state of the internal organs. In a hypervigilant condition such as chronic anxiety, the information from vagus nerve increases the activity of the locus ceruleus and the NE neurons. VNS may work through modulation of the locus ceruleus and the NE system.

NE is cleared from the synaptic cleft by a re-uptake transporter that is also capable of taking up DA—most likely due to the structural similarity of these two transmitters (see Figure 4.4). This may explain why atomoxetine, a NE reuptake inhibitor, results in an increase in DA (as well as NE) in the prefrontal cortex although it does not inhibit the DA reuptake pump.

Epinephrine. The *epinephrine* (or adrenaline) neurons are few and play a minor role in the CNS. Most of the epinephrine in the body is produced in the adrenal medulla and excreted with sympathetic stimulation. Therefore, epinephrine plays a much greater role outside of the brain as a hormone, than within as a neurotransmitter.

Indoleamines

Serotonin (5-hydroxytryptamine)

POINT OF INTEREST

No other neurotransmitter is more closely associated with modern neuropsychopharmacology than serotonin, also called *5-hydroxytryptamine (5-HT)*. In actuality, serotonin is found in many parts of the body outside of the CNS, such as platelets and mast cells. Only approximately 1% to 2% of the body's serotonin in located in the brain.

Serotonin is synthesized from tryptophan that must be obtained in the diet (see Figure 4.6). Unlike with the catecholamines, levels of serotonin in the brain can be lowered significantly with insufficient dietary tryptophan (grains, meats, and dairy products are good sources of tryptophan). In the pineal gland there are two additional enzymes that convert serotonin to *melatonin*, the other indoleamine.

The location of the cell bodies and distribution of the serotonin neurons are similar to that of the catecholamines (see Figure 4.7). The cell bodies are relatively few in number (approximately 200,000) and reside in the raphe nuclei in the brain stem. As with NE, the serotonin neurons project to virtually all areas of the brain.

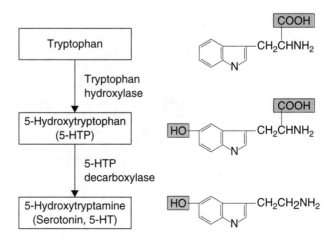

FIGURE 4.6 ● Serotonin synthesis. (Adapted from Bear MF, Connors BW, Paradiso MA, eds. *Neuroscience: exploring the brain*, 3rd ed. Baltimore: Lippincott Williams & Wilkins; 2007.)

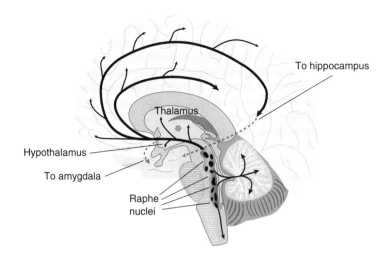

FIGURE 4.7 ● The serotonergic system. The cluster of Raphe nuclei along the brainstem has projections to most of the brain and spinal cord. These neurons play an important roll in mood, anxiety, and with the sleep–wake cycle.

DISORDERS

As we all know, the serotonin neurons play an important role in depression and anxiety, and are also implicated in the sleep–wake cycle. Serotonin, as with the catecholamines, is removed from the synaptic cleft by the reuptake of the transmitter with the serotonin transporter. It is the blockade of this process that is believed to result in the therapeutic effect of the commonly prescribed antidepressants. Although increasing the availability of serotonin in the synaptic cleft has proven therapeutic value for the treatment of depression, it remains unclear if insufficient serotonin is part of the etiology of the disorder.

Histamine. Histamine is not just for itching anymore. Although histamine is released from mast cells as part of an allergic reaction in the peripheral tissue, in the brain it is involved in arousal and attention. Most of the cell bodies start in the tuberomammilary nucleus of the posterior hypothalamus, with sparse but widespread projects to all regions of the brain and spinal cord. When animals are alert, the histamine neurons are active. Histamine neurons are quiet when animals are sleeping.

Acetylcholine. In the 1920s, acetylcholine (ACh) was the first molecule to be identified as a neurotransmitter (see Figure 1.6 in Chapter 1, Historical Perspective). ACh is the only small molecule transmitter that is not an amino acid or directly derived from one. ACh is actually not a monoamine, but is often grouped with these neurotransmitters due to similar size and distribution.

ACh plays a prominent role in the peripheral ANS and is the neurotransmitter at the neuromuscular junction. Its relative ease of accessibility outside the cranium is one reason it was discovered first. The neurons in the CNS arise from cell bodies in the brain stem and forebrain with prominent projects to the cortex and hippocampus. It is these later projections to the hippocampus that are involved with learning and memory and are disrupted in Alzheimer's disease.

TREATMENT

As prescribers, we are often struggling with unintended sedation due to blocking of the histamine neurons (antihistamines), for example, tricyclic antidepressants, clozapine, or olanzapine. More recently, there has been increased interest in activating the histamine neurons as a treatment for fatigue. Modafinil, the only agent in the class, indirectly activates the histamine neurons and has been used successfully as a treatment for narcolepsy, excessive sleepiness, and ADHD.

NEUROPEPTIDES

In late 1960s and early 1970s it was established that many peptides initially discovered in a variety of regions, for example, gut, heart, and so on, as well as the newly discovered endorphins and enkephalins, are also produced and are active in the brain. This is another example of the parsimonious evolution of neurotransmitters: The same transmitter has different functions in various organs or brain region depending on its location.

These peptides such as adrenocorticotropic hormone (ACTH), luteinizing hormone, somatostatin, and vasopressin (to name a few) have important endocrine functions in the body, such as the regulation of reproduction, growth, water intake, salt metabolism, temperature control, and so on. In the last 30 years, it has been established that these same peptides are synthesized in nerve cells and have effects on behaviors such as learning, attachment, mood, and anxiety. This has generated tremendous interest in further analysis of the effects of these neuroactive peptides on behavior. Table 4.1 gives examples of neuropeptides from the five classes.

The neuropeptides are small chains of amino acids, which one can see in Figure 4.1, and are considerably larger than the classic neurotransmitters. Furthermore the formation, release, and inactivation of the neuropeptides differ from that of the monoamines. Figure 4.8 shows the life of a neuropeptide in relation to a classic neurotransmitter. Peptides must be transcribed from mRNA on the ribosomes of the endoplasmic reticulum. Initially the peptide is a large *propeptide* precursor, which is cleaved into an active neuropeptide as it is moved from the Golgi apparatus into large dense core vesicles that are stored at the terminal bud of the neuron. Unlike the monoamines, neuropeptides are not recycled by the neuron, but are rather broken down by

TABLE 4.1

The Five Classes of Neuropeptides and Some Examples

Peptide Class	Example
Gut–brain peptides	Substance P
	Cholecystokinin
	Galanin
Pituitary peptides	Adrenocorticotropic hormone (ACTH)
	Luteinizing hormone (LH)
	Oxytocin
	Vasopressin
Hypothalamic releasing peptides	Corticotropin-releasing factor (CRF)
	Gonadotropin-releasing hormone (GnRH)Thyroidtropin-releasing hormone (TRH)
	Somatostatin
Opioid peptides	β-Endorphin
	Enkephalins
Other peptides	Angiotensin
	Bradykinin

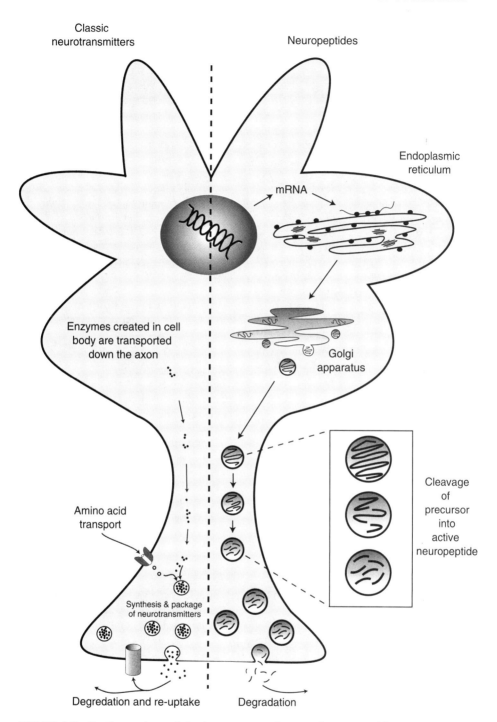

FIGURE 4.8 ● Comparison of classic neurotransmitters and neuropeptides.

degradative enzymes (*peptidases*) on the receptor membrane.

POINT OF INTEREST

In some cases the neuropeptides travel relatively long distances from their release to a receptor. This begs the question: Are they transmitters or hormones? Further complicating our understanding of the role of neuropeptides, it has been shown that they do not always evoke an action potential. They can play a gentle role—often called *modulation*—in facilitating or exacerbating the effects elicited by the classic neurotransmitters, and they are often stored in the same neuron as 5-HT, NE, or DA. It appears that neuropeptides act as transmitters, hormones, or modulators depending on the tissue, synapse, and frequency of stimulation.

UNCONVENTIONAL NEUROTRANSMITTERS

It would be foolish to think that we have discovered all the neurotransmitters—or even all the transmitter classes. For example, two unconventional neurotransmitters are being studied that are expanding our understanding of how the brain communicates and what constitutes being a neurotransmitter.

Gases

Most commonly associated with erectile dysfunction, *nitric oxide* (*NO*) is a gas that is formed in glutamate neurons when arginine is converted into citrulline and NO. NO has the ability to diffuse (without obstruction) out of the originating cell, through the extracellular medium and into any neighboring cell that it meets. NO converts guanosine triphosphate (GTP) into cyclic guanosine monophosphate (GMP) that acts as a second messenger. Cells containing the NO synthase (the enzyme that creates NO) constitute only approximately 1% of neuronal cells in the brain, but reach out so extensively that nearly every cell in the brain may encounter NO. It is hard to imagine this gas as a neurotransmitter in the traditional sense if for no other reason than it cannot be stored in vesicles to await for the appropriate signal to be released. But NO does send a message to the neighboring cells that signals an increase in activity—almost like turning the porch lights on shows our neighbors that we are home.

Endocannabinoids

The journey from recognizing an effect of a substance on behavior to identifying the endogenous substrate and receptor is a common and fascinating story. Reserpine and the monoamines, and morphine and the enkephalins, are two well-known examples of this process. Marijuana and the endocannabinoids are the latest in this history of searching for the mechanisms to explain an effect. The main active compound of marijuana is Δ^9-tetrahydrocannabinol (THC), which binds

---

TREATMENT

Since the serendipitous discovery in the 1950s that patients treated for tuberculosis with an agent that inhibited MAO showed improvement in mood, there has been an explosion in the manipulation of monoamines as treatment for depression and anxiety: tricyclic antidepressants (TCAs), selective serotonin reuptake inhibitors (SSRIs), and so on. Although this has resulted in incalculable relief for millions of patients, the newer medications are in many ways just refinements of the original concept. They all increase the monoamines in the synaptic cleft. The neuropeptides offer the possibility of a unique mechanism for the treatment of psychiatric disorders.

Several pharmaceutical companies are investigating neuropeptide systems as novel therapeutic targets for depression, anxiety, and pain. Unfortunately, none have come to market and some have been withdrawn from investigation. The problem may be that the desired effects are only mild, and are not robust enough to justify seeking full FDA approval. This may reflect the modulating role that neuropeptides have in the CNS. Additionally, the blood has circulating peptidases that chew up neuropeptides delivered by pills or even intravenously. This has been a major stumbling block in creating neuropeptide-based medications for psychiatric treatments.

DISORDERS

The question remains: What effect does NO have on behavior and mental disorders? Little is known about this, but NO may be involved with aggression and sexual behavior, as well as migraine headaches. Knock out mice, bred without NO synthase, are extraordinarily aggressive and sexual, although their behavior is mediated by testosterone and absent in females. These findings suggest that NO may restrain aggressive and sexual behavior. It is worth noting that the medications for erectile dysfunction have not been associated with any adverse effects on mental function. This may be due to the inability of these medications in their current form to cross the blood–brain barrier.

to the cannabinoid receptor and causes the well-known euphoria, calm, distorted cognition, and "munchies." Following the discovery of the receptor, there was an active search for the naturally occurring ligands that resulted in the identification of the endogenous cannabinoids known as the *endocannabinoids*.

The cannabinoid receptor (CB_1) is widely expressed throughout the brain on presynaptic terminals. The effect of activating CB_1 receptors results in inhibition of that neuron and in a simple way explains the calming effect of marijuana. The prospect of activating or blocking the CB_1 receptor for therapeutic reasons such as pain, anxiety, and nausea are being pursued vigorously. One fascinating prospect is the potential for a weight loss treatment. Some enterprising researchers speculated that if stimulating the cannabinoid receptor caused the "munchies," then blocking the same receptor might inhibit appetite. Rimonabant, a potent and selective blocker (antagonist) of the CB_1 receptor, has been shown in clinical studies to facilitate weight loss: a treatment that is vastly needed in industrial countries.

QUESTIONS

1. Which is an indoleamine?
   a. DA.
   b. NE.
   c. Melatonin.
   d. Aspartate.

2. Which pathway is believed to result in the negative symptoms of schizophrenia?
   a. Nigrostriatal.
   b. Mesocortical.
   c. Mesolimbic.
   d. Tuberoinfundibular.

3. Which pathway mediates prolactin?
   a. Nigrostriatal.
   b. Mesocortical.
   c. Mesolimbic.
   d. Tuberoinfundibular.

4. The cell bodies of the NE neurons are located in the locus ceruleus and the
   a. Medullary reticular formation.
   b. Raphe nuclei.
   c. Arcuate nucleus.
   d. Tuberomammilary nucleus.

5. Most of the cell bodies for histamine neurons reside in the
   a. Medullary reticular formation.
   b. Raphe nuclei.
   c. Arcuate nucleus.
   d. Tuberomammilary nucleus.

6. Which statement is not true regarding NO.
   a. It is quickly degraded.
   b. It converts GTP into cyclic guanosine monophosphate (cGMP).
   c. It is stored in dense core vesicles.
   d. It is formed from arginine.

7. All of the following are neuropeptides except
   a. Cannabinoid peptides.
   b. Pituitary peptides.
   c. Opioid peptides.
   d. Hypothalamic releasing peptides.

8. The most common neurotransmitter in the brain is
   a. Serotonin.
   b. DA.
   c. GABA.
   d. Glutamate.

See Answers section at end of book.

CHAPTER 5

Receptors and Signaling the Nucleus

INTRODUCTION

In this chapter we continue a discussion about events at the cellular level and explore what happens at receptors, after neurotransmitters have been released.

Electrochemical communication continues at the receptor on the postsynaptic membrane. Without a receptor, the neurotransmitter is like a tree falling in the woods with no one to hear it. The binding of the neurotransmitter with the receptor initiates a series of events that change the postsynaptic cell in some way. Receptors are protein units embedded in the lipid layer of the cell membrane. There are two basic types of receptors activated by neurotransmitters (more on this later), and the response generated depends on what type of receptor is activated.

Agonists and Antagonists

As physicians, much of what we attempt to do by prescribing medications involves enhancing or limiting the effects of the neurotransmitter at the receptor. Figure 5.1 shows an example of the various effects of neurotransmitters or medications on a receptor. Pharmacologists and neuroscientists use the terms *ligand, agonist,* and *antagonists* but in this book we will also use the more self-explanatory terms such as *transmitter, drug/medication, stimulate,* and *block.*

FAST RECEPTORS: CHEMICAL

There are two basic types of receptors for neurotransmitters. The one we usually think of is shown in Figure 5.1—an ion channel (also called *transmitter-gated ion channel*). A neurotransmitter or medication stimulates the opening of the pore inside the receptor and ions rapidly flow into the cell. Receptors that allow the entry of positive ions such as Na^+ or Ca^{2+} result in an excitatory postsynaptic potential (EPSP). Acetylcholine and glutamate result in such activation and are considered excitatory.

Receptors permeable to negative ions, such as Cl^-, will result in inhibitory postsynaptic potentials (IPSPs). γ-Aminobutyric acid (GABA) and glycine, both considered inhibitory, cause this kind of activation. The essential point regarding these transmitter-gated ion channels is that they are fast. These receptors are magnificent little machines that can rapidly allow the entry of large currents with great precision. The ions pour into the cell and the signal from the proceeding neuron, whether excitatory or inhibitory, is quickly propagated along the membrane of the target cell. As we reviewed in Chapter 3, Cells of the Nervous System, an action potential is only generated if enough EPSPs bring the resting potential of the postsynaptic cell above the threshold at the axon hillock.

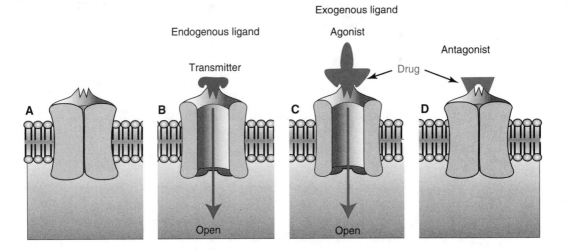

FIGURE 5.1 ● An unbound receptor in closed state (**A**). A natural ligand (neurotransmitter) stimulates the receptor, which then opens to allow entry of ions (**B**). Medication simulates the action of the natural ligand and the receptor opens (**C**). An antagonist blocks the action of the ligand so the receptor cannot be opened (**D**).

Amino Acid Receptors

The amino acid receptors mediate most of the fast transmitter-gated channels in the brain. The two prominent ones are glutamate and GABA, which are reviewed in the subsequent text.

POINT OF INTEREST

The receptors, unlike the transmitter, come in a variety of styles—a relationship that is much like feet and shoes. You only have two feet, but many shoes. Serotonin is one example: there are 14 different receptor subtypes for this one neurotransmitter. Some receptors are categorized as different classes whereas others are just different subtypes within a class. It is not entirely clear why some differences constitute a new class and others just warrant a new subtype. Most likely a committee decides.

Glutamate. There are three prominent glutamate receptors: *N-methyl-d-aspartate (NMDA)*, *α-amino-3-hydroxy-5-methyl-4-isoxazole propionate (AMPA)*, and *kainate*, each with several subtypes. They are named after the artificial agonist that selectively activates them. For example, NMDA activates the NMDA receptor, but not the AMPA, or kainate receptors. NMDA and AMPA mediate the bulk of fast excitatory synaptic transmission in the brain. The role of kainate is not clearly understood.

NMDA and AMPA receptors, which often coexist on the same postsynaptic receptor, both allow the rapid entry of Na^+ into the cell (and the simultaneous exit of K^+) that generates the depolarization of the postsynaptic cell. NMDA receptors are unique in that they also allow the entry of Ca^{2+} that can act as a second messenger inside the cell. This can have a profound impact on the cell resulting in lasting changes, as will be shown at the end of this chapter when we discuss long-term memory.

The NMDA receptor is further unique in that it requires both the glutamate transmitter and a change in the voltage to open before it will allow the entry of Na+ and Ca^{2+}. This property is due to the presence of Mg^{2+} ions, which clog the NMDA receptor at resting voltage. Figure 5.2 shows how the AMPA receptor works in conjunction with the NMDA receptor to depolarize the cell and bring Ca^{2+} into the cell. This property has a significant impact on the capacity of the neurons to change.

γ-**Aminobutyric Acid.** GABA and *glycine* are the primary inhibitory neurons in the brain; inhibition is a process that must be tightly regulated. Too much inhibition causes the brain to slow down—even lose consciousness; too little inhibition can result in overall brain excitation and result in seizures. The GABA receptor is unique in that it has several other sites where chemicals can modulate its function (see Figure 5.3). For example, *barbiturates* and *benzodiazepines* have their own

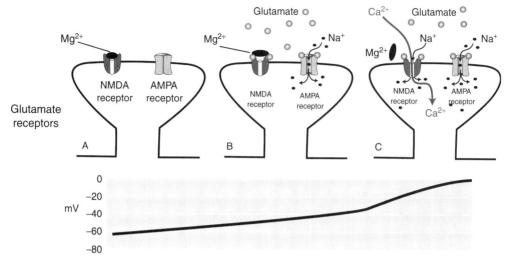

FIGURE 5.2 ● **A:** A postsynaptic glutamate terminal with both receptors closed. **B:** The presence of glutamate transmitters opens the AMPA receptor but not the NMDA receptor. **C:** When the voltage in the postsynaptic neuron gets above −35 mV, the magnesium ion blocking the receptor falls off and Na$^+$ as well as Ca^{2+} ions pour into the cell. AMPA, α-amino-3-hydroxy-5-methyl-4-isoxazole propionate; NMDA, N-methyl-D-aspartate.

distinct sites on the GABA receptor. These medications by themselves do not open the GABA channel, but they can enhance the strength or frequency of the opening. Hence, more Cl$^-$ enters the cell and a greater inhibitory effect is elicited.

Ethanol is another popular drug that enhances the function of the GABA receptor. Long-term use of ethanol decreases the expression of the GABA receptor, which may explain the tolerance that develops with alcoholism. Whether the receptor alterations contribute to the propensity for seizures when the alcohol is withdrawn remains unclear.

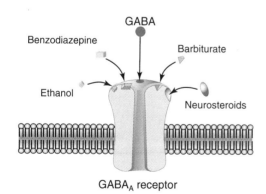

FIGURE 5.3 ● The GABA receptor showing the other drugs that can modify and enhance the inhibitory effect of these receptors. GABA, γ-aminobutyric acid. (Adapted from Bear MF, Connors BW, Paradiso MA, eds. *Neuroscience: exploring the brain*, 3rd ed. Baltimore: Lippincott Williams & Wilkins; 2007.)

The steroid hormones can also modulate GABA receptors (sometimes called *neurosteroids* when they have effects on neurons). This may explain the psychiatric symptoms that develop at times of drop in sex hormone levels, for example, premenstrual syndrome (PMS), menopause, and andropause. Additionally researchers have found that some steroid hormone levels drop in patients who panic during an attack. Others have shown that medications such as olanzapine and fluoxetine—known to decrease anxiety—increase steroid hormone levels. We will review this in greater detail in the Chapter 6, Hormones and the Brain, and Chapter 13, Sex and the Brain.

SLOW RECEPTORS: METABOLIC

Starting in the 50s, researchers teased out the details of a second type of receptor—one that activates a cascade of biochemical events in the cytosol of the receptor cell that ultimately modifies the function of target proteins or the DNA. This type of receptor, called a *G-protein–coupled receptor*, is perhaps even more relevant to the effect of psychiatric medications than the transmitter-gated ion channel. G-protein is the short form for guanosine triphosphate (GTP)–binding protein. Although there are many types of G-protein–coupled receptors, the basic style involves three steps.

1. A neurotransmitter binds to the receptor.
2. The receptor activates the G-protein, which moves along the intracellular membrane.
3. The G-protein activates the "effector" protein.

TREATMENT: ANTIEPILEPTIC DRUGS

The background about inhibitory and excitatory receptors helps one understand the major mechanisms of action of the antiepileptic drugs (AEDs). The goal of treatment with these medications is to modify the aberrant bursting properties, synchronization, and spread of abnormal firing without affecting ordinary electrical activity. These effects, although intended to control seizure disorders, have wide-ranging applications to other neuropsychiatric disorders such as bipolar affective disorder (BPAD), anxiety, pain, and alcohol dependence, to name a few.

The major effects of the well-known AEDs fall into three categories and are shown in the table. The first involves the voltage-gated sodium channel discussed in Chapter 3, Cells of the Nervous System. Remember that these are the pores that allow rapid entry of sodium into the cell to propagate the action potential along the axon. Modulation of the gating of these channels is believed to account for some of the effectiveness of several AEDs. The second category involves the voltage-gated calcium channels (also reviewed in Chapter 3, Cells of the Nervous System), which are located on the terminals of the neuron and instigate the release of neurotransmitters into the synaptic cleft. Blockade of these channels decreases the neurotransmitter release and ultimately decreases excitability.

The final mechanism of action involves the GABA receptor and increasing inhibition. We already discussed the enhanced effect that barbiturates and benzodiazepines can have on the GABA receptor. Additionally, valproate and gabapentin increase GABA synthesis and turnover with the net effect of increased activity of these inhibitory neurons. Hypothetically, a fourth mechanism of action is possible: blocking the glutamate receptors and decreasing neuronal excitability. Unfortunately, with glutamate receptor–blocking agents, clinical trials have been disappointing and none have made it to the market yet.

The Mechanisms of Action for Some of the Well-known Antiepileptic Drugs

	Sodium Channels $\geq$	Calcium Channels $\geq$	GABA System
Phenytoin	X	—	—
Carbama-zepine	X	—	—
Lamotrigine	X	X	—
Valproate	X	X	↑ turnover
Gabapentin	—	X	↑ turnover
Phenobarbital	—	X	X
Benzodia-zepines	—	—	X

GABA, γ-aminobutyric acid.

Although effector proteins can be G-protein–gated ion channels, which allow the entry of ions, the more interesting effector proteins are enzymes that trigger a process called the *secondary messenger cascade*. Figure 5.4 shows an example of this cascade. The neurotransmitter activates the G-protein, which slides along the membrane and stimulates the effector protein—in this case, adenylyl cyclase. The activated adenylyl cyclase then converts adenosine triphosphate (ATP) into cyclic adenosine monophosphate (cAMP): the second messenger, which will diffuse away into the cytosol where it can alter neuronal function. With the exception of serotonin type 3 receptor (5-hydroxytryptamine$_3$ [5-HT$_3$]), all the monoamine receptors belong to the G-protein–coupled family.

Serotonin Receptors

The original discovery of the serotonin receptor led to two subtypes: 5-HT$_1$ and 5-HT$_2$. Further discoveries, especially the application of molecular cloning techniques, has resulted in multiple subdivisions of these two receptors, and the addition of several more for a total of 14. Although the prospect of activating or blocking the various receptors for further refinement of psychopharmacologic treatment is an enticing possibility, the clinical results with a few exceptions have been limited.

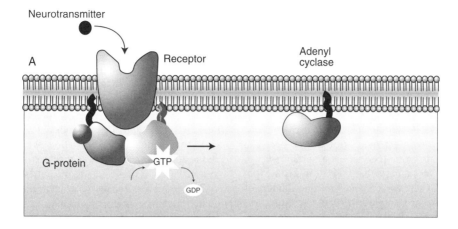

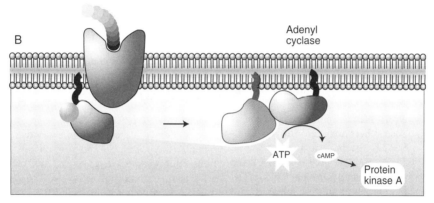

FIGURE 5.4 ● G-protein-coupled receptor. The initiation of the second messenger cascade starts with a neurotransmitter binding with G-protein receptor and ends with the conversion of ATP into cAMP. ATP, adenosine triphosphate; cAMP, cyclic adenosine monophosphate; GTP, guanosine triphosphate; GDP, guanosine diphosphate.

POINT OF INTEREST

Autoreceptors reside on the cell body or terminal of the *presynaptic neuron*. They sense the presence of the neurotransmitter and provide negative feedback to the neuron. That is, if too much of the neurotransmitter is present, these receptors activate a second messenger and turn off further release of the neurotransmitter—and in some cases reduce synthesis of the neurotransmitter. The figure shows an example of this type of receptor using the 5-HT$_{1A}$ (anxiety related) and 5-HT$_{1D}$ (migraine related) receptors. Similar autoreceptors are known for other transmitters such as dopamine and norepinephrine. Blocking these specific receptors may provide unique ways to alleviate specific symptoms.

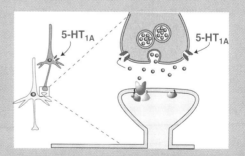

Autoreceptors such as 5-HT$_{1A}$ (which reside on the cell body) and 5-HT$_{1D}$ (which resides on the postsynaptic terminal) provide negative feedback to the neuron. In this example, too much serotonin turns off further release and/or synthesis of serotonin. 5-HT$_{1A}$, 5-hydroxytryptamine$_{1A}$

The 5-HT$_1$ receptors make up the largest subtype with 5-HT$_{1A}$, 5-HT$_{1B}$, 5-HT$_{1D}$, 5-HT$_{1E}$, and 5-HT$_{1F}$. 5-HT$_{1A}$ has received the most interest and seems to play a prominent role in depression and anxiety. It is an autoreceptor on the cell body. Stimulation of this receptor reduces cell firing and curtails the release of serotonin. How this would improve mood is unclear, but blocking this receptor has decreased the effectiveness of tricyclic antidepressants in rat models of depression. The anxiolytic buspirone (Buspar) is a partial 5-HT$_{1A}$ agonist, which suggests that 5-HT$_{1A}$ has some role in anxiety. The development and distribution of buspirone is an example of specific serotonin receptor targeting, which has had only a marginal effect on clinical practice.

The 5-HT$_{1D}$ receptor is also an autoreceptor but is located on the nerve terminal at the synapse. Here it appears to function to sense the serotonin in the synaptic cleft and turn off release of more serotonin when stimulated. The 5-HT$_{1D}$ receptor is stimulated by the antimigraine drug sumatriptan (Imitrex) although the importance of this effect in the overall efficacy of the medication is unclear. Some researchers are exploring the effectiveness of a 5-HT$_{1D}$ receptor antagonist for the treatment of depression. The goal is to block the negative feedback mediated through the 5-HT$_{1D}$ receptor so that more serotonin is released into the synapse.

Some other important serotonin receptors for the psychiatrist are 5-HT$_{2A}$ and 5-HT$_{2C}$. The 5-HT$_{2A}$ receptor has been identified as playing an important role in the "atypicalness" of the second-generation antipsychotic agents (clozapine, risperidone, olanzapine, etc.). These newer agents have a greater capacity to block 5-HT$_{2A}$ than the traditional agents such as haloperidol and it is speculated that this results in the observed decrease in extrapyramidal symptom (EPS) and greater cognitive improvements.

Dopamine Receptors

The dopamine receptors are involved in a wide range of functions including locomotion, cognition, psychosis, and even neuroendocrine secretion. It became clear after 1979 that there was more than one dopamine receptor: D$_1$ and D$_2$. More recently with molecular cloning they have identified three more receptors: D$_3$, D$_4$, and D$_5$. The D$_3$ and D$_4$ receptors are "D$_2$-like" and the D$_5$ receptor is "D$_1$-like." However, the D$_1$ and D$_2$ receptors remain the most important.

$$\text{"D}_2\text{-like"} = \text{D}_3 \text{ and } \text{D}_4$$

$$\text{"D}_1\text{-like"} = \text{D}_5$$

The D$_1$ and D$_2$ receptors have been distinguished by their differing affinity for binding with traditional antipsychotic agents such as haloperidol: The D$_2$ receptor has high affinity whereas the D$_1$ receptor has low affinity. Increased D$_2$ receptor antagonism correlates with the therapeutic efficacy and EPS side effect with the traditional antipsychotics. There is great interest in the "D$_2$-like" receptors (D$_3$ and D$_4$) as possible alternative sites for therapeutic potentiation with antipsychotic agents, but as yet these receptors have failed to translate into clinically significant benefits.

The psychostimulants (cocaine, amphetamine, methylphenidate, etc.) work in part by blocking the reuptake of dopamine and leaving more dopamine in the synapse to stimulate the dopamine receptors. The effects are increased energy, improved cognition, and even psychosis. The effects on reward and cognition seem to be more prominently mediated by the D$_1$ receptor. Augmenting D$_1$ and D$_2$ receptors (agonists) are the mainstay of treatment for Parkinson's disease.

Adrenergic Receptors

The adrenergic receptors are divided into three main subtypes α_1, α_2, and β. Each one of these has three subtypes: α_{1a}, α_{1b}, α_{1d}, α_{2a}, and so on. We will focus on the three main subtypes. The α_1 receptor is believed to play a role in smooth muscle contraction and has been implicated in effecting blood pressure, nasal congestion, and prostate function. Although widely expressed in the central nervous system (CNS), the central role of the α_1 receptor remains to be determined. Locomotor activation and arousal have been suggested by some studies. Stimulation of the α_1 receptor may synergistically increase the activity of the serotonin neurons in the raphe nucleus although stimulation of the α_2 receptor may have just the opposite effect.

The α_2 receptor subtypes in the CNS inhibit the firing of the norepinephrine neurons through autoreceptors. This mechanism of action is believed to mediate the sedative and hypotensive effects of the α_2 receptor agonist clonidine. Additionally, stimulation of the α_2 receptors decreases sympathetic activity that may explain the therapeutic utility of clonidine for suppressing the heightened sympathetic state for patients in opiate withdrawal.

The β receptor subtypes are more famous for their part in slowing cardiac rhythm and lowering blood pressure. The functions of the β receptors in the CNS, although widely distributed, are not well understood. It is not uncommon to use a β blocker, for example, propranolol, for treating performance anxiety or antipsychotic-induced akathisia. Whether these benefits come from a central or peripheral blockage of the β receptor, or both, is not known.

Histamine Receptors

There are now four histamine receptors although H_4 is predominately in the periphery and only recently discovered. The H_1 receptor is the target for the classic antihistamines, which highlights its role in sedation and conversely arousal. Of great interest to psychiatrists is the role of H_1 in weight gain. Recent analysis has shown that the potential to gain weight with antipsychotic agents correlates with the antagonism for the H_1 receptor, for example, clozapine and olanzapine have the most affinity and weight gain, whereas aripiprazole and ziprasidone have the least.

The H_2 receptor is more traditionally associated with the gut. Blockade of the H_2 receptor has been a widely used treatment for peptic ulcer disease. The H_3 receptor functions as an inhibitory receptor on the histamine neurons as well as other nonhistamine nerve terminals. The role of this receptor is not clearly understood, but may be involved in appetite, arousal, and cognition.

Cholinergic Receptors

It was with the cholinergic receptor that scientists first realized that one neurotransmitter (acetylcholine [Ach]) could have different receptors. The initial subtypes were identified and named after the drug that distinguished its effect. For example, nicotine will stimulate cholinergic receptors in skeletal muscle, but not in the heart. Conversely, muscarine will stimulate the heart, but has no effect on skeletal muscle. Therefore, the two receptors can be identified by the actions of different drugs and the receptors were named after those drugs: nicotinic and muscarinic. Unfortunately, it has been hard to find a drug with unique action on each receptor subtype, so we are stuck with designations such as 1A, 2B, and so on.

Many more subtypes of the nicotinic and muscarinic receptors have been identified since the early days of receptor delineation, but the significance of these various subtypes for the psychiatrist remains obscure. Clearly, ACh is important in cognition and memory as noted by the benefits of inhibiting acetylcholinesterase as a treatment for Alzheimer's disease. Likewise the blockage of the muscarinic receptor by tricyclic antidepressants and antipsychotic medications results in troublesome dry mouth, constipation, and urinary hesitancy (which we generically call the anticholinergic side effects). However, the importance of one receptor subtype over another has not been shown.

SIGNALING THE NUCLEUS

After the neurotransmitter has stimulated the G-protein to slide across the membrane and activate an enzyme (which is the case with most of the catecholamines) a cascade of events with second messengers transpires to modify neuronal function. Neurons use many different second messengers as signals within the cytosol—two of which we have discussed: Ca^{2+} and cAMP. The second messengers regulate neuronal function by activating enzymes that will add a phosphate group (*phosphorylation*) to other proteins in the cell. The *protein kinases*, of which there are wide varieties, are the enzymes that add a phosphate group to other proteins. Protein kinase A and calcium/calmodulin protein kinase (CaMK) are two examples of this sort of enzyme. Once proteins are phosphorylated they are "turned on" and can execute a broad range of cellular functions such as regulating enzyme activity or ion channels.

Alternatively, the protein kinases can elicit broader changes in neuronal functioning by activating the DNA and promoting the synthesis of messenger ribonucleic acid (mRNA) and proteins—*gene expression*. This process takes longer but can have large and relatively stable effects on the cell, for example, upregulation of receptors or the production of growth factor proteins. Figure 5.5 shows an example of how two different types of

DISORDERS

Myasthenia gravis is an autoimmune disease in which the body produces antibodies to the nicotinic ACh receptor. Patients complain of weakness and fatigue in the voluntary muscles resulting from the interruption of the chemical signal at the neuromuscular junction. Muscarinic receptors in the heart and CNS are unaffected.

ACh, unlike the monoamines, is cleared from the synaptic cleft by an enzyme, acetylcholinesterase. One treatment for myasthenia gravis is with the acetylcholinesterase inhibitors such as edrophonium (Tensilon) that prolong the life of the released ACh.

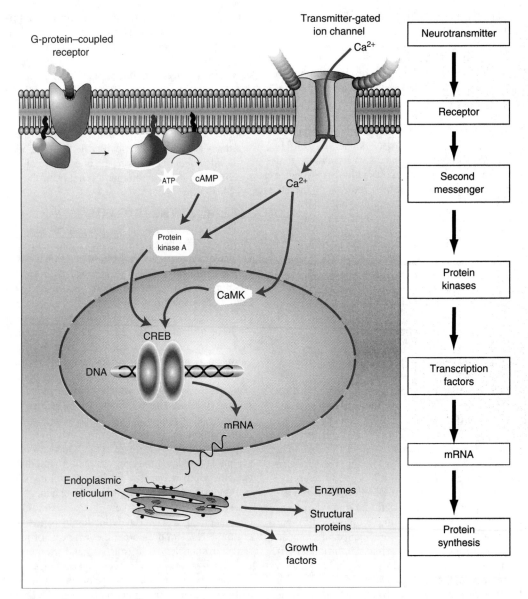

FIGURE 5.5 ● Signaling the nucleus. The neurotransmitters stimulate a cascade of events that ultimately leads to activation of the DNA (gene expression) and the synthesis of proteins that can modify the function of the cell. ATP, adenosine triphosphate; cAMP, cyclic adenosine monophosphate; CaMK, calcium/calmodulin protein kinase; CREB, cyclic adenosine monophosphate response element binding; mRNA, messenger ribonucleic acid.

receptors—a G-protein–coupled receptor and a transmitter-gate ion channel—can activate a second messenger that will stimulate the production of new proteins.

LONG-TERM POTENTIATION: A SUMMARY EXAMPLE

Understanding long-term potentiation (LTP) is a way to apply what has been discussed in the past few chapters to a topic of great relevance to

neuroscience: learning and memory. LTP is a laboratory example of learning that was discovered accidentally. As we have seen, applying a single stimulus to a neuron generates an excitatory impulse (EPSP) in the cell. Applying high-frequency stimuli—hundreds of impulses within a second—generates a higher EPSP in the cell. What was found accidentally was that once a neuron has been exposed to high-frequency stimulation, something changes, and now a single stimulus will

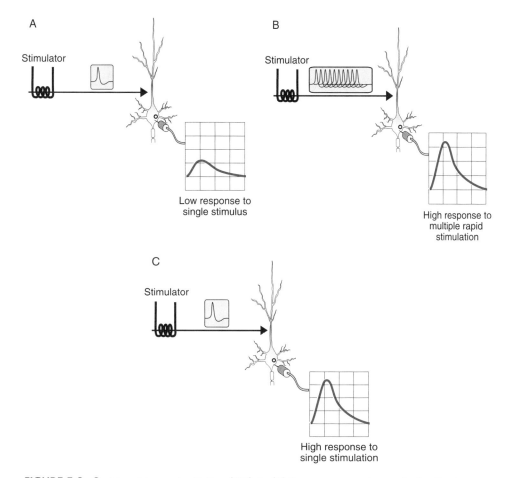

FIGURE 5.6 ● Long-term potentiation (LTP). In (**A**) the neuron receives a single stimulus that generates a small impulse in the cell body. In (**B**) a high-frequency stimulus generates a big response in the cell body. This process changes something in the cell, and following this high-frequency testing, the original single stimulus (**C**) generates a big response in the cell body.

generate a high EPSP. This sort of change has been shown to last for several months if not longer. Figure 5.6 shows these three steps.

LTP sounds like one of those topics that neuroscientists discuss ad nauseam, but which has little relevance to practicing clinicians. *Oh contraire*! LTP is a demonstration—although artificial—that neurons can incorporate lasting changes, which is an essential step to developing memories and skills. And what is life without memories? Likewise, problems with memories are diagnostic for several of the disorders we frequently encounter, for example, Alzheimer's disease and post-traumatic stress disorder (PTSD).

The interesting aspect of LTP comes when we start looking at the molecular changes that take place when LTP occurs. Researchers have shown that both glutamate receptors (NMDA and AMPA

as shown in Figure 5.2) must be operational for the process to work. Likewise others have shown that calcium (a second messenger) and the kinases are required for LTP. Of even greater interest is the demonstration that protein synthesis (gene expression) is an essential part of the development of LTP. All the processes shown in Figure 5.5 are involved in LTP.

What happens inside the cell with the induction of LTP? Clearly there is some strengthening of the connection between the two cells that are communicating when LTP occurs. Figure 5.7 depicts the events that transpire when the presynaptic cell is hyperstimulated, the postsynaptic cell signals its nucleus, and the connection between the two cells is enhanced by the insertion of more glutamate receptors. Additional evidence has shown that a retrograde signal such as nitric oxide diffuses back

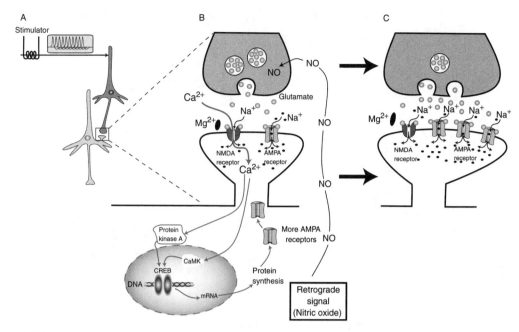

FIGURE 5.7 ●   The process of LTP inducing a change at the synapse. **A:** Hyperstimulation of the presynaptic neuron. **B:** The NMDA and AMPA receptors open, allowing the entry of the second messenger, calcium, which signals the nucleus to synthesize more receptors. **C:** The new AMPA receptors are inserted into the membrane that has the effect of increasing the cell's responsiveness to future stimulation. LTP, long-term potentiation; NMDA, *N*-methyl-D-aspartate; AMPA, α-amino-3-hydroxy-5-methyl-4-isoxazole propionate; NO, nitric oxide.

across the synaptic cleft and induces the presynaptic neuron to release more transmitters. The combined result is increased sensitivity and responsiveness at the synapse: more transmitters and more receptors resulting in a stronger signal.

TREATMENT: ANXIETY

Some of the anxiety disorders, particularly those involving avoidance of a specific situation or memory, can improve with the emotional learning that results from behavior modification. Recent research has shown that exposure therapy plus a partial NMDA agonist (D-cycloserine) resulted in superior reduction in symptoms when compared to exposure treatment alone. The stimulation of the NMDA receptor is believed to enhance the learning process induced by psychotherapy. The prospect of medications to activate the NMDA receptor in combination with psychotherapy as a way to accelerate healing is exciting.

Amazingly, the structural changes to the synapse can actually be seen under the right experimental circumstances. Engert and Bonhoeffer filled neurons from the hippocampus with fluorescent dye and then induced LTP. They captured the development of new spines on the postsynaptic dendrite as shown in Figure 5.8. This research is consistent with other data that suggests that the development of spines is potentially the structural manifestation of learning and memory.

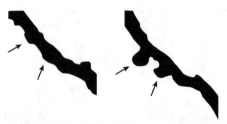

A Spines before LTP   B Spines 1 hour after LTP

FIGURE 5.8 ●   With the induction of LTP in neurons from the hippocampus, new spines developed on the dendrite within an hour as shown by the *arrows*. LTP, long-term potentiation. (Adapted from Engert F, Bonhoeffer T. Dendritic spine changes associated with hippocampal long-term synaptic plasticity. *Nature*. 1999;399[6731]:66–70.)

LTP demonstrates that electrical, molecular, and structural changes are involved in the process of storing information. It is not too much of a leap to assume that highly emotional events—such as high-frequency stimulation—leave lasting memories in a manner similar to LTP.

TREATMENT: TMS

LTP has not been established in humans for obvious ethical reasons. Repetitive transcranial magnetic stimulation (rTMS) offers a possible noninvasive method of stimulating conscious human subjects that can mimic the effects of LTP. The prospect of inducing long-lasting changes to the human cortex through noninvasive stimulation offers the prospect of a new kind of treatment applicable to a wide range of mental disorders.

Preliminary studies have demonstrated changes in motor skills consistent with changes seen with LTP when subjects receive continuous stimulation at the motor cortex. The changes lasted up to 60 minutes beyond the period of stimulation. Although the utility of a change lasting only 60 minutes is of little clinical value, the prospect of altering the function of the cortex without breaching the blood brain barrier is an exciting possibility.

QUESTIONS

1. Which equation is correct?
   a. Antagonist = stimulate.
   b. Agonist = block.
   c. Agonist = transmitter.
   d. Antagonist = endogenous ligand.

2. Which is not a glutamate receptor?
   a. NMDA.
   b. cAMP.
   c. AMPA.
   d. Kainate.

3. The strength of the GABA inhibitory signal is enhanced by all of the following except
   a. Ethanol.
   b. Phenobarbital.
   c. Carbamazepine.
   d. Neurosteroids.

4. The AEDs exert their major effects through all of the following except
   a. Decreasing glutamate activity.
   b. Modulation of the voltage-gated sodium channels.
   c. Blockade of the voltage-gated calcium channels.
   d. Increasing GABA activity.

5. Which of the following is true?
   a. Mg^{2+} is a common second messenger.
   b. Most monoamine receptors are fast receptors.
   c. Fast receptors typically lead to gene expression.
   d. Autoreceptors give negative feedback to the neuron.

6. Gene expression stimulated by a neurotransmitter involves all of the following except
   a. Phosphorylation.
   b. Long-term potentiation.
   c. Protein kinases.
   d. G-protein–coupled receptor.

7. All of the following about LTP are true except
   a. Enhanced EPSP.
   b. Increased receptors.
   c. Gene expression.
   d. Enhanced ligand binding.

8. Which describes LTP best?
   a. It was discovered by accident.
   b. Neuroscientists love to pontificate on this topic.
   c. It is an example of learning.
   d. All of the above.

See Answers section at end of book.

CHAPTER 6

Hormones and the Brain

CHARACTERISTICS OF A HORMONE

As described in the preceding chapters, electrochemical signaling is the brain's primary method of communication. The other way the brain signals its intentions is through hormones, which are molecules sent to the target cells by way of the blood stream.

Neurons and neurotransmitters can be compared to telephone wires connecting one phone to another. Hormones are like TV signals that are broadcast across the skies and only recognized by appropriate receivers. With the advent of cell phones and cable TV, the distinction between direct and broadcast communication has blurred. This blurring has also occurred in the brain. Increasingly, we are finding that traditional neurotransmitters sometimes function as hormones and hormones sometimes function as neurotransmitters. For example, epinephrine can be a neurotransmitter, but functions as a hormone when released from the adrenal medulla with a signal from the sympathetic division of the autonomic nervous system (ANS).

Although they can act in a similar manner, hormones differ from neurotransmitters in several key ways. Hormones tend to do the following:

1. Effect behavior and physiology in a gradual manner over days and weeks.
2. Receive reciprocal feedback.
3. Secrete in small pulsatile bursts.
4. Vary the levels on a circadian rhythm.
5. Have different effects on different organs.

The last point (no. 5) is of great interest to us and will be a large part of the focus of this chapter.

TREATMENT: GnRH AGONIST

Clinicians can override the pulsatile nature of a releasing hormone to effectively treat problems such as endometriosis, prostate cancer, and early-onset puberty.

This treatment has also been used with sex offenders as a form of "chemical castration." In this process, a long-acting gonadotropin-releasing hormone (GnRH) agonist, leuprolide (Lupron Depot), inhibits the release of luteinizing hormone (LH) and follicle-stimulating hormone (FSH), although it stimulates the receptor. This effect is achieved because the continuous stimulation—in contrast to the usual intermittent stimulation—causes the desensitization of receptors in the pituitary. As a result, LH and FSH are not produced, which subsequently reduces the production of sex hormones.

Figure 5.3 in Chapter 5, Receptors and Signaling the Nucleus, showed that γ-aminobutyric

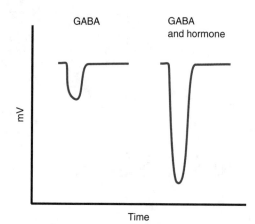

GABA   GABA
              and hormone

mV

Time

FIGURE 6.1 ● The Cl⁻ current is enhanced when a progesterone metabolite is added to γ-aminobutyric acid (GABA). Cl, (Adapted from Rupprecht R, Holsboer F. Neuroactive steroids: Mechanisms of action and neuropsychopharmacologic perspectives. *Trends Neurosci.* 1999;22[9]:410–460.)

acid (GABA) receptors are influenced by steroid hormones, although they are clearly not the primary target of these hormones. Figure 6.1 shows how the addition of a progesterone metabolite enhances the GABA elicited Cl⁻ current. This may explain the emergence of psychiatric symptoms with fluctuations in the sex hormones.

The difference between hormones and neurotransmitters is further blurred by the existence of *neuroendocrine* cells (sometimes called *neurosecretory cells*). Neuroendocrine cells are hybrids of neurons and endocrine cells (see Figure 6.2). They receive neural signals, but also secrete a hormone into the blood stream. The hypothalamus signals the pituitary with neuroendocrine cells.

Classification

There are three types of hormones, which can be grouped by their chemical structure: (a) protein, (b) amine, and (c) steroid (see Table 6.1). Protein hormones, such as neuropeptides, are large molecules composed of strings of amino acids. Amine hormones are small molecules derived from amino acids. Steroid hormones are composed of four interlocking rings synthesized from dietary cholesterol.

Effecting Target Cells

Hormones have two primary effects on target cells:

1. They promote differentiation and development.
2. They modulate the rate of function.

Hormones bind to specific receptors on or in the target cell in three ways. Most of the protein and amine hormones exert their effects by binding with receptors imbedded in the cell wall (as is the

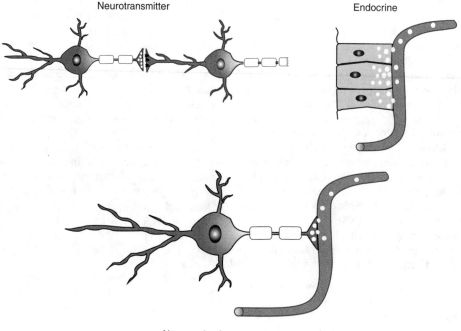

Neurotransmitter   Endocrine

Neuroendocrine

FIGURE 6.2 ● Chemical communication systems in humans.

TABLE 6.1

The Major Classes of Hormones

Protein Hormones
  Oxytocin
  Vasopressin
  Releasing Hormones
    Corticotropin-releasing hormone (CRH)
    Thyrotropin-releasing hormone (TRH)
    Gonadotropin-releasing hormone (GnRH)
    Growth hormone-releasing factor (GHRF)
  Tropic Hormones
    Adrenocorticotropic hormone (ACTH)
    Thyroid-stimulating hormone (TSH)
    Luteinizing hormone (LH)
    Follicle-stimulating hormone (FSH)
    Growth hormone (GH)
    Prolactin
Amine Hormones
  Epinephrine
  Norepinephrine
  Thyroid hormone
  Melatonin
Steroid Hormones
  Estrogens
  Progestins
  Androgens
  Glucocorticoids
  Mineralocorticoids

case with the classic neurotransmitters). The steroid hormones and thyroid hormone are lipophilic and can pass directly through the cell wall. They bind with receptors inside the cell. The steroid hormones bind with a receptor in the cytoplasm, which initiates protein synthesis when the complex couples with the DNA. The thyroid hormone receptor belongs to a family of nuclear hormone receptors. These receptors reside in the nucleus on the gene and suppress gene expression until activated by thyroid hormone (specifically T3). Figure 6.3 shows these three different receptors.

In all cases, the hormones change the function of the target cell by stimulating gene expression. This process is called a *genomic effect*. Some hormones effect neurons without stimulating the transcription of genes by modulating ion receptors. This process is called a *nongenomic effect*.

CENTRAL NERVOUS SYSTEM AND HORMONES

The primary endocrine glands in the brain are the hypothalamus and the pituitary gland. The hypothalamus appears to be the command center that integrates information about the state of the brain and the body by way of neuronal projections and intrinsic chemosensitive neurons. The hypothalamus coordinates the actions of the pituitary gland to maintain homeostasis in response to changes in the body and environment. Some of the essential somatic functions controlled by the hypothalamus and pituitary gland are as follows:

1. Control of blood flow (e.g., drinking, blood osmolarity, and renal clearance).
2. Regulation of energy metabolism (e.g., feeding, metabolic rate, and temperature).
3. Regulation of reproductive activity.
4. Coordination of response to threats.
5. Control of circadian rhythms.

The remarkable number of functions governed by these relatively small glands is possible due to the diversity of neuronal projections sent to the hypothalamus from the brain, as well as up the spinal cord. Additionally, the hypothalamus and pituitary gland have a multitude of intrinsic chemosensitive neurons that respond to circulating levels of various hormones. The pituitary gland, as well as some areas of the hypothalamus, is an area of the brain not protected by the blood-brain barrier. This allows for quicker feedback about the current status of target organs.

Of particular interest to behavioral neuroscientists are the direct afferent projections the hypothalamus receives from areas of the brain with well-known psychiatric functions. Four of these important projections are as follows:

1. Corticohypothalamic fibers: frontal cortex.
2. Hippocampohypothalamic fibers: hippocampus.
3. Amygdalohypothalamic fibers: amygdala.
4. Thalamohypothalamic fibers: thalamus.

These afferent fibers play a large role in the stimulation, or lack of stimulation, to the hypothalamus and the pituitary gland in the course of psychiatric disorders that result in many of the endocrine abnormalities found with mental illness.

Figure 6.4 shows the complex relationship between the cortex, hypothalamus, pituitary gland, and target organs for the neuroendocrine system. The figure illustrates the central location of the hypothalamus, the two sides of the pituitary, the variety of target organs affected, and the feedback

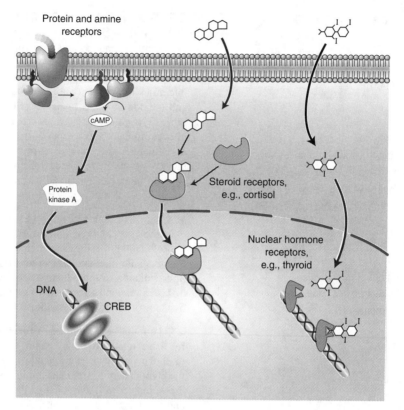

FIGURE 6.3 ● The three types of receptors utilized by different hormones. CREB, cyclic adenosine monophosphate response element binding; cAMP, cyclic adenosine monophosphate.

mechanisms. Figure 6.5 shows most of the hormones associated with the anterior pituitary gland, particularly the releasing hormones excreted by the neuroendocrine cells of the hypothalamus, which stimulate the release of the tropic hormones.

Although we will not review the endocrine system extensively, it is important to mention its importance because of the effects that the hormones (see Figures 6.4 and 6.5) have on the brain. Most of these will be addressed in their specific chapter in the middle section of this book. We will, however, discuss hypothalamic-pituitary-adrenal (HPA) axis and hypothalamic-pituitary-thyroid (HPT) axis in more detail here before moving on.

THYROID: THE HYPOTHALAMIC-PITUITARY-THYROID AXIS

Thyroid hormones are involved in maintaining optimal metabolism in nearly every organ system and are integral to the temperature regulation of the body. The secretion of thyroid hormones is controlled by the HPT axis shown in Figure 6.6. The neuroendocrine cells in the hypothalamus secrete

thyrotropin-releasing hormone (TRH) into the portal circulation of the pituitary. The TRH binds with receptors on the thyrotroph cells of the anterior pituitary and stimulates the release of thyroid-stimulating hormone (TSH). The hypothalamic neuroendocrine cells also synthesize and release somatostatin, which inhibits the release of TSH (as well as growth hormone).

TSH stimulates the synthesis and release of two thyroid hormones from the thyroid gland: (a) triiodothyronine (T_3) and (b) tetraiodothyronine (T_4). T_4 is the predominant form of thyroid released by the gland, but T_3 is the more biologically potent form. T_4 is converted into T_3 by the target organs as well as the brain.

In humans, congenital hypothyroidism causes severe structural and functional neurologic abnormalities. This disorder is easily corrected, but so horrid when missed. It is one of the few medical conditions routinely screened in the newborn nursery.

The role of thyroid hormones in the maintenance of the mature brain is less understood. The brain maintains tight control over the level

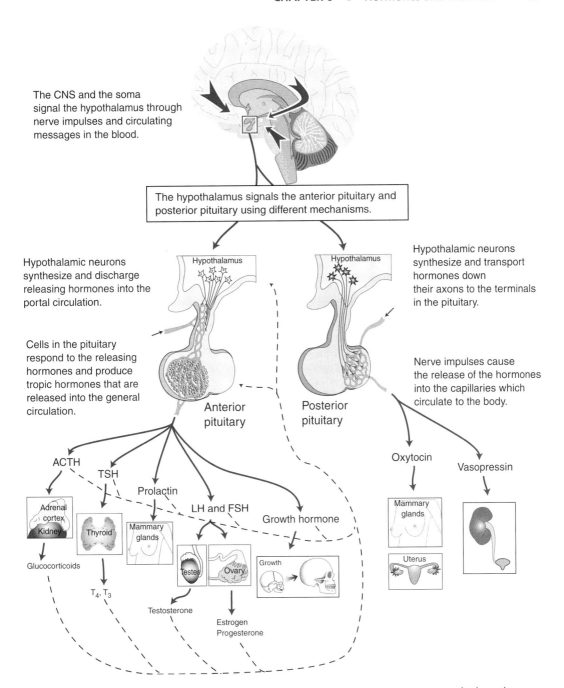

The CNS and the soma signal the hypothalamus through nerve impulses and circulating messages in the blood.

The hypothalamus signals the anterior pituitary and posterior pituitary using different mechanisms.

Hypothalamic neurons synthesize and discharge releasing hormones into the portal circulation.

Cells in the pituitary respond to the releasing hormones and produce tropic hormones that are released into the general circulation.

Hypothalamic neurons synthesize and transport hormones down their axons to the terminals in the pituitary.

Nerve impulses cause the release of the hormones into the capillaries which circulate to the body.

FIGURE 6.4 ● Information from the cerebral cortex and blood stream converges on the hypothalamus, which instigates a cascade of actions and in turn responds to feedback from the target organs. CNS, central nervous system; ACTH, adrenocorticotropic hormone; TSH, thyroid-stimulating hormone; T_4, tetraiodothyronine; T_3, triiodothyronine; LH, Luteinizing hormone; FSH, follicle-stimulating hormone.

of thyroid hormone in the central nervous system (CNS) and thyroid nuclear receptors are highly expressed throughout the brain, particularly within the hippocampus. Clinical features of hypothyroidism and hyperthyroidism, including significant neuropsychiatric symptoms, are described in Table 6.2.

Additionally, clinical studies have shown that the T_3 hormone can augment treatment resistant depression, as well as accelerate the response to antidepressants when initiating treatment for depression. However, meta-analysis of augmenting and accelerating studies found the trials to be small in number and not uniformly positive.

Thyroid hormones are important for the function of the adult brain, but the underlying molecular mechanism by which the HPT axis influences neuropsychiatric conditions remains unclear. Many authors on psychiatry postulate that the cognitive and emotional symptoms associated with thyroid disorders are related to changes in serotonin, norepinephrine (NE), and dopamine. Indeed, studies on rats have found increased serotonergic transmission concomitant with decreased 5-HT_{1A} sensitivity and increased 5-HT_{2A} sensitivity with exogenous thyroid. With regard to NE, Gordan et al. have demonstrated anterograde transport of T_3 from the cell bodies in the locus coeruleus to the nerve terminals in the hippocampus and cerebral cortex. They believe that T_3 functions as a cotransmitter along with NE. This suggests that sufficient T_3 is needed for proper NE activity.

An alternative explanation for the influence of thyroid hormones on the psychiatric status of the mature brain revolves around their role with nerve growth factors. Nerve growth factor genes are activated by T_3 during development, although growth factors, such as brain-derived neurotropic factor (BDNF), are unaltered by thyroid hormone in the adult brain. Recently, Vaidya et al. established that 5-HT_{1A} stimulation with chronic T_3 administration altered the production of BDNF in the hippocampus, although neither did so alone. They postulate a synergistic relationship between 5-HT_{1A} receptors and thyroid hormones in the expression of BDNF (see Chapter 18, Depression, for more on the role of BDNF in depression).

The most compelling explanation for the correlation between mood disorders and thyroid

Releasing hormones	CRH	TRH	PRH	GnRH	GHRH	Hypothalamus
Tropic hormones	ACTH	TSH	Prolactin	LH and FSH	Growth hormone	Anterior pituitary
Target organs	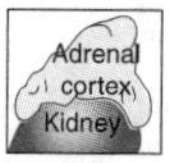 Adrenal cortex Kidney	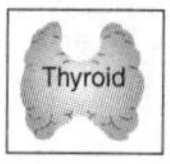 Thyroid	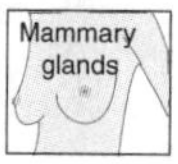 Mammary glands	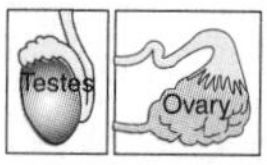 Testes Ovary	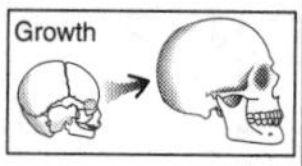 Growth	
Peripheral hormones	Gluco-corticoids	T4, T3		Testosterone Estrogen Progesterone		

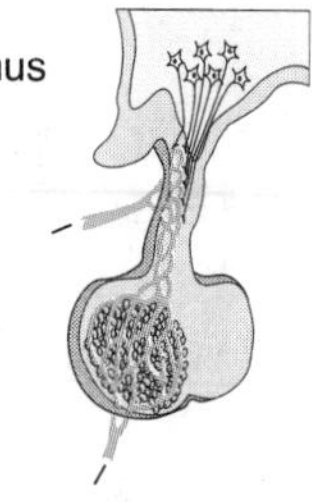

FIGURE 6.5 ● The anterior pituitary. Releasing hormones excreted by the hypothalamus stimulate the release of tropic hormones from the anterior pituitary. The tropic hormones then stimulate the target organ to change or release its own hormone. CRH, corticotropin-releasing hormone; TRH, thyrotropin-releasing hormone; PRH, prolactin-releasing hormone; GnRH, gonadotropin-releasing hormone; GHRH, growth-hormone-releasing hormone; ACTH, adrenocorticotropic hormone; TSH, thyroid-stimulating hormone; LH, luteinizing hormone; FSH, follicle-stimulating hormone; T4, tetraiodothyronine; T3, triiodothyronine.

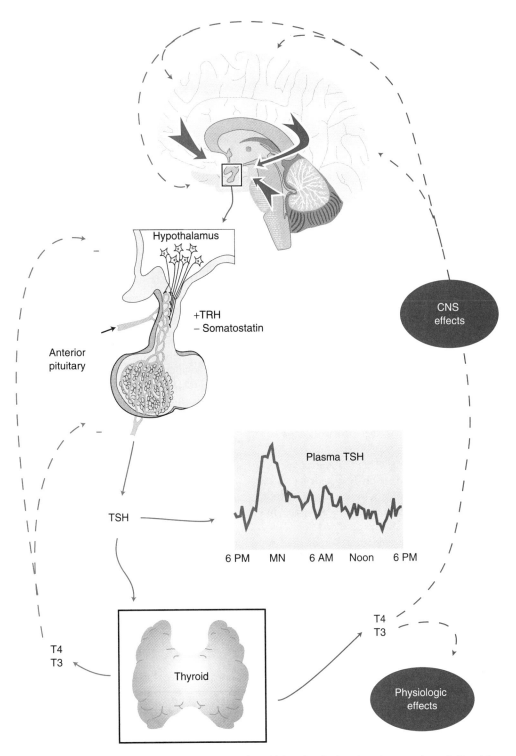

Hypothalamus

+TRH
− Somatostatin

Anterior
pituitary

CNS
effects

Plasma TSH

TSH

6 PM   MN   6 AM   Noon   6 PM

T4
T3

T4
T3

Thyroid

Physiologic
effects

FIGURE 6.6 ● The hypothalamic-pituitary-thyroid (HPT) axis showing the complex relationship between the brain and thyroid hormones. The important point is that tetraiodothyronine (T4) and triiodothyronine (T3) have direct effects on the brain as well as the body. TRH, thyrotropin-releasing hormone; TSH, thyroid-stimulating hormone.

TABLE 6.2

Common Clinical Features of Abnormal Thyroid Function

	Physical Symptoms	Psychiatric Symptoms
Hypertyroidism	Tachycardia	Anxiety
	Weight loss	Irritability
	Heat intolerance	Trouble in concentrating
	Sweating	Emotionally labile
		Psychomotor agitation
Hypertyroidism	Fatigue	Depressed mood
	Weight gain	Decreased libido
	Cold intolerance	Psychomotor retardation
	Dry skin	Poor memory
		Severe forms: delusions and hallucinations

hormones appears to be related to the general effect that thyroid has on brain metabolism, much like the effect on peripheral metabolism. Positron emission tomography (PET) studies on patients with hypothyroidism show global reduction in brain activity and as much as a 23% reduction in cerebral blood flow in the patients compared to controls. In a remarkable study at the National Institutes of Mental Health, Marangell et al. examined TSH in medication free patients with mood disorders, none of whom had overt thyroid disease. The study found an inverse relationship between TSH and global cerebral blood flow. Additionally, the areas with the greatest reduction in blood flow were the areas of the brain associated with depression: Left dorsolateral prefrontal cortex (PFC) and medial PFC.

One can postulate that the hypothalamus responds to the reduced metabolism of the PFC (by way of the afferent fibers) as a result of the depression and reacts by stimulating the release of TSH. In essence, the HPT axis is seeking to correct the brain disorder.

HYPOTHALAMIC-PITUITARY-ADRENAL AXIS AND STRESS

The HPA axis controls the synthesis and release of the corticosteroids. The corticosteroids are derived from dietary cholesterol in the adrenal cortex and include the mineralocorticoids, sex hormones, and glucocorticoids (see Figure 6.7). The mineralocorticoid aldosterone assists in the maintenance of the proper ionic balance by stimulating the kidney to conserve sodium and excrete potassium. The sex

DISORDER: MOOD DISORDERS

Although it is clear that thyroid disorders cause neuropsychiatric symptoms and that adding thyroid hormone can accelerate and augment the treatment of mood disorders, relatively few psychiatric patients have thyroid disease. Two analyses of clinical patients with depression found a 2% to 2.5% incidence of thyroid disease. The researchers concluded that routine screening for thyroid disease was not justified. Furthermore, although some patients with affective disorders can have mild laboratory changes, often referred to as subclinical thyroid disease, almost all anomalies resolve with effective treatment of the psychiatric disorder.

DISORDER: ANOREXIA NERVOSA

Women with anorexia nervosa, when purging and undernourished, often have symptoms that resemble hypothyroidism (cold intolerance, bradycardia, low resting metabolic rate, etc.). Thyroid studies of patients in this condition have found low normal T_4, low T_3, and normal TSH. Additionally, reverse T_3, the metabolically inactive enantiomer of T_3, is increased. This thyroid profile is called *euthyroid sick syndrome*. It can be produced by starvation in normal volunteers and is corrected with weight gain.

This decrease in active T_3 thyroid profile seems like a physiologic adaptation to malnutrition, with the goal of preserving calories and limiting the expenditure of energy. Some patients with eating disorders will take exogenous thyroid to stimulate their metabolism.

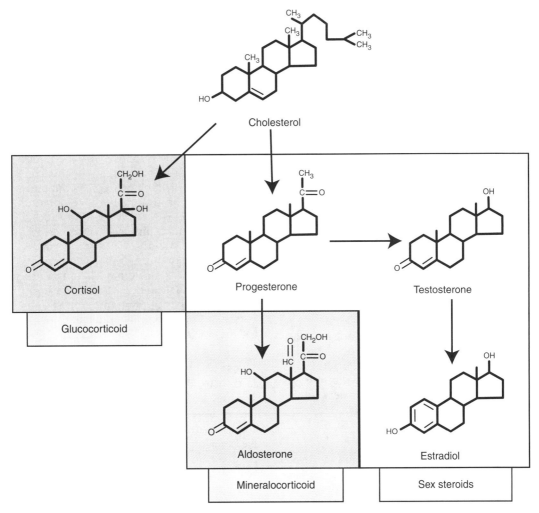

FIGURE 6.7 ● The corticosteroids are built from the sterol backbone of cholesterol by the addition or removal of side groups.

hormones are secreted in negligible amounts, but have physiologic significance, and are covered in more detail in Chapter 13, Sex and the Brain. The hormone of greatest interest to the mental health community is the glucocorticoid cortisol.

Cortisol is of great interest to us because it mobilizes energy (by promoting catabolic activity) and increases cardiovascular tone. At the same time, cortisol suppresses anabolic activity, such as reproduction, growth, digestion, and immunity. The release of cortisol varies through out the day, with maximal secretion in the early morning hours to effectively prepare the brain and body for the rigors of the day. Cortisol also plays a large part in acute and chronic stress, which we will discuss subsequently.

The secretion of the adrenal cortex is controlled by the hypothalamus (see Figure 6.8). The hypothalamus, with input from the cortex and feedback through the blood, synthesizes and releases corticotropin-releasing hormone (CRH) into the portal circulation of the pituitary, which in turn stimulates the release of adrenocorticotropic hormone (ACTH) from the anterior pituitary. The input to the hypothalamus from the cortex includes inhibitory signals from the hippocampus and activating signals from the amygdala. In other words, a healthy hippocampus turns down the HPA axis, while an active amygdala turns it up. This is important in understanding the endocrine role in depression and anxiety.

DISORDER: ANXIETY

CRH is an example of a hormone that has multiple effects on the body. The primary role of CRH is the stimulation of ACTH, but CRH receptors can be found throughout the brain, not just on the anterior pituitary, suggesting other functions for this hormone. Blocking of the CRH receptors may have a role to play in the treatment of anxiety (see Chapter 19, Anxiety).

ACTH is released into the systemic circulation from the anterior pituitary. ACTH starts as a large propeptide precursor that is cleaved into smaller segments, some of which (such as ACTH) are biologically active (i.e., β-endorphin and alpha-melanocyte-stimulating hormone [α-MSH]). ACTH stimulates the release of cortisol from the

adrenal cortex. This has a variety of physiologic effects, including changes in the CNS. The high incidence of psychiatric symptoms in patients with primary endocrine disorders, such as Cushing's disease and Addison's disease, is supportive evidence of the direct effects of cortisol on the brain.

DISORDER: ADDISON'S AND CUSHING'S DISEASES

Addison's disease, first described by Thomas Addison in 1855, results from a loss of cortisol and aldosterone secretion due to the near total or total destruction of both the adrenal glands. Classic symptoms include anorexia, nausea, and hypotension, along with neuropsychiatric symptoms of apathy, fatigue, irritability, and cognitive impairment.

Cushing's disease is named after neurosurgeon Harvey Cushing, who in 1932 linked adrenal hyperplasia and hypercortisolaemia with a pituitary adenoma. The somatic effects of excessive cortisol include easy bruising, truncal obesity, muscle atrophy, osteoporosis, and impaired immune response. The psychiatric symptoms are similar to endogenous depression: irritability, depressed mood, insomnia, and trouble with memory/concentration. Patients can also experience euphoria and even hypomania, as well as psychosis. However, these symptoms are more common in patients taking glucocorticoid medications. With both Addison's and Cushing's diseases, most psychiatric symptoms remit with the resumption of normal endocrine status.

Stress

In his book, *Why Zebras Don't Get Ulcers*, Sapolsky uses a clever example to illustrate the difference between the acute physical stress that a zebra experiences when running from a lion and the chronic psychological stress that many people experience in modern industrial societies. The acute response is the biologic equivalent of mobilizing troops to handle a perceived threat. The sympathetic activation by ANS and the liberation of cortisol bring the body and brain to an alert, fight or flight orientation. Cortisol has the effect of mobilizing energy, increasing cerebral glucose,

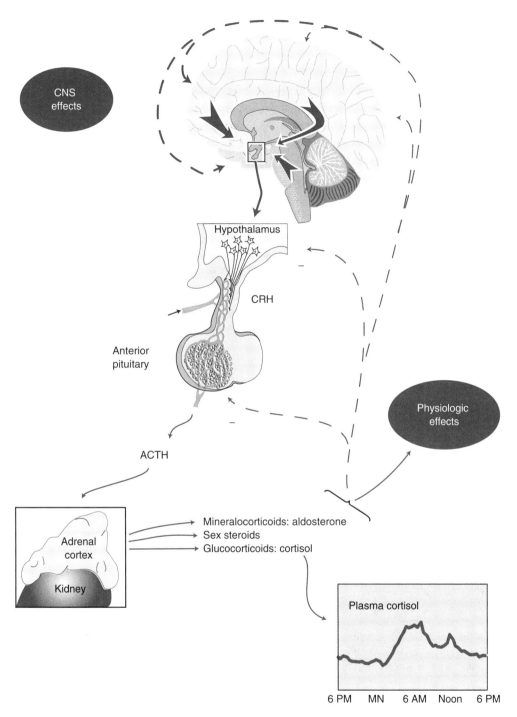

CNS effects

Hypothalamus

CRH

Anterior pituitary

Physiologic effects

ACTH

Adrenal cortex

Kidney

Mineralocorticoids: aldosterone
Sex steroids
Glucocorticoids: cortisol

Plasma cortisol

6 PM   MN   6 AM   Noon   6 PM

FIGURE 6.8 ●   The hypothalamic-pituitary-adrenal (HPA) axis. Note that adrenocorticotropic hormone (ACTH) releases an array of hormones with a diurnal variation. As with all hormones, there are direct effects on the cerebral cortex. CNS, central nervous system; CRH, corticotropin-releasing hormone.

and turning down the nonessential functions (i.e., erections, digestions, etc.). Ultimately, the brain becomes more focused and vigilant.

The body and brain pay a price for maintaining a heightened state of alertness when the stress persists and the person cannot adapt. As seen with Addison's and Cushing's diseases, too little or too much cortisol is pathologic. The benefits of cortisol can be graphed as an upside-down "U." Moderation is best.

Chronic stress is best defined as an adverse experience that induces heightened arousal over which one has little control. One of the effects of chronic stress is that the brain is unable to turn down the HPA axis, which exposes the brain and body to excess glucocorticoids. Although most of the data comes from patients on glucocorticoid medications with Cushing's disease or from laboratory animal studies, the adverse consequences are believed to be similar to that of the harried stressed-out individual.

Pathologic consequences of heightened sympathetic activity and HPA activation are hypertension, formation of atherosclerotic plaque, diabetes, ulcers, and impaired immune function. In the brain, the most dramatic negative effect involves the hippocampus, a structure with ample glucocorticoid receptors and afferent fibers to the hypothalamus. The hippocampus is well known for its role in memory, and excess glucocorticoids have indeed been shown to have the following effects:

1. Impair memory performance.
2. Disrupt long-term potentiation (LTP).
3. Induce atrophy of hippocampal dendrites.
4. Shrink the hippocampus.
5. Decrease neurogenesis.

These cognitive changes do not develop without an active amygdala. The amygdala, well known for its role in anxiety, is stimulated by glucocorticoids, which in turn potentiates the hippocampus (see Figure 6.9). Chronic stress increases the dendritic arborization of neurons in the basolateral amygdala, which may be a reason people have trouble forgetting traumatic events.

Cushing's Disease
Excessive glucocorticoid levels, for any reason, have been shown to cause impairments in declarative memory as well as hippocampal atrophy. In a remarkable analysis of patients with Cushing's disease who underwent neurosurgical resection, Starkman et al. showed that decreasing urinary cortisol correlated with increase in the hippocampal volume. In a follow-up study, they showed that a greater improvement in memory (word list

learning) was associated with greater increase in the hippocampal volume.

Aging
There is evidence that glucocorticoids may contribute to age-related neuronal atrophy and cognitive decline. An essential aspect of a healthy, adaptive stress response is the ability to shut off the system when the threat has passed. Studies on rats have shown that the HPA axis is slower to turn off as the animals age. Therefore, as the animal ages, it is exposed to more continuous high levels of glucocorticoids. In humans, the ability to turn off the HPA axis and the sympathetic nervous system in tranquil times is a variable trait. Some people are able to do this more effectively than others.

Lupien et al. followed up 51 healthy volunteers over 6 years and annually measured 24-hour plasma cortisol. They assessed memory and hippocampal volume in sub-groups of those with high levels of cortisol and compared those findings to the groups with lower levels of cortisol. They found greater impairments in memory and a 14% reduction in the volume of the hippocampus in the group with high cortisol levels. These results suggest that prolonged exposure to glucocorticoids either reduces the ability of neurons to resist insults, or directly damages the neurons.

TREATMENT: DEPRESSION

Patients with depression exhibit the triad of hypercortisolaemia, hippocampal atrophy, and cognitive impairment (we will cover this in greater detail in Chapter 18, Depression). Of note is a recent study of patients with psychotic depression that showed an improvement in symptoms when treated with mifepristone (a glucocorticoid receptor antagonist blocker known as *RU-486*—the "abortion pill"). In this open-label trial, mifepristone was given in low doses as well as high doses to patients with psychotic major depression. No new medications were started and patients were allowed to remain on their antidepressant and/or antipsychotic medications. Most of the patients given adequate mifepristone showed a 50% reduction in depression and psychotic scores. These findings suggest that hormone dysregulation may play a role in the cause or expression of depression.

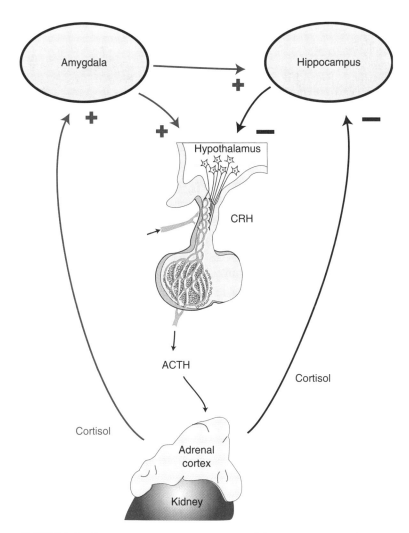

FIGURE 6.9 ● A schematic representation of the connections and feedback between the hypothalamic-pituitary-adrenal (HPA) axis and the amygdala and hippocampus. CRH, corticotropin-releasing hormone; ACTH, adrenocorticotropic hormone.

DISORDER: POST-TRAUMATIC STRESS DISORDER

It is not surprising that one can find neuroendocrine abnormalities in patients with post-traumatic stress disorder (PTSD). What is remarkable is that the findings are the opposite of what one would expect: decreased cortisol levels. It has been suggested that a low cortisol level is the result of inadequate feedback to the pituitary due to excessive glucocorticoid receptors. This may be a genetic vulnerability and could help explain why individuals have varying responses to the same trauma. The insufficient cortisol response that some individuals mount to a stressor may predispose them to excessive sympathetic and inflammatory activity. This results in symptoms such as pain, fatigue, and anhedonia. Conditions such as chronic fatigue syndrome and fibromyalgia also exhibit decreased plasma cortisol.

QUESTIONS

1. How can a GnRH agonist reduce the production of sex hormones?
   a. By blocking the FSH and LH receptors.
   b. Secondary to deactivation of the neuroendocrine cells of the hypothalamus.
   c. By continuous stimulation of the GnRH receptors.
   d. By enhancing negative feedback to the hypothalamus.

2. Which of the following is true?
   a. Thyroid hormone can enhance the GABA current.
   b. Protein hormones bind a receptor on the DNA.
   c. Hormones are used for fast signals.
   d. Neuroendocrine cells excrete directly into the circulation.

3. Which of the following is correct?
   a. GnRH → LH → Estrogen.
   b. GHRH → LH → Testosterone.
   c. TRH → TSH → Prolactin.
   d. CRH → TSH → Cortisol.

4. Possible explanations for the role of thyroid hormone in mood disorders include all of the following except
   a. Changes in brain metabolism.
   b. Effects on growth hormones.
   c. Changes in glucocorticoid receptors.
   d. Effects on 5HT receptors.

5. Women in the acute phase of anorexia nervosa exhibit a thyroid profile called "euthyroid sick syndrome," which includes all of the following except
   a. Low T3.
   b. Low Reverse T3.
   c. Low to normal T4.
   d. Normal TSH.

6. The triad of hippocampal atrophy, hypercortisolaemia, and cognitive impairment have been found with all the following except
   a. Cushing's disease.
   b. Addison's disease.
   c. Alzheimer's disease.
   d. Major depression.

7. All of the following go together except
   a. Amygdala atrophy.
   b. Hippocampal atrophy.
   c. Memory deficit.
   d. LTP disruption.

See Answers section at end of book.

Adult Development and Plasticity

In a video produced in 1996 by Robert Sapolsky for the Teaching Company entitled *Biology and Human Behavior*, Dr. Sapolsky stated,

"To the greater extent you've got all the neurons you're ever going to have to deal with by the time we're 4 or 5 years old and, unfortunately, all you do from there is lose them."

This belief—stated by Dr. Sapolsky such a short time ago—was shared by almost all clinicians and neuroscientists until recently. We are not criticizing Dr. Sapolsky, whose outstanding contributions to the field were cited in the previous chapter. Rather, we wish to show that even astute Stanford Professors just a short time ago believed the brain was a static organ. The authors of this book were no more enlightened at that time.

An abundance of new research has established that the brain is not the fixed structure we used to envision. Although the rate of change and development is especially prominent early in life, altering the structure of the brain in response to environmental factors remains a feature across the entire life span.

The almost unbelievable prenatal development of the central nervous system (CNS) is a fascinating topic beyond the scope of this text. Suffice it to say that a single fertilized egg develops into 100 billion neurons with 100 trillion connections in a short amount of time. In utero, this process is largely activity-independent and genetically driven. After birth, interactions with the environment begin to modify development and play a greater role.

PHASES OF DEVELOPMENT
The cellular events that transpire can be divided into four phases.

1. *Neurogenesis*: The production, migration, and development of distinct new cell types—nerve or glial—from undifferentiated stem cells.
2. *Cell expansion*: The branching of axons and dendrites to make synaptic connections.
3. *Connection refinement*: The elimination of excessive branching and synaptic connections.
4. *Apoptosis*: Programmed neuronal cell death.

Neurogenesis
The cells of the intestinal epithelium are turned over every 2 weeks whereas skin cells are replaced every 1 to 2 months. The adult brain is not nearly this prolific, but is not barren either. Unequivocal newborn neurons have been identified in the hippocampus of elderly subjects whose brains were examined shortly after death. One group has estimated that 270,000 new cells are generated in the dentate gyrus of the adult rat each *month*. In contrast, others have estimated that 250,000 new neurons are generated each *minute* during the peak of fetal development. So neurogenesis continues, but at a slower pace.

Undifferentiated neural stem cells remain in the CNS and continue to divide throughout life, as shown in Figure 7.1. They divide into more neural stem cells as well as neural precursors that grow into neurons or support cells. However, they must migrate away from the influence of the stem cells before they can differentiate, and only about half the cells successfully move and transform.

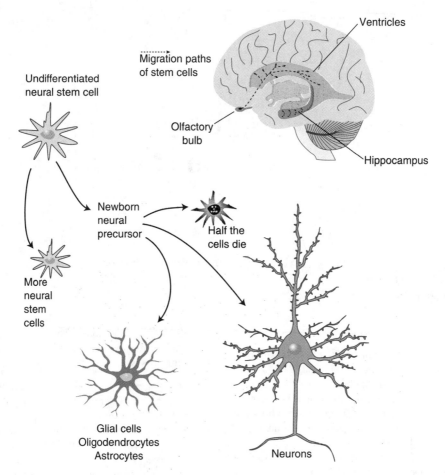

FIGURE 7.1 ● The process of neurogenesis starts with an undifferentiated neural stem cell that has the capacity to migrate and transform into functioning nerve cells. (Adapted from Gage FH. Brain, repair yourself. *Sci Am.* 2003;289[3]:46–53.)

The locations and potential for division of the remaining stem cells in the adult human brain are a hot, controversial topic. Clear evidence for adult neurogenesis has been limited to the granule cells of the dentate gyrus and olfactory bulb (see Figure 7.2). Newborn cells are identified by tagging them with a molecule such as bromodeoxyuridine (BrdU), a thymidine analog that can be incorporated into newly synthesized DNA. A florescent antibody specific for BrdU is then used to detect the incorporated molecule and thereby indicate DNA replication.

In 1999, Gould et al. identified newborn nerve cells in the neocortex (prefrontal, temporal, and parietal) of adult monkeys. They established that neural stem cells migrated through the white matter and differentiated into neurons and extended axons (see Figure 7.3). Unfortunately, the number of new cells are less than that found in the hippocampus or olfactory bulb, and inadequate for significant CNS repair. However, the future of neurological treatment may lie in finding methods (medications, exercise, magnetic stimulation, etc.) to invigorate the limited primate neurogenesis to replace damaged tissue.

Rate of Neurogenesis

The rate of neurogenesis is modulated by various factors. It is known that enriched environments and exercise will increase neurogenesis (see Figure 7.4). Additional research suggests that gonadal steroid hormones may also enhance new cell production. There is more research showing the positive effects of estrogen on mammal brains, but testosterone will stimulate nerve cell production in songbirds (and possibly middle-aged men seeking to recapture the vigor of youth). The point is that various factors may promote neurogenesis and could be utilized as a part of treatment for neurological disorders.

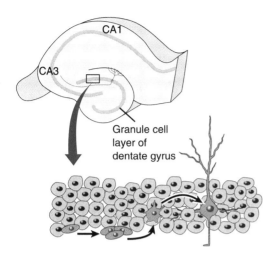

FIGURE 7.2 ● The granule cell layer of the dentate gyrus is the most studied location of neurogenesis. (Adapted from Gage FH. Mammalian neural stem cells. *Science.* 2000;287[5457]:1433–1438.)

POINT OF INTEREST

The studies establishing an increase in neurogenesis with enriched environments for mice have also documented increased size of the dentate gyrus of the hippocampus. Additionally, they have shown improved memory performance on hippocampal dependent memory tasks (water maze) in these mice. These findings validate the link between neurogenesis, neuronal growth, hippocampal size, and memory.

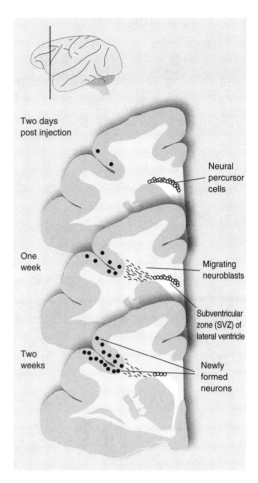

FIGURE 7.3 ● Adult macaque monkeys were injected with BrdU and sacrificed 2 hours, 1week, and 2 weeks later. These sections from the prefrontal cortex show the development and migration of neural precursor cells from the subventricular zone (SVZ), through the white matter to the neocortex. Additional tests established that some of the cells were newly formed neurons. (Adapted from Gould E, Reeves AJ, Graziano MS, et al. Neurogenesis in the neocortex of adult primates. *Science.* 1999;286[5439]:548–552.)

Stress, on the other hand, has an inhibitory effect on neurogenesis. Extended maternal separation is a well-characterized model of early life stress for a rodent. As adults, such rodents will show protracted elevations of CRF, ACTH, and corticosterone (cortisol in a rat), as well as behavioral inhibition in response to stress. Recent work from Gould's laboratory has shown that rats exposed to prolonged maternal separation will have a long-lasting blunting of neurogenesis. When the corticosterone is experimentally lowered, the neurogenesis rebounds to normal levels—suggesting that hypersensitivity to corticosterone may be the mechanism of action that suppresses neurogenesis.

The relation between early stress, the HPA axis, and neurogenesis is particularly interesting because of the role of the hippocampus in modulating the HPA axis. We can conceptualize that a healthy hippocampus is necessary to put the brakes on an activated HPA axis after the stressful event dissipates. This research suggests that early stress (an unavailable mother) leads to a smaller hippocampus due to insufficient neurogenesis, which results in an overactive HPA axis and all those secondary problems discussed in the previous chapter.

Stem cells

One potential way to rebuild a damaged brain is to implant human embryonic stem cells that

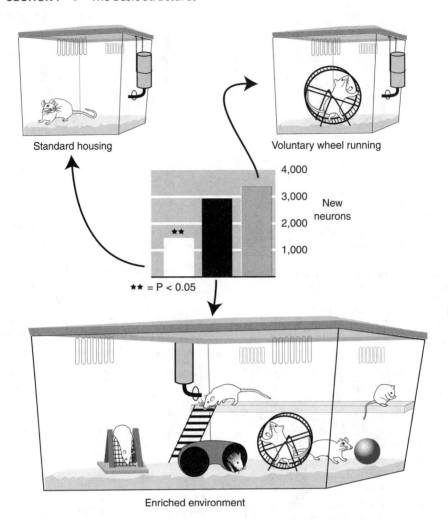

Standard housing

Voluntary wheel running

4,000

3,000   New
          neurons
2,000

1,000

★★ = P < 0.05

Enriched environment

FIGURE 7.4 ● A study by Brown, et al., showed that an enriched environment and physical exercise stimulated neurogenesis in the hippocampus
but not in the olfactory bulb in mice. (Graph adapted from Brown J, Cooper-
Kuhn CM, Kempermann G, et al. Enriched environment and physical activity
stimulate hippocampal but not olfactory bulb neurogenesis. *Eur J Neurosci.*
2003;17[10]:2042–2046.)

have been isolated from a very immature embryo
(only 100–200 cells). So far it was difficult to
get these immature cells to differentiate into functioning neurons outside the olfactory bulb and
hippocampus. The problem may be the absence
of biochemical signals that normally prompt the
developing stem cell to migrate and differentiate.

A group in Japan recently reported a successful
intervention in monkeys with chemically induced
Parkinson's disease. The important difference may
have been a "cocktail" of several growth factors
that coaxed the undifferentiated cells to develop
into neurons and then into authentic dopamine
(DA) neurons. These cells were then injected
into the bilateral putamen of the "Parkinsonian"

monkeys. Figure 7.5 shows a diagram of the
procedure and some results.

Cell Expansion

The second phase of neuronal growth, often called
synaptogenesis, describes the extensive growth of
axons and dendrites to make synaptic
connections—a process that primarily occurs early
in life. The tips of axons and dendrites have
growth cones that appear to reach out with fin-
gerlike structures, *filopodia*, and literally pull the
growth cone to its destination. The axon is guided
in a specific direction by chemical signals that
attract and repel the growth cone, that is, *chemoat-
tractants* and *chemorepellents*.

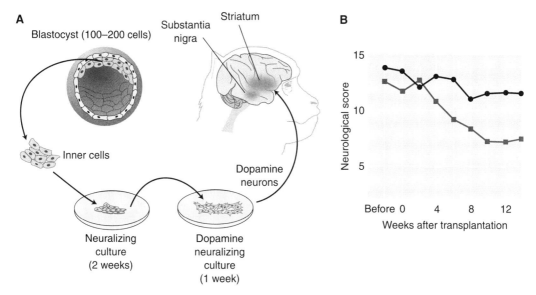

FIGURE 7.5 ● A: Shows the process of harvesting embryonic stem cells, stimulating the development of dopamine neurons in several cultures, and injecting them into a monkey with chemically induced Parkinson's disease. B: Shows the improved neurological scores over 14 weeks. (Adapted from Takagi Y, Takahashi J, Saiki H, et al. Dopaminergic neurons generated from monkey embryonic stem cells function in a Parkinson primate model. *J Clin Invest.* 2005;115[1]:102–109.)

In a comprehensive postmortem analysis, Huttenlocher determined synaptic density across the life span in two regions of the human brain from 14 individuals. Using an electron microscope and special stains, he counted synaptic connections from thin sections of the visual cortex and prefrontal cortex after autopsies. The results, displayed graphically in Figure 7.6, show that the greatest synaptogenesis takes place shortly after birth and occurs sooner for the visual cortex.

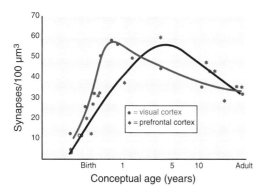

FIGURE 7.6 ● Synaptic densities from two areas (visual and prefrontal cortex) were calculated from 14 postmortem analyses from individuals who died of non-neurological diseases. (Adapted from Huttenlocher PR, Dabholkar AS. Regional differences in synaptogenesis in human cerebral cortex. *J Comp Neurol.* 1997;387[2]:167–178.)

Maximum synaptic density is reached before the first year in the visual cortex, but not until 3.5 years in the prefrontal cortex. Synaptogenesis is accompanied by an increase in the size of the nerve cell to support the increased metabolic needs created by the expanded axons and dendrites.

Connection Refinement

The third phase of neuronal cell development often referred to as *pruning*, or *synaptic elimination*, entails retraction and elimination of excessive connections. This process is a pattern that is repeated frequently in nature—many connections are created and the weak or unlucky dies. The process proceeds at different rates for different regions of the brain, as shown in Figure 7.6. Other researches suggest that the refinement occurs in an order based on need. For example, sensory and motor areas go through refinement first and executive functions last.

Most remarkable to the mental health clinician is the late and extensive reduction of the frontal cortex through adolescence into adulthood, as shown in Figure 7.6. These data correlate with psychological tests measuring executive function. It is almost paradoxical that the maturing process that our adolescents struggle through is actually a refinement and reduction of the gray matter and not growth. Most likely, the maturing brain is making better connections, not more.

Disordered pruning may be the pathological basis for such conditions as autism and schizophrenia. A consistent finding in patients with autism is greater total brain volume, which is not present at birth but develops during the first few years of life. It has been suggested that this is due to abnormal connectivity and a lack of pruning. Schizophrenia, which typically develops in late adolescence and is associated with a loss of gray matter, may be the result of excessive pruning (see Chapter 20, Schizophrenia).

Apoptosis

Programmed cell death, *Apoptosis*, is the final phase of the sculpting of the brain. It is called *programmed*, which reflects the fact that the cells actually carry genetic instructions to self-destruct. Neurotrophins, discussed next, save the neuron by turning off the genetic program. When the intracellular cascade has been activated, apoptosis proceeds in a characteristic process: cell shrinkage, fragmentation, and phagocytosis of the cellular remnants. This is distinguished from necrotic cell death, which results from trauma and is characterized by rapid cell membrane lysis.

Modifications of any of these four phases—for example, enhancing neurogenesis or retarding apoptosis—are potential targets for treatment interventions for such conditions as depression and Alzheimer's disease. Active research for such treatments is going on.

Brain Imaging Studies

The postmortem studies by Huttenlocher provided an in-depth analysis of synaptic connections, but were limited by the number of brains—particularly young adult brains—that he could analyze. Brain imaging studies, on the other hand, allow the examination of a larger number of subjects and can be repeated as the subjects age. Unfortunately, brain imaging currently does not have the resolution to the level of the synapse, so the studies must focus on larger structures, such as the volume of white and gray matter.

Two groups, one from UCLA and the other at NIMH, have conducted an extensive research of brain development during childhood and adolescence using MRI scans. One study, shown in Figure 7.7, scanned 145 healthy subject, 99 of whom had at least two scans. The results for the gray matter show the same developmental pattern of increase in childhood and decrease in adolescence—consistent with a pattern of cell growth followed by connection refinement—reinforcing the perception of the brain as an organ undergoing change, at least into young adulthood.

NEUROTROPHIC GROWTH FACTORS

Neurotrophic factors—literally growth factors for nerve cells—are best defined as any molecule that affects the nervous system by influencing the growth or differentiation of neurons or glia. Neurotrophic factors, affectionately called "brain fertilizers", are the stimulus behind neurogenesis and synaptogenesis (see Figure 7.8). Rita Levi-Montalcini et al. accidentally discovered the first growth factor 40 years ago (see Chapter 1, Historical Perspective). They were able to isolate a protein from a mouse sarcoma that stimulated the growth of nerve cells as well as increased the size and branching of the cells. Although called *nerve growth factor* (NGF)—implying that it stimulates all nerve cells—this particular neurotrophin only affects sympathetic neurons and some sensory ganglion cells. Several decades of research have established four rules regarding the cells affected by NGF.

1. NGF mediates cell survival.
2. Cells that do not receive enough NGF die.
3. Target organs produce NGF.
4. Specific NGF receptors are present on innervating nerve terminals.

Because NGF is specific for a limited subset of peripheral nerves, it was assumed for many years that there were a host of other neurotrophic factors following similar rules waiting to be discovered. Unfortunately, the fortuitous discovery of NGF has not been repeated with other factors. Identifying and purifying factors that are excreted in such minute quantities has turned into an arduous task. Several factors have been discovered and are being studied, such as neurotrophin-3

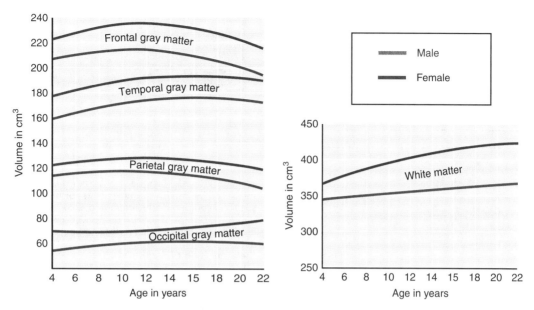

FIGURE 7.7 • MRI analyses from 145 healthy subjects showing the changing gray and white matter volumes for different regions of the brain for males and females. (Adapted from Giedd JN, Blumenthal J, Jeffries NO, et al. Brain development during childhood and adolescence: A longitudinal MRI study. *Nat Neurosci.* 1999;2[10]:861–863.)

(NT-3), glial cell line-derived neurotrophin factor (GDNF), and insulinlike growth factor (IGF), to name a few, but the one that is of most interest to mental health is brain-derived neurotrophic factor (BDNF).

The actions of neurotrophins such as BDNF are mediated primarily through Trk (for tyrosine kinase) receptors on the nerve cell membrane. The extracellular portion of the receptor binds with the neurotrophic factor, which in turn initiates an intracellular cascade that leads to biological effects. As yet, there are no small molecule agonists or antagonists for these receptors, which hinders a better understanding of the action of the neurotrophic factors.

Signaling the Trk receptor can lead to changes in three aspects of the cell state:

1. Cell survival or death.
2. Synaptic stabilization or elimination.
3. Process growth or retraction.

The affect is determined by the specific neurotrophic factor, the combination of receptors signaled, and the intracellular pathways expressed in that cell. Disruption of the neurotrophic factor signaling is presumably an explanation (and possible treatment) for some neurodegenerative diseases, for example, Huntington's, Parkinson's, and Alzheimer's diseases.

TREATMENT: NEUROTROPHINS

Medicating with neurotrophins or stimulating their increased production is an exciting prospect for future neuropsychiatric treatment. Some studies suggest that this may be the mechanism by which lithium, ECT, and antidepressants resolve depression (see Chapter 18, Depression). If this is true, future treatments for depression will focus on more effective ways to stimulate growth factors. Other researchers have examined the therapeutic benefits of growth hormones for such disorders as amyotrophic lateral sclerosis (ALS) and multiple sclerosis (MS). The biggest difficulty is finding effective yet unobtrusive methods to deliver the neurotrophins to the CNS.

CRITICAL PERIODS

In utero, the development of the CNS is directed by genes, although toxins or infectious agents can impede the process. After birth, interaction with one's environment plays a synergistic role with the genes to sculpt the CNS. Early interactions

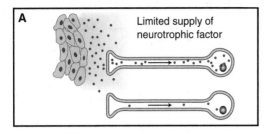

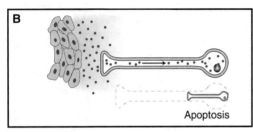

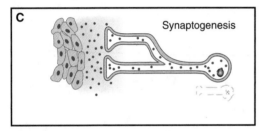

FIGURE 7.8 ● Neurotrophic factors mediate cell proliferation and elimination by promoting cell growth, stimulating synaptogenesis, and preventing apoptosis.

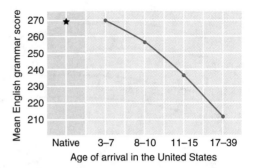

FIGURE 7.9 ● Language acquisition as measured by English grammar tests for native speakers compared to Korean and Chinese immigrants. (Adapted from Johnson JS, Newport EL. Critical period effects in second language learning: The influence of maturational state on the acquisition of English as a second language. *Cognit Psychol.* 1989;21[1]:60–99.)

during the time of great cellular expansion mold the brain's anatomy with an ease and permanence that can never be repeated or undone. These stages in development when the environmental input is so crucial to determining the structure of the brain are called *critical periods.*

Language acquisition is an example of the importance of a critical period. Early exposure to native sounds has a lasting impact on speech, which is hard to alter later in life. Johnson and Newport demonstrated this by examining English proficiency in Korean and Chinese speakers who arrived in the United States between the ages of 3 and 39. They found that subjects who arrived in the United States before the age of 7 had equivalent fluency to native speakers, whereas those who arrived after the age of 7 had a linear decline in performance until puberty (see Figure 7.9).

The development of the visual cortex provides an excellent example of critical periods. David Hubel and Torsten Wiesel (who later received the Nobel Prize for this work) established the importance of normal visual experience early in life for proper development of the visual cortex in cats and monkeys. In a series of experiments, they sutured one eyelid shut in kittens and later monkeys for short lengths of time during various weeks after birth. They established, down to the level of the neuron, the profound effect of visual deprivation at critical periods of development.

Figure 7.10 shows how the experiments by Hubel and Wiesel were conducted. Radioactive proline was injected into an eye where it was transported down the axons to the lateral geniculate nucleus of the thalamus. Some of the labeled proline that spilled out of the terminal would be taken up by the lateral geniculate nucleus (LGN) neurons and transported to the visual cortex. The location of the radioactive molecules can be visualized using autoradiography.

Figure 7.11 shows the results—both real and schematic—of suturing one eye shut for differing periods of time early in life. The autoradiographs in the second row show a normal cat compared with a cat whose eye was closed from 2 weeks until 18 months. This demonstrates—as do the drawings in the third row—how the neurons from the occluded eye regress and the neurons from the good eye expand. The bottom row shows the terminal branching, *arborization*, of the LGN neurons in the visual cortex for a normal eye and one that was occluded for just 1 week at 30 days of age. Hubel and Wiese have estimated that the critical period for ocular deprivation in a cat is 3 to 4 months.

In humans, the critical period for vision extends out to 5 or 6 years of age. For example, children with congenital cataracts can have substantial and permanent visual deficits if the occluded lens is

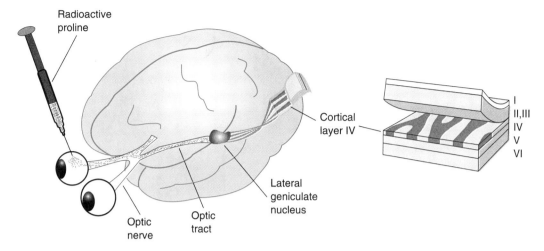

FIGURE 7.10 ● Injecting radioactive proline into an eye allows visualization of the cortical innervation in layer IV from that eye when the animal is sacrificed several weeks later. (Adapted from Bear MF, Connors BW, Paradiso MA, eds. *Neuroscience: exploring the brain*, 3rd ed. Baltimore: Lippincott Williams & Wilkins; 2007; Purves D, Augustine GJ, Fitzpatrick D, et al. *Neuroscience.* Sunderland, MA: Sinauer; 2004.)

not corrected early enough. However, adults with cataracts regain their pre-existing visual acuity when the lens is replaced because their visual cortex is already developed.

Strabismus, often called *lazy eye*, is a misalignment of the eyes due to improper control by the eye muscles. Children with this condition experience double vision. The response of the brain to receiving two images is to suppress the input from one eye. This can result in low acuity or even blindness in the suppressed eye due to developmental impediments during the critical period. One form of treatment is to patch the good eye and force the brain receiving input from the suppressed eye to develop.

DISORDER: PERSONALITY

Extrapolating these studies to behavior, one wonders about critical periods and personality development. For example, what is the effect of early exposure to TV? Recent studies suggest that too much time in front of the TV leads to attentional problems for children, poorer academic achievement, and increased aggression. One wonders what neuronal connections fail to develop when children spend too much time watching TV.

ADULT NEUROPLASTICITY

This description of critical periods suggests a bleak picture for changes in the adult brain, but there is more hope for your old cortex than we used to think. Even Hubel and Wiesel described one monkey whose one eye was occluded between days 21 and 30 and who appeared blind in the deprived eye. However, 4 years later he had an estimated acuity of 20/80 in the bad eye and 20/40 in the normal eye.

Plasticity is defined as the capability of being formed or molded. Neuroplasticity enables the brain to adapt to environmental factors that cannot be anticipated by genetic programming. The size and organization of the cortical representations of stimuli are continually reshaped by experience.

Studies with monkeys have shown a significant reorganization of the cortical maps with changes in sensory input. In one experiment, the researchers measured the representation of the fingers on the cortex before and after amputation of the middle finger. Figure 7.12 shows how the cortex adapted to the change. Neurons deprived of their normal sensory input now respond to stimulation from the closest fingers. Similar changes have been observed with humans with phantom limbs. For example, some patients experience sensation on their amputated lower arm when their face is scratched—a phantom sensation. Functional imaging scans performed during such stimulation have shown activation of the somatosensory region for both the face and where the lower arm was.

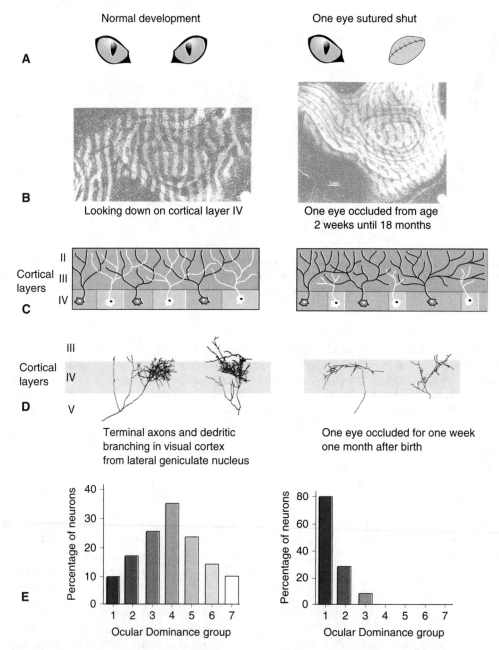

FIGURE 7.11 ● **A–E:** Comparing the normal development of the visual cortex on the left with development on the right when one eye has been sutured shut for varying lengths of time. Electrodes inserted horizontal to the cortex show distinctive patterns of ocular dominance depending on which eyes developed properly (**E**). (**B:** From Wiesel TN. Postnatal development of the visual cortex and the influence of environment. *Nature.* 1982;299[5884]:583–591. **D:** From Antonini A, Stryker MP. Rapid remodeling of axonal arbors in the visual cortex. *Science.* 1993;260[5115]:1819–1821. Reprinted with permission from AAAS.)

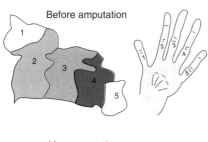

Before amputation

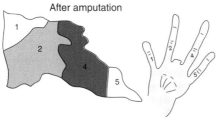

After amputation

FIGURE 7.12 ● After amputation of a monkey's finger, the cortical neurons reorganize. The neurons formally responding to stimulation of the third finger now respond to stimulation from the 2nd and 4th fingers. Similar "re-mapping" also occurs in the thalamus. (Adapted from Merzenich MM, Nelson RJ, Stryker MP, et al. Somatosensory cortical map changes following digit amputation in adult monkeys. *J Comp Neurol.* 1984;224[4]:591–605.)

Other studies have shown expansion of the cortical representation with increased input. Monkeys, from the same laboratory that performed the experiments described here were taught to rotate a disc using only digits 2, 3, and sometimes 4 to receive banana-flavored pellets. After several months of practice, the cortical region activated by those fingers was enlarged (see Figure 7.13). The cortical representations expand with use and regresses without use.

The Musician's Brain

Learning to play a musical instrument is a complex task that requires practice, practice, and practice. Because of this, musician's brains have served as a model of neuroplasticity. Figure 7.14 shows the enhanced signals from the somatosensory and auditory cortex for highly skilled musicians compared to controls. Figure 7.14 (a) shows the representation of the cortical signal from the little finger on the left hand for string musicians and controls when the fingers were stimulated. This difference did not exist for the thumb or the fingers on the right hand. In Figure 7.14 (b), the musicians had a 25% greater neuronal excitation for the piano tones than the controls. In both cases, the musicians who had started playing at the youngest age displayed the largest signal.

Taken in total, these studies suggest that starting early is best, but even the late bloomers can change their brains and develop new skills. Clearly, as anyone who has tried to learn a new language, instrument, or sport knows, it requires work and diligence to change the brain.

Maladaptive Neuroplasticity

Prolonged practice has its dark side. Approximately 1% of professional musicians will develop a condition called *focal dystonia*: loss of control of skilled movements in the performing hand. It is usually a career-ending disorder and is believed to result from maladaptive neuroplasticity stimulated by long hours of repetitive movements. Neuroimaging studies show a fusion of the digital representations in the somatosensory cortex (see Figure 7.15). It is almost as though the neurons fuse together such that separate individual movements are no longer possible.

Cellular Changes

The cellular mechanisms that accompany the cortical changes seen with monkeys rotating discs and musicians playing instruments (and hopefully readers of this book) are poorly understood. Some similar processes that may play a role in

TREATMENT: STROKE

After a stroke, many patients will avoid using the affected limb and preferentially use the intact limb. Functional imaging studies of stroke patients have shown contraction of the cortical representation of the affected limb, which is consistent with lack of use. A new kind of rehabilitation for stroke patients called *constraint-induced* *movement therapy* corrects this problem and improves function even in chronic conditions. Patients have their good limb restrained with a mitt or harness and are forced to use their impaired limb. Controlled trials have shown this treatment to improve motor skills as well as increase the cortical activity in the affected area.

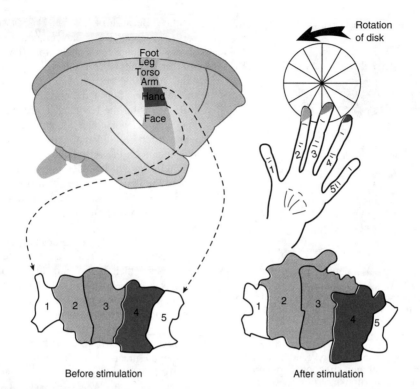

FIGURE 7.13 ● The expansion of cortical representation of the dorsal fingers of a monkey before and after several months of stimulation. (Adapted from Jenkins WM, Merzenich MM, Ochs MT, et al. Functional reorganization of primary somatosensory cortex in adult owl monkeys after behaviorally controlled tactile stimulation. *J Neurophysiol*. 1990;63[1]:82–104.)

the dynamics of the neocortex were discussed in earlier chapters of this book. A good model is Long Term Potentiation (LTP), discussed in the last section of Chapter 5, Receptors and Signaling the Nucleus. Figure 5.8 shows an example of new spine development induced with LTP. Such spine development along with branching of the dendrites are seen with enriched environments, as shown in Figure 3.3. It is tempting to speculate that successful learning involves production of growth factors that stimulate arborization of dendrites in the cortex.

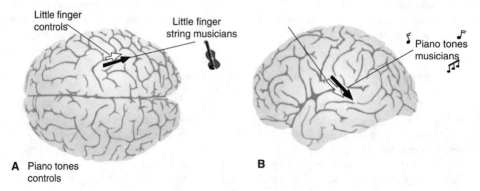

FIGURE 7.14 ● Musicians (black arrow) and controls (white arrow) show differences in the somatosensory (**A**) and auditory (**B**) cortex. (Adapted from Pantev C, Engelien A, Candia V, et al. Representational cortex in musicians. Plastic alterations in response to musical practice. *Ann N Y Acad Sci*. 2001;930:300–314.)

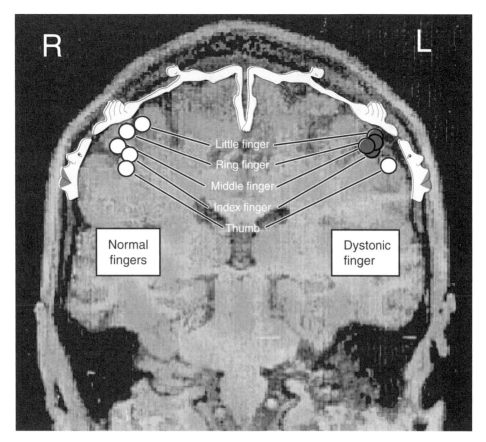

FIGURE 7.15 ● Functional representation of the fingers from the right and left hands of a musician with focal dystonia of the left hand. The response from the somatosensory cortex is superimposed on an MRI. Note the fusion of the representations for the fingers from the affected left fingers that is not seen with the separated fingers from the right hand. The thumb—a digit not requiring as much movement when playing—is unaffected. (Adapted from Elbert T, Candia V, Altenmuller E, et al. Alteration of digital representations in somatosensory cortex in focal hand dystonia. *Neuroreport.* 1998;9[16]:3571–3575.)

This sort of treatment is consistent with the focus of this chapter: that the brain has the capacity to change, but it must be exercised.

Adult Nerve Regeneration

Why is it that the nerves in the peripheral nervous system (PNS) can regenerate while those in the CNS cannot? Likewise, why can amphibians regrow long nerve connections, but mammals cannot? How come the most complex organ in the universe is less capable of repair than more primitive organs? It appears that the brain responds to injuries with actions that are intended to preserve the complex connections, but this ultimately also prevents regeneration.

Oligodendrocytes and astrocytes respond to CNS injury by forming what is called a *glial scar*. This scar limits cellular damage by preserving the blood–brain barrier and mediating the inflammatory response. Unfortunately, the glial scar is full of molecules (not found in the PNS) that inhibit the growth cone and prevent regeneration. The neurons have the capability of growing after an injury but cannot get through the glial scar. The current thinking is that an effective treatment to regenerate functional long axons will utilize a combination of enzymes to dissolve the inhibitory molecules along with methods to stimulate intrinsic growth hormones.

The Controversy Continues

As this book was being wrapped up, a remarkable study was published that warrants inclusion. The new research seems to establish that neurogenesis does *not* occur in adult human brain. Researchers utilized a remnant of the cold war to determine the age of neurons and non-neural brain cells in postmortem cortical biopsies.

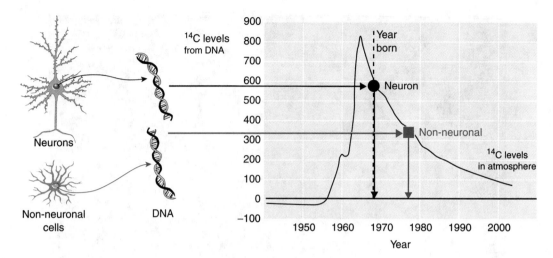

FIGURE 7.16 ● Post-mortem analysis of ^{14}C levels in DNA from neurons and non-neuronal brain cells shows that the neurons were created at the time of this individual's birth. (Adapted from Bhardway RD, Curtis MA, Spalding KL, et al. Neocortical neurogenesis in humans is restricted to development. *Proc Natl Acad Sci U S A.* 2006;103[33]:12564–12568.)

The amount of ^{14}C carbon in the atmosphere remained almost constant until the above-ground nuclear bomb testing during the 50s and 60s. Then there was a huge increase in ^{14}C, which rapidly distributed around the globe. The amount of ^{14}C in the atmosphere has steadily decreased since the 1963 Test Ban Treaty.

The amount of ^{14}C in a cell can be used to give an accurate date of the cell's birth when plotted on the known curves of ^{14}C available in the atmosphere over the last 50 years. For example, the ^{14}C in rings in a tree will match the ^{14}C in the atmosphere at the time that ring was formed. The neuroscientists in Sweden used this technique to determine the age of brain cells in seven individuals who died suddenly.

The researchers were able to separate nuclei from neurons and non-neuronal cells from different regions of the cortex. Then the DNA was extracted, analyzed for ^{14}C, and plotted on the known levels of ^{14}C in the atmosphere. The results are shown in Figure 7.16.

These results seem to establish that all the adult human neurons in the *neocortex* were created perinatally and none since then. Non-neuronal brain cells continue to form and are born, on average, 5 years after the birth of the individual. However, neurons are born in the hippocampus and olfactory bulb throughout the life of mammals, but their functional status remains a mystery.

So, if the brain does not in fact create new cortical neurons, how does it adapt, change, and learn? Well, much of the plasticity of the brain can still occur with modulation of pre-existing cells and their connections. Likewise, the existence of neurogenesis after brain trauma remains to be determined. Finally, the role of the glial cells in pathology and remission may be more important than we have typically thought.

No one said understanding the brain and how we think was going to be easy!

QUESTIONS

1. Brain fertilizer.
   a. Apoptosis.
   b. Critical period.
   c. Focal dystonia.
   d. Neurotrophins.

2. Programmed cell death.
   a. Apoptosis.
   b. Critical period.
   c. Focal dystonia.
   d. Neurotrophins.

3. Maximum synaptogenesis.
   a. Apoptosis.
   b. Critical period.
   c. Focal dystonia.
   d. Neurotrophins.

4. Inappropriate neurogenesis.
   a. Apoptosis.
   b. Critical period.
   c. Focal dystonia.
   d. Neurotrophins.

5. Not one of the phases of development.
   a. Neurogenesis.
   b. Synaptogenesis.
   c. Neuroplasticity.
   d. Pruning.

6. Factors that do not enhance CNS neurogenesis.
   a. Amputation.
   b. Antidepressants.
   c. Enriched environments.
   d. Exercise.

7. Cannot develop from neural stem cells.
   a. More neural stem cells.
   b. Oligodendrocytes.
   c. Astrocytes.
   d. Schwann cells.

8. Possible explanation for schizophrenia.
   a. Focal dystonia.
   b. Excessive pruning.
   c. Altered neurotrophins.
   d. Dopamine receptor apoptosis.

See Answers section at end of book.

Behaviors

Pain

Pain and pleasure are the greatest driving forces of human behavior. We will cover pain in this chapter and pleasure in the following one.

ACUTE PAIN

Pain-producing stimuli are detected by specialized afferent neurons called *nociceptors*. The receptors are free nerve endings—not an identifiable structure as we have for touch and vibration. These cells respond to a broad range of physical and chemical stimuli, but only at intensities that are capable of causing damage.

Peripheral Tissue

The nociceptors in peripheral tissue are activated by injury or tissue damage that results in the release of bradykinins, prostaglandins, and potassium (see Figure 8.1). These molecules in turn cause the secretion of substance P from other branches of the axon, which stimulates the release of histamine and promote vasodilation.

Aδ and C fibers send the signal to the dorsal horn of the spinal cord by way of the dorsal root ganglion. The Aδ fibers are myelinated axons that quickly send the first, sharp signals of pain. The C fibers are unmyelinated and send a slower, dull pain signal (see Figure 8.2). The cell bodies of the nerves reside in the dorsal root ganglion, which becomes important for treatments that seek to modify damaged nerves.

Spinal Cord

The nociceptive afferent nerve fibers synapse in the dorsal horn of the spinal cord. Information about tissue injury is passed on to the next neurons, which then cross to the contralateral side and ascend to the brain.

The signal can be modified at this point by descending fibers (discussed later) or from simultaneous activity by nonpain neurons (mechanoreceptors: Aβ fibers). The Aβ fibers can dampen the pain signal in what is called the *gate theory of pain*. Figure 8.3 shows how a signal from the larger mechanoreceptor activates an inhibitory interneuron in the dorsal horn, which results in a smaller signal conveyed to the brain. The gate theory explains why rubbing an injury seems to reduce the pain and is the rationale for the use of transcutaneous electrical stimulation (TENS).

Ascending Pathways

There are a variety of ways to describe the different nociceptive pathways that ascend to the brain in the spinal cord. Unfortunately, there is no consensus on the proper nomenclature for these tracts and no two authors seem to use the same terms. Recently, the perception of pain—and the areas participating, in the CNS—has been divided into two prominent domains: sensory-discriminative and affective-motivational. This dichotomy (summarized in Table 8.1) is a good way to understand the ascending pathways.

TREATMENT: DELETING C FIBERS

A fascinating study suggests that it is possible to selectively delete the C fibers as a treatment for chronic pain. The C fibers have a receptor on their cell wall that is not found with any great frequency on other neurons. This receptor—called the *VR1 receptor*—is a sodium/calcium ion channel. Resiniferatoxin (RTX) is an old medication that attaches to the VR1 receptor and causes a large, prolonged increase in Ca_2^+. The resulting calcium cytotoxicity rapidly destroys and "deletes" the neuron.

In a study with eight dogs affected by arthritis and/or cancer pain, the authors injected RTX directly in the CSF and noted a profound decrease in pain (as measured by the owners assessment on a visual analogue scale—see Figure). The owners also noted improved activity and great reduction in the use of analgesics. This treatment has the potential to selectively ablate the aching quality of chronic pain while preserving

sensations of touch, proprioception, and locomotor function. Studies in humans are needed.

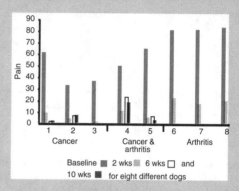

Dogs in pain before and after experimental treatment to "delete" C fibers, as measured by the owners using a visual analogue scale. (Adapted from Karai L, Brown DC, Mannes AJ, et al. Deletion of vanilloid receptor 1-expressing primary afferent neurons for pain control. *J Clin Invest*. 2004;113[9]:1344–1352.)

Sensory-Discriminative

The sensory-discriminative domain encompasses the traditional pathway we learned in our training. The signal travels up the *spinothalamic tract*, synapses in the lateral thalamus, and proceeds to the somatosensory cortex. Figure 8.4 is a diagram of this pathway. This type of pain allows the subject to become aware of the location of the pain and answer the question, "where does it hurt?" However, the perception of pain is much more

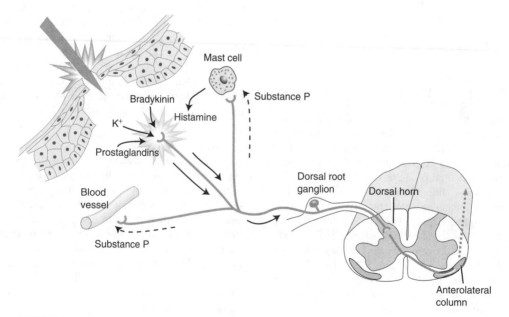

FIGURE 8.1 ● Peripheral nociceptive responses to acute trauma. (Adapted from Kandel ER, Schwartz JH, Jessell TM, eds. *Principles of neural science*, 4th ed. New York: McGraw-Hill; 2000.)

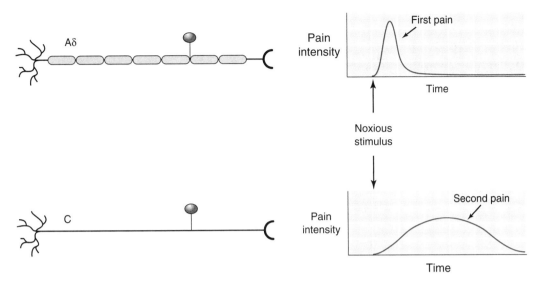

FIGURE 8.2 ● Aδ and C fibers transmit pain signals at different rates. (Adapted from Bear MF, Connors BW, Paradiso MA, eds. *Neuroscience: exploring the brain*, 3rd ed. Baltimore: Lippincott Williams & Wilkins; 2007.)

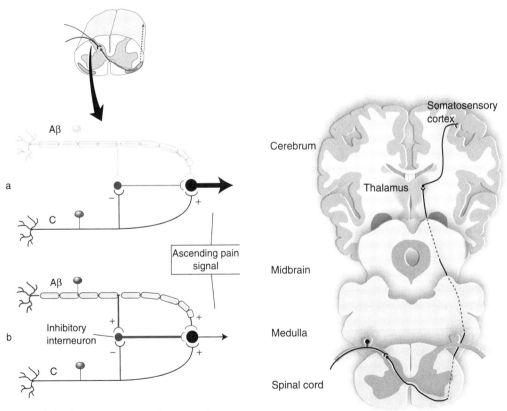

FIGURE 8.3 ● Gate theory of pain in the dorsal horn of the spinal cord. **A:** Without input from Aβ fibers a large signal is transmitted to the brain, **B:** a smaller signal is transmitted with input from Aβ fibers.

FIGURE 8.4 ● Spinothalamic tract transmitting the sensory-discriminative pain signal from the periphery to the somatosensory cortex.

TABLE 8.1

The Two Afferent Pathways Bringing Pain Signals from the Periphery to the CNS

Sensory-Discriminative	Affective-Motivational
Where does it hurt?	How much does it hurt?
Lateral thalamus	Medial thalamus
Somatosensory cortex	ACC, insula, PFC, amygdala

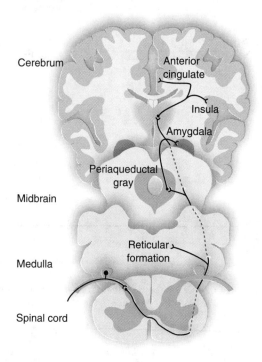

FIGURE 8.5 ● Affective-motivational pain tracts.

than just identifying the location of a noxious sensation and withdrawing the injured limb.

Affective-Motivational

The other signals communicate the intensity of a noxious sensation. There are several tracts that transport these signals, such as the spinoreticular tract or the spinomesencephalic tract—just to name a few. The important point is that all the signals travel in the anterolateral region of the spinal cord and terminate in different locations such as the reticular formation, periaqueductal gray matter (PAG), and the amygdala. The rest of the signals synapse in the medial thalamus before proceeding to other areas of the cerebral cortex (see Figure 8.5).

The affective-motivational signals communicate the unpleasantness of the sensation and answer the question, "how much does it hurt?" In the cortex, these signals activate areas associated with emotional feelings, such as the anterior cingulate cortex (ACC), insula cortex, and prefrontal cortex—as well as the amygdala. Functional brain imaging studies over the past two decades have documented activity in these areas during pain perception—areas we typically associated with mood, attention, and fear. Activity in these regions of the brain helps us understand the concomitant depression, hyper-focus, and anxiety we see with patients in pain.

Figure 8.6 shows drawings of some of the areas that become active with acute pain. In this study, subjects were scanned at rest and later with a hot probe (approximately 50°C) applied to the upper right arm. The scan at rest was later subtracted from the stimulated scan and the resulting areas of activation were superimposed on an MRI. Note the diverse areas that become active with acute pain—thalamus, anterior cingulate cortex, prefrontal cortex, and insula, as well as others.

The experience of pain is more than just identifying where it hurts.

It is also important to note that some of the activation is on both sides of the brain. This shows that there is more to the processing of pain signals in the CNS than implied by our simplified figures 8.4 and 8.5.

CONGENITAL INSENSITIVITY TO PAIN

Congenital insensitivity to pain, a term used to describe rare genic conditions in which people lack the ability to sense pain, initially sounds like a blessing but is actually a nightmare. Individuals with this condition fail to identify or respond to noxious, injuring stimuli and suffer excessive burns, fractures, and soft tissue damage. Ultimately the unrecognized injuries and secondary complications lead to an early death.

The spectrum of congenital insensitivity to pain provides an example of the distinction between sensory and affective components of pain. Subjects with frank congenital insensitivity to pain are without the peripheral Aδ and C fibers. These patients lack the sensory-discriminative as well as affective components of pain and are the most at risk for harm and premature death.

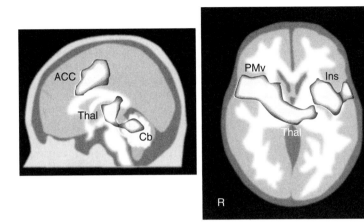

FIGURE 8.6 ● PET scans showing activity in the brain with acute pain. ACC, anterior cingulate cortex, Thal, thalamus, Cb, cerebellum, Ins, insula, PMv, ventral premotor cortex. (Adapted from Coghill RC, McHaffie JG, Yen YF. Neural correlates of interindividual differences in the subjective experience of pain. *Proc Natl Acad Sci U S A.* 2003;100[14]:8538–8542.)

A milder condition, termed *congenital indifference to pain*, is found in individuals who can distinguish sharp, and dull pain, but are indifferent to the sensation. They lack the emotional responses and normal withdrawal movements; they can feel the pain, but are not concerned. Subjects with this disorder have normal peripheral nerve fibers but seem to have an as yet unidentified central impairment of the affective-motivational component of pain.

Congenital insensitivity to pain with anhidrosis (CIPA) is a specific rare autosomal recessive disorder characterized by absence of pain (along with inability to sweat, unexplained episodes of fever, and mental retardation). It is of particular interest that the genetic basis of this disorder has been identified as a mutation in the gene for the Trk receptor—the receptor that binds with nerve growth factor (NGF). As we saw in the last chapter, nerves need to receive some nerve growth factor to survive. Cells lacking the receptor are unable to incorporate the growth factor and wither away (or fail to develop). The patient lacks pain fiber and therefore does not experience pain.

Pain Tolerance Spectrum

People have different abilities to tolerate pain. This has been shown in multiple psychological studies and observed by most us in our clinical population. More recently, brain imaging studies have documented that subjects with less pain tolerance have greater activation of the cortical areas discussed earlier (anterior cingulate cortex [ACC], insula cortex, and prefrontal cortex, along with the somatosensory cortex).

The genetic factors that determine pain tolerance are becoming increasingly apparent. A recent study examined pain tolerance in 202 women and genetic variants for the gene encoding for catecholamine-O-methyltransferase (COMT), an enzyme involved in the regulation of catecholamines and enkephalins. After initially measuring pain tolerance with a noxious thermal stimuli, the researchers assessed the genetic make up of each participant. They found that three genetic variants for COMT accounted for 11% of the variation in pain perception (a large percentage in genetic studies). Figure 8.7 shows how five different combinations of these genetic variants accounted for differing pain responsiveness.

One wonders if subjects who excel at physically demanding professions are more tolerant to pain than those of us with more sedentary jobs. Surprisingly, little has been done to study this phenomenon (although watching the NFL, NHL, and *Tour de France* provides ample case material). A study with ballet dancers found increased pain tolerance in the dancers compared to nondancer and men compared to women (see

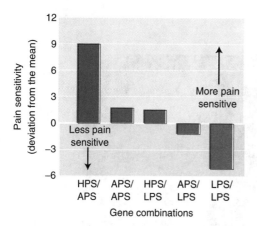

FIGURE 8.7 ● Pain responsiveness categorized by three major combinations of genetic variations for the COMT enzyme. LPS, low pain sensitivity, APS, average pain sensitivity, HPS, high pain sensitivity. Subjects with the LPS variation were 2.3 times less likely to develop temporomandibular joint disorder (TMJ). (Adapted from Diatchenko L, Slade GD, Nackley AG, et al. Genetic basis for individual variations in pain perception and the development of a chronic pain condition. *Hum Mol Genet.* 2005;14[1]:135–143.)

Figure 8.8). It is possible that individuals who are successful in physically demanding professions were born with, or developed, better tolerance to pain—along with being highly motivated, exceptionally coordinated, and creative.

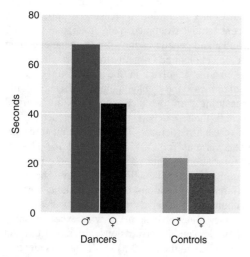

FIGURE 8.8 ● Increased pain tolerance, measured in seconds, until pain became intolerable in a bowl of ice water for ballet dancers compared to controls, for both men and women. (Adapted from Tajet-Foxell B, Rose FD. Pain and pain tolerance in professional ballet dancers. *Br J Sports Med.* 1995;29[1]:31–34.)

DISORDERS: SCHIZOPHRENIA

There is a long history of noting increased pain tolerance in patients with schizophrenia, dating back to Kraepelin and Bleuler. More recently, surgeons and internists have written anecdotal reports of patients with schizophrenia who appear to experience little pain despite suffering from extremely painful physical conditions. It is not clear if the pain tolerance is a consequence of the illness, the psychotropic medications, or simply a lack of affect, i.e., the patient feels the pain but fails to express it appropriately.

Hooley and Delgado sought to avoid these complicating factors by measuring pain sensitivity in the relatives of patients with schizophrenia. They found that subjects with a family history of schizophrenia showed elevated pain thresholds and tolerance. Of interest, the pain correlated with measures of self-referential thinking, magical ideation, and perceptual disturbances. The pathology of this aberrant pain sensitivity is unknown, but may be part of the genetic makeup of schizophrenia.

DESCENDING PATHWAYS AND OPIOIDS

The discovery of the opioid-mediated pain-modulation circuits is one of the great stories in neuroscience. In the late 1960s it became apparent that the brain exerts a top–down control of pain. A big break came in 1969 with the discovery that electrical stimulation of the *periaqueductal gray* (PAG), the gray matter surrounding the third ventricle and the cerebral aqueduct in the midbrain, results in considerable analgesia. Reynolds implanted electrodes in the PAG of rats and performed abdominal surgery without problems when the electrodes were stimulated. Although the animals did not respond to the pain, they were able to move about the cage (before and after surgery) and displayed a startle response to visual or auditory stimuli while the electrodes were active.

Subsequent work has led to a detailed knowledge of the descending pain-modulating circuits. Figure 8.9 shows a drawing of the important features of these pathways. Input from the prefrontal

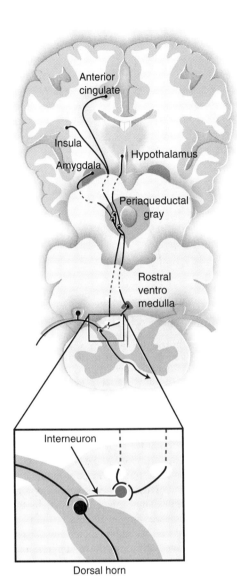

Opium

It is likely that opium was used as early as 4000 B.C. by the ancient Sumerians. By the 17th century, the therapeutic value of opium was well known. Morphine was first isolated in 1806 and codeine in 1832. Heroin was introduced to medicine in 1896. The uses and abuses of opium and its analogues have permeated most cultures of the world. Yet, how does morphine relieve pain?

It was established that microinjections of morphine into the PAG or the dorsal horn produced a powerful analgesia and that the opioid antagonist naloxone could block this effect. Furthermore, transection of the axons from the RVM reduces the morphine induced analgesia.

Opioid Receptors

The discovery of the opioid receptors was a major breakthrough in understanding the pain modulatory system. Three major classes of opioid receptors have been identified: μ, δ, and κ. However, most of the focus has been on the μ receptor because its activation is required for most analgesics. Indeed the affinity that a medication has for the μ receptor correlates with its potency as an analgesic. *Naloxone* also binds with the μ receptor but acts as the quintessential antagonist for it blocks activation and can precipitate withdrawal.

The opioid receptors are concentrated in the PAG, RVM, and dorsal horn—areas well known for pain modulation. However, the receptor can be found throughout the body, including skin, muscles, and joints, which help explain the benefits as well as typical side effects associated with opioids, for example, constipation, and respiratory depression.

Endogenous Opioids

Clearly, animals did not evolve a receptor so that drug abusers could enjoy heroin. In the mid-1970s the race was on to find the neurotransmitter that the body produces to activate the opioid receptor. The result was the discovery of the β-endorphin, enkephalins, and dynorphins: the three major classes of endogenous opioid peptides. The genes for these peptides are distributed throughout the CNS

Figure 8.10 gives an example from the dorsal horn of the enkephalins and the μ receptors working together to decrease the pain signal sent to the brain. Note that the μ receptors are on both the presynaptic as well as the postsynaptic neurons.

FIGURE 8.9 • Descending pain-modulating pathways that enable the brain to inhibit the intensity of the ascending pain signals

areas of the anterior cingulate and insular cortex as well as hypothalamus and amygdala converge on the PAG. The PAG does not send neurons directly on to the dorsal horn, but rather projects by way of intermediary nuclei such as the *rostral ventral medulla* (RVM). Other serotonergic and noradrenergic neurons (not shown) also project down on to the afferent pain neurons. The end result is inhibition and diminution of the pain signal that is sent up the ascending anterolateral tracts to the brain.

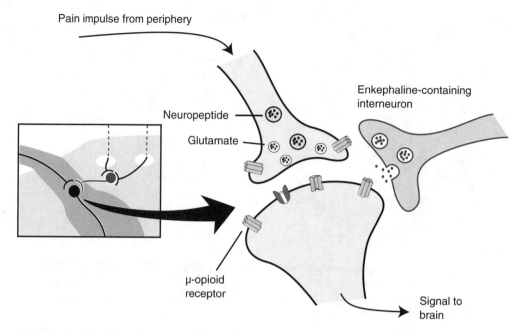

Pain impulse from periphery

Enkephaline-containing interneuron

Neuropeptide

Glutamate

μ-opioid receptor

Signal to brain

FIGURE 8.10   ● Descending pathways stimulate an interneuron in the dorsal horn to release enkephalins, that activates the μ receptors. The effect on the presynaptic neuron is to decrease the release of glutamate and neuropeptides. With the postsynaptic neuron, stimulation of the μ receptors hyperpolarizes the membrane. These two actions result in a smaller signal coming out of the dorsal horn.

POINT OF INTEREST

β-endorphin is a derived from a larger precursor molecule called *proopiomelanocortin* (POMC), found primarily in the pituitary. POMC contains other biologically active peptides, including ACTH. Consequently, the stress response—discussed in a previous chapter—includes the release of ACTH as well as β-endorphin into the bloodstream. One wonders about the evolutionary advantage of these two peptides being released together.

Placebo

The use of placebos, substances with no intrinsic therapeutic value, is the oldest treatment known to man. In the modern era of medicine, the placebo response has been equated with the statement "all in your head." More recently, it has been recognized that the placebo response is real—and actually in our heads. After the discovery of the endogenous opioid, it was shown that placebo anesthesia could even be reversed with naloxone.

Brain imaging studies of subjects anticipating an effective treatment for pain but given a placebo have shown reduced activity in the pain perception areas and increased activity in the pain-modulation areas—those associated with endogenous opioids (see Figure 8.11). Thus, placebos work in two ways. First, by decreasing awareness in the pain-sensitive regions and second by increasing activity in regions involved with top–down suppression.

Acupuncture

Acupuncture has been used for thousands of years in China, Korea, and Japan, but only recently has been introduced to the West. The healing power of acupuncture is believed to work by re-establishing the proper "energy balance" in disordered organs. The treatment is conducted by inserting a needle into specific locations along meridians established through ancient clinical experience. The lack of scientific correlation or good clinical trials can be troubling to those of us who subscribe to a Western orientation to physiology and illness.

One of the difficulties in conducting good clinical trial with acupuncture is separating the specific effect of stimulating the acupoints from the placebo effect. A recent study in London sought to overcome this problem by including two placebo arms along with active acupuncture treatment. The

Placebo induced decrease

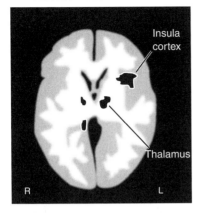

Placebo induced activation

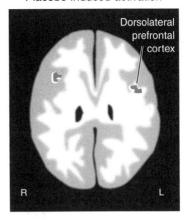

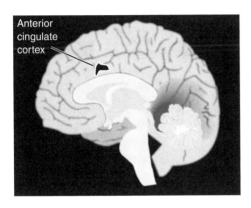

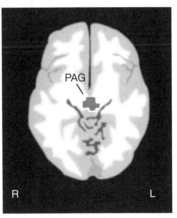

Decreased activity in pain-sensitive regions

Increased activity in pain-suppressing regions

FIGURE 8.11 ● The brain imaging studies of the placebo response showing two aspects to the brain's reaction. On the left, control minus placebo shows decreased activity in those areas that perceive pain. On the right, placebo minus control shows increased activity in areas that suppress pain from the top down. (Adapted from Wager TD, Rilling JK, Smith EE, et al. Placebo-induced changes in FMRI in the anticipation and experience of pain. *Science*. 2004;303[5661]:1162–1167.)

first placebo treatment was with a blunt needle and the patients were aware they were being given an "inert" treatment. The second placebo arm intervention utilized what can best be described as a "stage needle"—when poked, the needle retracted into the handle, giving the appearance that the skin had been pierced. Surprisingly, few of the subjects were aware of the difference between the "stage needle" and real acupuncture.

While these patients—all with osteoarthritis—were being stuck, they were also being scanned with a PET. The results showed that areas of the brain associated with top–down modulation of pain—dorsolateral prefrontal cortex, anterior cingulate cortex, and midbrain—were active with "stage needles" as well as real needles. Only

the ipsilateral insula was solely activated by real acupuncture. These results suggest that acupuncture works by way of a large placebo response and also a distinct, but as yet unknown, unique physiological effect.

Stress-Induced Analgesia

Perhaps the most impressive demonstration of top–down modulation of pain is the extreme analgesia shown by individuals at times of stress, for example, the athlete or performing artist who does not appreciate the pain until much later. The classic example was described by Beecher regarding men wounded in battle during the Second World War. He examined 215 men brought to a forward hospital with serious injuries: long bone fractures,

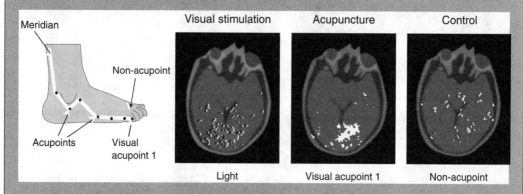

Meridian

Visual stimulation   Acupuncture   Control

Non-acupoint

Acupoints   Visual acupoint 1

Light   Visual acupoint 1   Non-acupoint

Light and acupuncture (at the visual acupoint 1) stimulate activity in the visual cortex whereas sham acupuncture does not. (Adapted from Cho ZH, Chung SC, Jones JP, et al. New findings of the correlation between acupoints and corresponding brain cortices using functional MRI. *Proc Natl Acad Sci U S A*. 1998;95[5]:2670–2673.)

penetrating wounds, etc. He found that only 25%, on being directly questioned regarding pain relief, said their pain was severe enough to make them want morphine. Beecher believed the relief the men experienced, when taken from the battle and brought to a safe location, blocked the pain.

The modern belief is that stress stimulates opioid dependent pathways that inhibit the pain signal. However, a group at the University of Georgia has revealed a role for the endocannabinoids in stress-induced analgesia independent of the opioid pathways. Several endocannabinoids rapidly accumulate in the PAG in the midbrain with stress. The group in Georgia demonstrated that stress-induced analgesia rats could be inhibited with endocannabinoid blockers. Their results suggest that higher cortical regions such as the amygdala release endocannabinoids into the PAG during stressful times to suppress pain perception. We can understand the brain's wisdom in having several mechanisms (endocannabinoids and opioids) to put pain on hold when other events are more important.

CHRONIC PAIN

Until the last half of the past century, pain was thought to be produced by a passive, direct-transmission system from peripheral receptors to the cortex. This is called *nociceptive pain* (which we have already discussed earlier) and examples include acute trauma, arthritis, and tumor invasion. There is a veritable medical industry based on locating and correcting the source of the nociceptive pain for patients who are suffering. Unfortunately, most evaluations fail to turn up a cause that explains the pain. One reason is that the traditional model of pain fails to take into account changes in the nerves. Clearly, many patients in pain—particularly chronic, persistent pain—have developed autonomous, maladaptive pain perception independent of tissue damage.

Neuropathic pain is a heterogeneous term used to describe pain that arises from an injured nerve—either centrally or peripherally. Examples of this type of pain are postherpetic neuralgia, diabetic neuropathy, and phantom limb. The distinction between neuropathic and nociceptive pain is important when choosing proper treatment. For instance, neuropathic pain may not respond as well to nonsteroidal anti-inflammatory agents, or opioids, and is better managed with antidepressants and anticonvulsants.

Neuropathic pain is frequently persistent, does not resolve with time, and is resistant to treatment. The pain often disables patients. The

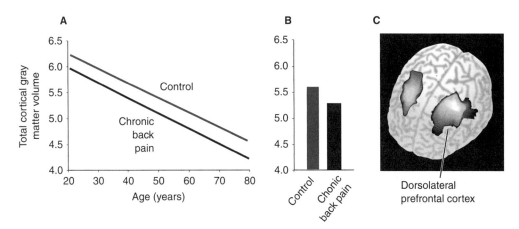

FIGURE 8.12 ● Gray matter loss with chronic back pain. **A:** Decrease in total gray matter volume for patients with chronic back pain compared to controls. **B:** Average for both groups. **C:** The dorsolateral prefrontal cortex is the specific region with decreased gray matter density. (Adapted from Apkarian AV, Sosa Y, Sonty S, et al. Chronic back pain is associated with decreased prefrontal and thalamic gray matter density. *J Neurosci.* 2004;24[46]:10410–10415.)

pathophysiological mechanism that underlie these neuropathic pain conditions are beginning to be teased out. One promising area of research is looking at the role of neurotrophic factors in the development of pathologic pain states.

Evidence suggests that the inflammatory state resulting from an injury results in the recruitment of immune system cells (mast cells and macrophages) that release cytokines (tumor necrosis factor and interleukins) that initiate and maintain sensory changes. One result of this process is the interruption of the retrograde transport of neurotrophins from the periphery, which support normal cell functioning. One neurotrophic factor in particular (glial cell line-derived neurotrophic factor [GDNF]) has been implicated. Several studies have shown that exogenous GDNF can prevent the development of experimental neuropathic pain.

Pain Memory

A striking example of the brain's elaboration of pain without sensory input can be found in patients after limb amputation. Many will continue to experience pain from lesions that existed on the limb before the surgery—what some call pain memory. For example, a person with an ulcer on the foot at the time of the operation will still feel the presence of the ulcer many months after the limb has been removed.

Several clever clinicians have shown that sufficient local anesthesia of the affected limb several days prior to the amputation significantly reduces the incidence of pain memories. These results suggest that pain has some lasting effect on the

brain, which can be attenuated with appropriate treatment.

Gray Matter Loss

A study by a group at Northwestern University enhances our understanding of the role of the CNS with chronic pain. Apkarian et al. scanned 26 patients with chronic back pain that had persisted for at least 1 year. They compared the results with age-matched controls and found a 5% to 11% loss of gray matter in patients with chronic back pain (see figure 8.12). Further regional analysis showed that the dorsolateral prefrontal cortex (DLPFC) was the specific area with greatest decrease in gray matter density. These results suggest that one explanation for chronic pain may be the loss of top–down modulation of pain, because we know that the DLPFC is involved in the inhibition of the ascending signals (see Figure 8.11).

What causes the gray matter loss with chronic pain? Several explanations are possible. First, the patients could be genetically predisposed to have less gray matter. Small injuries result in persistent pain because the patients lack sufficient CNS modulation of the ascending pain signal. Second, medications, or abused substances have a toxic effect on the gray matter. Third, the unremitting pain signal with the associated negative affect and stress results in an excitotoxic and inflammatory state that essentially wears out the brain circuitry.

Regardless of the etiology, the data shows that there is more to chronic back pain than just having a "bad back."

TMS, PFC & POST-OPERATIVE PAIN.

Transcranial Magnetic Stimulation (TMS) is a noninvasive procedure that can stimulate the cerebral cortex. The PFC has been implicated as a region that modulates pain tolerance. A cleaver collaboration between anesthesiology and psychiatry shows that activation of the PFC with TMS can decrease pain perception.

Patients undergoing gastric bypass surgery were randomized to receive 20 minutes of either active of sham TMS immediately after surgery. Total morphine administer by patient-controlled analgesia pumps was tracked as an indirect measurement of pain. The figure shows that patients who received active TMS used approximately 40% less morphine in the 48-hours after the operation.

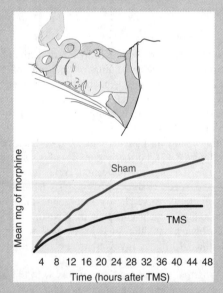

One 20-minute session of TMS applied to the left PFC postoperatively greatly reduced the total morphine administered by the patients. (Adapted from Borckardt JJ, Weinstein M, Reeves ST, et al. Postoperative left prefrontal repetitive transcranial magnetic stimulation reduces patient-controlled analgesia use. *Anesthesiology.* 2006;105[3]:557–562.)

DEPRESSION AND ANTIDEPRESSANTS

There is a long and well-documented correlation between depression and pain. Patients with chronic pain have a high incidence of depression and patients with depression have an increased expression of painful physical symptoms. Recently, studies have shown that patients with depression and pain are less likely to achieve remission of their depression.

There is also a long history of using antidepressants for many pain conditions and have shown to be effective in decreasing pain for low back pain, diabetic neuropathy, postherpetic neuralgia, fibromyalgia, and migraines as well as other pains. Traditionally, the tricyclics were used, but with the development of cleaner medications, other agents were tried. Of interest, the SSRIs have been disappointing—often not separating from placebo in controlled trials. It appears that only agents that inhibit the reuptake of norepinephrine as well as serotonin are effective for pain reduction. Recently the newer agents that tout a dual mechanism of action (venlafaxine and duloxetine) have been shown to reduce pain due to diabetic neuropathy. Duloxetine even has an FDA indication for peripheral diabetic neuropathy.

How do the antidepressants decrease pain? One possibility could be the beneficial effect of correcting the mood. Yet, SSRIs give disappointing results. Likewise, patients without depression will show some pain reduction. Another possibility is the enhancement of the descending pathways. Some of the fibers projecting from the brain stem down onto the dorsal horn of the spinal cord are serotonergic and noradrenergic. More action from these neurons would further dampen the signals from the periphery.

A final possibility for understanding the effectiveness of antidepressants for pain is a cortical mechanism. PET scans of depressed patients and patients with pain both show decreased activity in the prefrontal cortex and increased activity in the insula and anterior cingulate cortex. It is possible that antidepressants moderate the pain perception by correcting the cortical imbalance associated with depression and pain.

Epidemic of Unexplained Pain

Let us not forget that pain is highly influenced by one's psychosocial expectations. A good example is the epidemic of vague upper limb pain, from Australia called *repetitive strain injury* (RSI). This condition was attributed to repetitive keyboard movements by telegraphists, but failed to follow the usual medical model. Reports in the medical literature and sensational media coverage as well as union and legal advocacy produced a dramatic increase in reports of RSI (see Figure 8.13). The condition peaked in 1984 and then declined, as

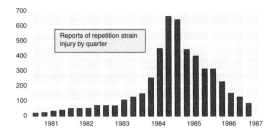

FIGURE 8.13 ● A psychosomatic pain epidemic. The graph shows reports of repetition strain injury at Telecom in Australia by quarter. (Adapted from Hocking B. Epidemiological aspects of "repetition strain injury" in Telecom Australia. *Med J Aust*. 1987;147[5]:218–222.)

the condition came to be perceived as psychosomatic and the courts went against the litigants. Similar epidemics have occurred in the UK and Japan.

Another classic study analyzed the development of late whiplash syndrome in Lithuania—a country where few drivers have car insurance or seek legal compensation after an accident. The authors questioned the subjects involved in known rear-end car collisions, one to three years after the accident, regarding neck pain and headaches, and compared their symptoms with matched control subjects. There was no significant difference between the groups. The authors concluded that "expectation of disability, a family history, and attribution of preexisting symptoms to the trauma may be more important determinants for the evolution of the late whiplash syndrome."

The important point is that the perception of pain is a product of the brain's abstraction and elaboration of sensory input. Many factors affect that process—not just nociceptive signals from the periphery.

QUESTIONS

1. Slow aching pain signals.
   a. Aδ fibers.
   b. Aβ fibers.
   c. C fibers.
   d. D fibers.

2. Simultaneous input from these nerve fibers explain the inhibitory effect of the gate theory of pain.
   a. Aδ fibers.
   b. Aβ fibers.
   c. C fibers.
   d. D fibers.

3. Not associated with the affective-motivational pathways of pain.
   a. Somatosensory cortex.
   b. "How much does it hurt?"
   c. Medial thalamus.
   d. Anterior cingulate and insula cortex.

4. Condition associated with increased pain tolerance.
   a. Depression.
   b. Anxiety.
   c. Fibromyalgia.
   d. Schizophrenia.

5. Not part of the descending pathways of pain.
   a. Periaqueductal gray.
   b. Dorsal horn.
   c. Spinothalamic tract.
   d. Rostral ventral medulla.

6. The primary opioid receptor.
   a. β receptor.
   b. δ receptor.
   c. κ receptor.
   d. μ receptor.

7. Unlikely explanation for chronic persistent pain.
   a. Genetic predisposition.
   b. Diminished placebo response.
   c. Changes in the gray matter.
   d. Damaged nerves.

8. Lacks significant analgesic effects.
   a. SSRIs.
   b. Opioids.
   c. NSAIs.
   d. Anticonvulsants.

See Answers section at end of book.

Pleasure

SEEKING PLEASURE

Voluntary behavior in animals is motivated by the avoidance of pain and the pursuit of pleasure. In this chapter we will focus on the neuronal mechanisms that guide our choices in the direction of stimuli that give a little reward to the brain.

Our existence—as individuals and as a species—is dependent on using the five senses to recognize and pursue actions necessary for survival. The motivation to pursue a beneficial act is driven in part by giving the brain a brief squirt of euphoria. This reward system has evolved over millions of years to enable an individual to sort through the variety of stimuli that bombard the senses and choose the ones that are appropriate.

The orbital aspect of the prefrontal cortex is known to play a critical role in goal-directed behavior. Figure 9.1 shows that the relative appeal of an item can be recognized in the brain even down to the level of a single neuron. In this study, electrodes placed in a single neuron in the orbitofrontal cortex registered different levels of activity based on the appeal of the food reward. A raisin generated the largest signal and was the most desired object; cereal was least active and least desired.

Many of our patients, family, and friends struggle with problems that they have created by pursuing the wrong rewards. Clearly, the addicted individual has lost control over his choices (more on this later), but what about the promiscuous college student, the young adult who accumulates excessive debt on new credit cards, or the child who plays video games instead of doing homework? These people are choosing pleasurable activities that are not to their benefit and even harmful.

The problems are related to how our reward system is designed. We are built for acquiring rewards that were historically in short supply. Now with the extraordinary success of the human race and industrialized civilization, we are exposed to abundance beyond what our wiring has evolved to handle. Junk food, pornography, shopping malls as well as alcohol, stimulants, and opioids usurp the mechanisms developed to enhance the survival of the hunter-gatherer in all of us.

DISORDER: MARITAL CONFLICT

Disparity in what brings joy is the major source of conflict in most relationships. Married couples frequently argue about sex, money, and how to spend leisure time. With each conflict, one partner wants to spend more time and money involved in some activity. For example, he wants to golf and buy a big boat for fishing; she wants to vacation with her family and fix up the house. He wants more sex; she wants more romance. The conflict really heats up when one partner is hurt by the others joy.

Happiness

There is clinical evidence to suggest that one's level of happiness remains remarkably fixed. For

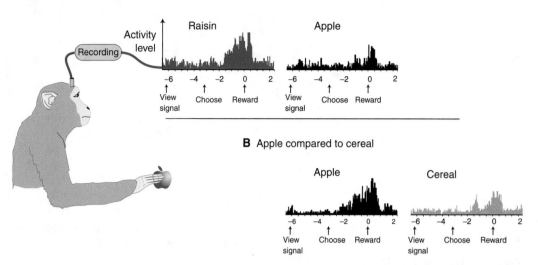

A Raisin compared to apple

B Apple compared to cereal

FIGURE 9.1 ●   A monkey is taught to view a signal, wait, then make the appropriate choice and be rewarded with designated food morsel. **A:** Shows the activity in an individual neuron in the orbitofrontal cortex when the monkey is offered a reward of either a raisin or an apple. **B:** Rewarded with either an apple or cereal. The size of the signal is believed to represent the motivational value, i.e., Raisin > Apple; Apple > Cereal. (Adapted from Tremblay L, Schultz W. Relative reward preference in primate orbitofrontal cortex. *Nature*. 1999;398[6729]:704–708.)

example, the person winning a lottery or the one suffering the loss of a limb tends to revert to their preexisting level of happiness after a period of euphoria or depression. It seems that happiness is hard-wired and closely fluctuates around a genetic "set-point" for each person. Unfortunately, there is surprisingly little neuroscience research on this topic.

ANATOMY OF REWARD

Pursuing a reward can be conceptualized as a ball rolling down hill. Animals will gravitate toward the most enjoyable activity the way a ball rolls to the lowest point. It seemingly happens without effort. However, although we cannot visualize the force of gravity pulling on a moving ball, we continue to tease out the neuroanatomy of the mammalian reward system.

The initial studies came in the mid 50s when Olds and Milner accidentally discovered that a rat would seek to continue stimulation from a thin electrode implanted in certain parts of his brain. Figure 9.2 shows the relative placement of an electrode in a rat's skull and the apparatus that Olds and Milner used to document the animals efforts to stimulate themselves. Remarkably, the rats exceeded all expectation in what they were willing to sacrifice to receive stimulation. Depending on where the electrode was placed, they would press

the lever up to 5,000 times in an hour, chose stimulation over food even when starving, and crossed an electrified grid for a chance to press the lever.

Fifty years of research has established that the mesolimbic dopamine system including the ventral tegmental area (VTA) and nucleus accumbens (NAc) (also called the *ventral striatum*) are the central structures of reward. These old but effective nuclei lie at the base of the brain (see Figure 9.3) and are the structures that were being indirectly stimulated in the Olds and Milner experiments. The NAc and VTA receive signals from a multitude of sources—the most prominent of which are the prefrontal cortex, amygdala, and hippocampus. It is significant that the input to the NAc and VTA are from areas involved in attention, executive decisions, and emotional memories. Aspects that are important when assessing a pleasurable activity.

Converging lines of evidence have shown that dopamine (DA) is the primary neurotransmitter that modulates the reward system. Using an implanted microdialysis apparatus, Pettit, and Justice were able to regularly sample dopamine concentration at the NAc. They found a correlation between the amounts of cocaine a rat would self-administer and the extracellular DA at the NAc (see Figure 9.4). Alternatively, blocking the effect of cocaine either with a dopamine antagonist (e.g., haloperidol) or

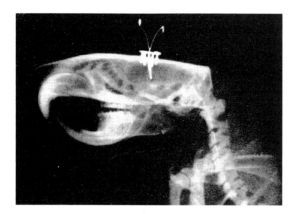
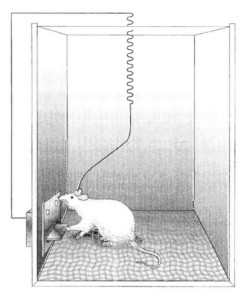

FIGURE 9.2 ● Above is an x-ray showing the placement of an electrode through the skull into the brain of a rat. On the right is a rat receiving a mild stimulus—and seemingly enjoying it—when he presses the lever. (From Olds J. Pleasure centers in the brain. *Sci Am*. 1956;195:105–112.)

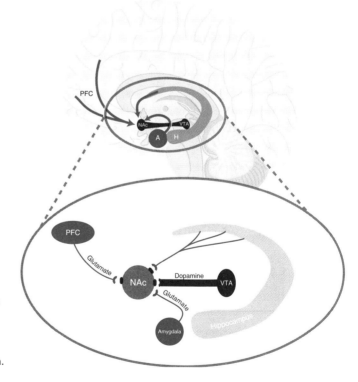

FIGURE 9.3 ● The anatomy of pleasure and reward is mediated in the nucleus accumbens with input from a variety of structures, only a few of which are shown here. NAc, nucleus accumbens; PFC, prefrontal cortex; VTA, ventral tegmental area.

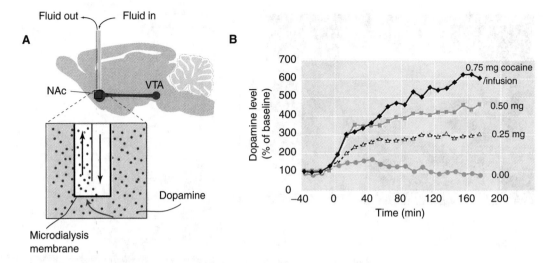

FIGURE 9.4 ● Using microdialysis in rats, Pettit and Justice found that increasing self-administered doses of cocaine resulted in greater extracellular dopamine at the nucleus accumbens. (Adapted from Pettit HO, Justice JB Jr. Effect of dose on cocaine self-administration behavior and dopamine levels in the nucleus accumbens. *Brain Res.* 1991;539[1]:94–102.)

lesioning the dopaminergic cells in the NAc eliminated the self-administration and drug-seeking behavior.

Brain Imaging

More recently, brain-imaging studies with human volunteers have further established the link between dopamine and pleasure. Volkow administered IV methylphenidate (Ritalin) and established a correlation between the dose of the medication and the occupancy of the dopamine transporter (stimulants work in part by blocking the dopamine reuptake pump). Additionally by asking the participant how they felt, a correlation between feeling "high" and occupancy of the dopamine transporter was established (see Figure 9.5).

Creative studies with functional imaging scanners have shown that it is not just drugs of abuse (amphetamines, alcohol, nicotine, etc.) that result in enhanced dopamine at the NAc, but many

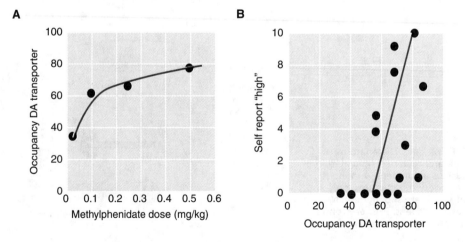

FIGURE 9.5 ● Methylphenidate and occupancy of the dopamine reuptake transporter. Higher doses of methylphenidate result in increased occupancy of the dopamine transporter, which results in increased dopamine available to the nucleus accumbens and—at strong enough levels—feeling "high". (Adapted from Volkow ND, Fowler JS, Wang GJ, et al. Role of dopamine in the therapeutic and reinforcing effects of methylphenidate in humans: Results from imaging studies. *Eur Neuropsychopharmacol.* 2002;12[6]:557–566.)

Drugs

1. Cocaine
2. Alcohol
3. Amphetamines
4. Methylphenidate
5. Nicotine

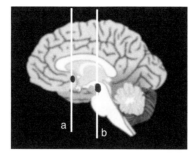

Feelings

6. Romantic love
7. Listening to music
8. Humor
9. Expectation of $$$
10. Inflicting punishment
11. Looking at beautiful faces
12. Social co-operation
13. Eating chocolate

a. Nucleus accumbens

b. Ventral tegmental area

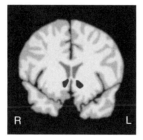
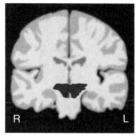

Drugs

1. Acute effects of cocain on human brain activity and emotion. *Neuron.* 1997;19:591–611.
2. Alcohol promotes dopamine release in the human nucleus accumbens. *Synapse.* 2003;49:226–231.
3. SPECT imaging of srtiatal dopamine release after amphetamine challenge. *J Nucl Med.* 1995;36:1182–1190.
4. Role of dopmaine in the therapeutic and reinforcing effects of methylphenidate in humans: Results from imaging studies. *Eu Neuropsychophar.* 2002;12:557–566.
5. Nicotine induce limbic cortical activation in the human brain: A functional MRI study. *Am J Psych.* 1998;155:1009-1015

Feelings

6. Reward, motivation, and emotion systems associated with early-stage intense romantic love. *J Neurophysiol.* 2005;94:327–337.
7. Intensely pleasurable responses to music correlate with activity in brain regions implicated in reward and emotion. *Proc Natl Acad Sci USA.* 2001;98:11818–11823.
8. Humor modulates the mesolimbic reward centers. *Neuron.* 2003;40:1041–1048.
9. Functional imaging of neural responses to expectancy and experience of monetary gains and losses. *Neuron.* 2001;30:619–639.
10. The neural basis of altruistic punishment. *Science.* 2004;305:1254–1258
11. Beautiful faces have variable reward value: fMRI and behavioral evidence. *Neuron.* 2001;32:537–551.
12. A neural basis for social cooperation. *Neuron.* 2002;35:395–405.
13. Changes in brain activity related to eating chocolate. *Brain.* 2001;124:1720–1733.

FIGURE 9.6 ● Drugs of abuse as well as good feelings will light up the mesolimbic dopamine pathway in functional imaging studies in humans. The studies documenting these findings are listed at the bottom of the Figure.

pleasurable activities. Figure 9.6 gives examples of feelings (looking at beautiful faces, eating chocolate, revenge, etc.) as well as the drugs that have all demonstrated increased dopamine at the NAc and/or VTA in functional scans in humans.

Figure 9.6 shows only the studies with humans. There are additional hedonic experiences that show similar findings with animals. For example, sexual behavior, violence, opioids, marijuana all increase dopamine at the NAc in animals. Furthermore, we can speculate that other pleasurable behaviors—those that would be difficult to investigate in a scanner, such as shopping, gambling, extreme sports, and defeating ones arch enemy—also may deliver a dollop of dopamine

to the NAc. The key point is this: Behaviors that people enjoy seem to precipitate an increase in the dopamine produced at the NAc.

One particularly interesting study conducted at the primate laboratory at Wake Forest University looked at the effect of social rank on dopamine in monkeys. The monkeys were initially housed individually and scanned for dopamine D_2 receptors, which were found to be similar for all monkeys. Next they were housed together in groups of four. After 3 months, the researchers determined who were the dominant and subordinate monkeys and then re-scanned them. The results are shown in Figure 9.7. Note that the dominant monkey now has significantly greater dopamine D_2 receptors in the striatum—an area that includes the NAc.

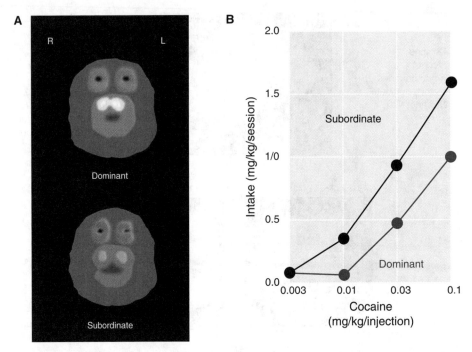

FIGURE 9.7 ● A: drawings of PET scans showing the prevalence of dopamine D_2 receptors for monkeys after establishing social hierarchy. B: The graph shows that the dominant monkey always self-administered less cocaine at different strengths of the drug compared to the subordinate monkey. (Adapted from Morgan D, Grant KA, Gage HD, et al. Social dominance in monkeys: Dopamine D_2 receptors and cocaine self-administration. *Nat Neurosci.* 2002;5[2]:169–174.)

The researchers also allowed the monkeys to self-administer different doses of cocaine. The graph on the right of Figure 9.7 shows that the dominant monkeys gave themselves less cocaine than the subordinates at different strengths of the drug. This suggests that the "good feelings" that come from being the alpha monkey buffer against seeking external sources of pleasure and provide some insight into the correlation between increased substance abuse and lower socioeconomic groups.

Pleasure Versus Novelty

It is overly simplistic to call the NAc the pleasure center. Research with rodents has found that dopamine will increase at the NAc with adverse stimuli—for example, a foot shock. Likewise, addicts have reported that they have continued to seek their drug although it is no longer pleasurable.

Some have suggested that the NAc determines the "wanting" and motivation to seek a reward—not the pleasurable experience itself. Volkow, director of National Institute of Drug Abuse, prefers the term "saliency" to describe the function of dopamine at the NAc. By salience she means new and unexpected stimuli that focus attention and motivate to seek more.

Di Chiara has studied the effect of various substances on dopamine release at the NAc. His group has shown that dopamine release is strongest for positive, novel reinforcements. Figure 9.8 shows the bump in dopamine at the NAc when a rat is given chocolate. However, when given the same amount of chocolate on the following day, the bump in dopamine is no longer significant.

Di Chiara has shown in other studies that habituation does not occur with cocaine. Day after day, rats will have a jump in dopamine at the NAc when given cocaine. Not only is the increase stronger in magnitude (up to 400% over baseline compared to 150% for chocolate), but also does not attenuate like the natural reinforcers. This may in part explain why cocaine is so addictive.

Amygdala

The amygdala along with the frontal cortex influences the mesolimbic dopamine system. Although better known for its role in fear and avoidance (see Chapter 19, Anxiety), the amygdala plays a role in seeking pleasure. The amygdala is critically involved in the process of acquiring and

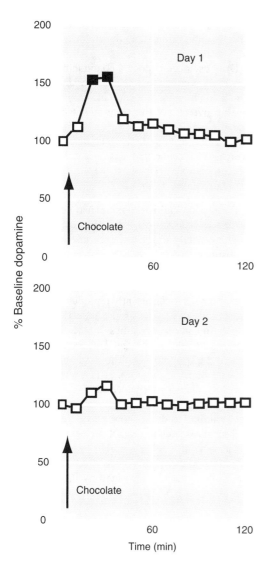

FIGURE 9.8 ● Habituation. When first given chocolate, a rat shows a significant increase (■) in its dopamine at the nucleus accumbens, which does not occur when given the same food on the following day. (Adapted from Bassareo V, De Luca MA, Di Chiara G. Differential expression of motivational stimulus properties by dopamine in nucleus accumbens shell versus core and prefrontal cortex. *J Neurosci.* 2002;22[11]:4709–4719.)

retaining lasting memories of emotional experiences whether they are pleasurable or traumatic. Studies have shown correlations between the activation of the amygdala during emotionally arousing events and subsequent recall. It is not known if the memories are actually stored in the amygdala or recalled from the cortex by the amygdala.

The process of associating emotional memories with particular events—a special song, helicopters flying overhead, or the smell of a cigarette—is classical conditioning. A demonstration of the role of the amygdala and seeking pleasure can be shown when a rat is conditioned to associate a sound or light with pressing a lever and receiving cocaine. If the rat no longer receives the cocaine when he presses the lever, he will almost completely stop pressing the lever—extinguishing the behavior. Later if he hears the conditioned sound or sees the light, he will resume pressing the lever as long as his amygdala is intact. A rat without an amygdala will fail to resume pressing the lever when stimulated with the tone or light. Clearly, the amygdala is essential to remembering the associations.

The Pursuit of Pleasure

People spend time doing what they enjoy. "Time sure flies when you're having fun" is the old saying. The propensity to get "lost" in an activity and lose track of time is a feature of rewarding activities—and something that can be a source of frustration for friends and family who do not enjoy the same activity.

The brain has several internal clocks. Circadian rhythms and the 24-hour clock are the best known. However, there are lesser-known circuits to manage milliseconds, which are essential for sports, dancing, music, and speech. Of relevance to this chapter, these circuits utilize dopamine and to some extent activate the VTA. Studies with rodents have found that D_2 agonists, such as methamphetamine, accelerate the internal clock whereas D_2 blockers, such as haloperidol, slow down the clock. This may explain why people inaccurately estimate the duration of a pleasurable activity.

POINT OF INTEREST

Albert Einstein is reported to have described his theory of relativity as such: "Put your hand on a hot stove for a minute, and it seems like an hour. Sit with a pretty girl for an hour, and it seems like a minute." Einstein eloquently described how our perception of the passage of time is affected by our feelings of pain and pleasure.

People who have the propensity to enjoy work have an adapted advantage over those who do not. We can imagine that nature selects for individuals the traits to enjoy activities that are beneficial, for example, hunting and gathering as well as communicating and planning. Alternatively, some people lose themselves in activities that are not healthy and continue to pursue them in spite of negative outcomes. This behavior and the effects on the brain are the focus of the next section.

ADDICTIONS CHANGE THE BRAIN

Most of the pleasurable activities that we are wired to pursue occur in nature in limited supply, making it hard to overindulge. Modern life, however, is full of many temptations that activate the mesolimbic pathway. Drugs of abuse, in particular, overwhelm and fundamentally alter the neurons that were never intended to experience such supraphysiologic levels of neurotransmitters. Addictions entail the persistent, destructive, and uncontrollable behaviors that involve obtaining the object of desire.

One simple definition of an addiction is the continued pursuit of a substance or activity in spite of negative consequences. This could apply to gambling, sex, alcohol, smoking, food, and even work. All these activities result in increased DA at the NAc. We will focus in this section on drugs of abuse and the changes they cause in the addicted brain. Figure 9.9 shows the location of several commonly abused drugs.

Some drugs have direct effects on the mesolimbic pathway while others work indirectly. The stimulants and nicotine result in increased dopamine at the NAc. The opioids, alcohol, and phencyclidine (PCP) (and to some extent nicotine) suppress the inhibitory neurons that modulate the NAc and VTA. With less inhibition, more dopamine is released to the NAc.

Drug use occurs along a continuum—from casual use to dominating one's life. Addictions result from a combination of genes and environment and develop over time. But once addicted, the drugs alter the architecture of the brain. Tolerance and withdrawal are two clinical manifestations of the changes that occur to the addicted brain. Other clinical examples that show the effects of persistent abuse are as follows:

1. Depression and anhedonia when not using.
2. Less responsive to natural rewards.
3. The capacity to relapse even many years after abstinence.

Global Impairments

One of the most consistently reproducible findings in the addictions field is the reduction in brain volume in chronic alcoholics. Studies have shown decreased total volume and gray matter, particularly in the frontal lobes. These findings co-occur with declines in cognition and memory. Alcoholics evaluated after a period of sobriety show some recovery of tissue volume whereas those who continue to drink show further reductions.

Recent research has established cigarette smoking as a confounding variable in brain volume reductions and cognitive decline. One study compared intelligence as measured by IQ in 172 men (see Figure 9.10). Alcoholism and smoking were

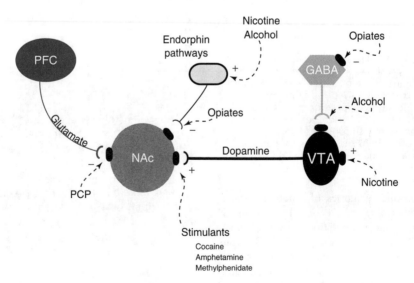

FIGURE 9.9 ● Possible sites of action by drugs of abuse on the mesolimbic pathway. PFC, prefrontal cortex; NAc, nucleus accumbens; VTA, ventral tegmental area; GABA, γ-Aminobutyric acid.

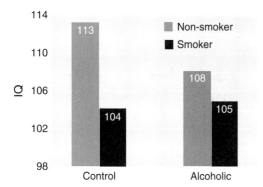

FIGURE 9.10 ● IQ is independently reduced in subjects with heavy alcohol or cigarette use. (Adapted from Glass JM, Adams KM, Nigg JT, et al. Smoking is associated with neurocognitive deficits in alcoholism. *Drug Alcohol Depend*. 2005; in press.)

independent risk factors for reductions in IQ. It is not known if smoking has a direct neurotoxic effect on cognition or an indirect effect from cardiovascular or pulmonary damage. Interestingly, smokers report that a cigarette enhances their attention and it has been shown that nicotine acutely improves cognitive performance. Yet, the long-term effect on cognition is detrimental.

Dopamine Receptors

The stimulants work by blocking the dopamine re-uptake pump as well as increasing the release of dopamine which results in more dopamine available to stimulate the NAc. Using positron emission tomography (PET) scans, Volkow has shown decreased D_2 receptors in cocaine addicts during withdrawal (see Figure 9.11), which persisted even

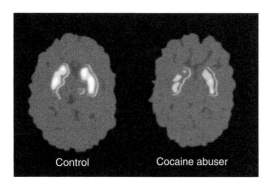

FIGURE 9.11 ● Horizontal PET scans at the level of the striatum. The cocaine abuser has less D_2 receptor binding compared to the control. (Adapted from Volkow ND, Li TK. Drug addiction: The neurobiology of behaviour gone awry. *Nat Rev Neurosci*. 2004;5[12]:963–970.)

when tested 3 to 4 months after detoxification. Similar findings have been demonstrated in subjects withdrawn from heroin, methamphetamine, and alcohol. These results imply that excessive use of hedonic substances results in a down-regulation of the D_2 receptor. This may explain the development of tolerance and need for the addict to take "more". Likewise, this helps us understand why the abstinent user has difficulty experiencing pleasure with the natural reinforcers of life.

Craving and the Frontal Cortex

The addict is someone who has moved from getting high to getting hooked. He is haunted by persistent, intrusive thoughts about his drug, and intensely desires to obtain more. He has lost control. In the literature and on the street, this is called *craving*.

The prefrontal cortex has been identified as a source of craving and also obsessions (see Chapter 19, Anxiety). Functional imaging studies have shown enhanced activity in the prefrontal cortex (PFC), particularly the orbital frontal cortex (OFC) and dorsolateral prefrontal cortex (DLPFC), when addicts are presented with drug related cues. For example, cocaine addicts shown pictures of white powder will light up their frontal lobes and will report "drug craving". It is noteworthy that the activity in the PFC correlates with the intensity of self-reported craving.

We discussed in the first section of this chapter the important role the PFC plays in making choices (Figure 9.1). An essential feature of addictions is the inability to make good choices. This problem can be demonstrated in the relative activity of the prefrontal cortex when addicts are shown various film clips.

In one important study, cocaine users were shown video clips of men smoking crack, sexually explicit scenes, and scenes of nature while in a functional brain scanner. Compared to the controls the cocaine users showed increased activation in the frontal cortex while viewing videos of men smoking crack but not when shown sexually explicit content. The authors concluded that the drug abusers had developed a heightened response to stimuli associated with drug use, but blunted response to other rewarding stimuli (see Table 9.1).

The persistence of cravings and the susceptibility to lose control even after years of abstinence suggest long-term changes in the neurons of the prefrontal cortex. Several findings with rats suggest the glutamatergic projections from the prefrontal cortex to the NAc (Figure 9.3) may be the culprit. The important findings are as follows:

1. Inactivation of the prefrontal cortex prevents relapse.

Reaction by Cocaine Users to Different Stimuli

Drug Related Cues	Natural Reinforcing Stimuli
Over-respond	Under-respond
Craving	Lack of interest
Increased activity in prefrontal cortex	Hypometabolism in prefrontal cortex

2. Glutamate receptor blockade at the NAc prevents relapse.
3. Increased glutamate is released in the NAc during relapse.

These results not only point to the glutamatergic projections as a source of craving, but also suggest a possible site to intervene for preventing relapse.

DISORDER: ANHEDONIA

One of the disturbing effects of a frontal lobotomy was a pervasive lack of motivation. The subjects were left with a general lack of interest in almost everything. While the procedure may have reduced interest in inappropriate activities, it also had a global effect on all interests. This is the challenge for treating the substance abuser. How to selectively eliminate the craving without altering the whole personality.

Synaptic Remodeling

The fact that drug induced adaptations are so permanent suggests that the drugs fundamentally alter the organization of the neuronal circuits and synaptic connectivity. In a series of experiments, Robinson et al. at the University of Michigan have studied the effects of amphetamine, cocaine, and morphine on the structure of pyramidal cells in various parts of the brain. Figure 9.12 shows the neurons from the parietal cortex.

The dendritic spines on the neuron are the postsynaptic receptors for input from other neurons. Presumably, changes in the number of spines reflect

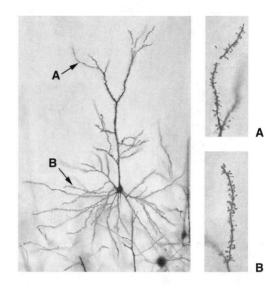

FIGURE 9.12 ● Photomicrograph of a Golgi-stained pyramidal cell from the parietal cortex. Multiple photographs at different focal planes were merged together to create this composite. The inserts on the right are from the apical (**A**) and basilar (**B**) regions. (From Kolb B, Gorny G, Li Y, et al. Amphetamine or cocaine limits the ability of later experience to promote structural plasticity in the neocortex and nucleus accumbens. *Proc Natl Acad Sci U S A*. 2003;100[18]:10523–10528.)

changes in the number of synapses on the neuron. In different experiments Robinson et al. has shown that amphetamine and cocaine will increase the number of spines whereas morphine results in a decrease. Figure 9.13 shows drawings of neurons from the NAc in rats exposed to morphine, saline, and amphetamine. Even to the naked eye one can see the opposite effects that morphine and amphetamine have on the number of spines.

Molecular Changes

Nestler et al. at the University of Texas Southwestern Medical Center have examined the molecular changes that underlie the long-term plasticity of addiction. As we discussed in Chapter 5, Receptors and Signaling the Nucleus, changes in the neuronal architecture are driven by gene expression. Nestler et al. identified two transcription factors in the NAc that contribute to gene expression and the resulting protein synthesis in the addicted state.

Cyclic adenosine monophosphate response element binding (CREB) is a transcription factor that is activated by increased dopamine concentrations during drug binges. CREB in turn promotes the production of proteins that dampen the

Morphine Saline Amphetamine

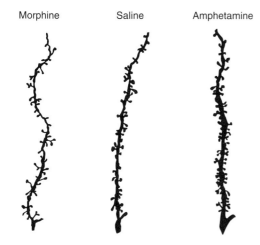

FIGURE 9.13 ● Changes in dendritic spines in the nucleus accumbens from rats exposed to morphine, saline, and amphetamine. Morphine decreases the number of spines whereas amphetamine induces an increase. (Adapted from Robinson and Kolb, 1997, 2002.)

reward circuitry and induce tolerance. The dampening effects stimulated by CREB are believed to be one of the reasons drug users need to take more of their substance to get the same effect. CREB may also mediate the depression and anhedonia felt by the addicts when unable to get drugs.

However, CREB is only part of the story. It is switched off within days of stopping drug use, yet the addict remains vulnerable to relapse for a long time. δ-FosB is another transcription factor that may explain the lasting effects of drug abuse. Unlike CREB, δ-FosB accumulates in the cells of the NAc and is remarkably stable. It remains active in the cells for weeks and months after drugs have stopped. Such long-lasting changes help us understand why addicts are susceptible to relapse even after years of abstinence.

Relapse

There are three well-known causes for relapsing.

1. Use of the drug or a similar drug.
2. Exposure to cues associated with drug use.
3. Stress.

All three causes result in increased release of dopamine at the NAc, which seems to impair the addicts will to remain abstinent.

The effects of stress on the mesolimbic dopamine system are mediated in part through the hypothalamic–pituitary–adrenal (HPA) axis. It appears that corticotrophin-releasing factor (CRF) and cortisol stimulate the release of dopamine. Studies with rats have shown that a stressor, such

as a foot shock, stimulates the HPA axis as well as reinstates drug-seeking behavior. Different studies have shown that the reinstatement for heroin, cocaine, and alcohol can be blocked by the administration of a CRF antagonist.

Developmental Disorder?

It is readily apparent that our joys and pleasures change as we age. A boy of latent age is not the least bit interested in sex, but a few years later as an adolescent he is bubbling-over with sexual excitement. The old saying, "the difference between men and boys is the price of their toys," describes the development of new sources of pleasure as men age. Changes in the brain most likely accompany the changes in what we seek for pleasure.

Adolescence is a time characterized by high levels of risk taking and impulsivity. This can be seen as enhanced approach behavior and reduced harm-avoidance behavior—or too much accelerator and not enough brake. In simple terms, the role of the NAc is to enhance approach behavior whereas one of the roles of the amygdala is to warn animals to avoid negative situations. A study looking at the activity in these brain areas during reward and loss, with adolescents and adults, sheds some light on this topic.

Ernst et al. examined the activity of the NAc and amygdala in adolescents and adults while they were playing a game with monetary reward. The subjects could win $4 if they made a correct choice. The authors looked at the relative activity of the NAc and amygdala when the subjects won compared to when they lost. Finally, they compared the regional activity for the adults and adolescents. The results (see Figure 9.14) show that all subjects had enhanced activity when they won and less when they did not. However, the adolescents showed greater activity in the NAc when winning and less decrease in the amygdala when losing. Specifically, the results show that the adolescent brain is different—more inclined to approach and less inclined to avoid.

The government restricts the use of legally available habit forming substances and activities to adults, for example, nicotine, alcohol, and gambling. There are many reasons for this policy, but in part it is driven by the belief that early exposure to these hedonic pleasures increases the risk of addiction. With nicotine there is some evidence that early exposure increases the likelihood of developing an addiction as an adult.

Epidemiological studies of adolescents suggest that smoking at a younger age leads to increased addiction to cigarettes. A recent study with rats has shown that early exposure has lasting

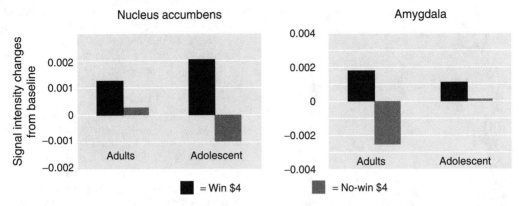

FIGURE 9.14 ● Activation in the nucleus accumbens and amygdala is different for adults and adolescents when they win or fail to win during a game with a reward of $4. (Adapted from Ernst M, Nelson EE, Jazbec S, et al. Amygdala and nucleus accumbens in responses to receipt and omission of gains in adults and adolescents. *Neuroimage.* 2005;25[4]:1279–1291.)

effects when compared to later exposure. Exposure to nicotine during the period that corresponds with preadolescence, but not as a postadolescent, increased the self-administration of nicotine as adults. Additionally, the adults who were exposed to nicotine at the younger age had greater expression of the nicotine receptor.

Adolescence is a time of great risk taking and novelty seeking. Unfortunately, many addictions commence during this period. Although more research is needed, the available studies suggest that early exposure to drugs of abuse may have long-lasting effects on behavior and the brain. These studies give credence to the cultural belief that keeping our adolescents involved in wholesome activities—sports, art, camping, and so on—may keep them away from drugs and alcohol until their brains are better able to handle the substances.

Treatment

Without a doubt, successful abstinence is most effective when the subject is motivated to stay clean, almost regardless of the treatment approach. A recent analysis of three psychological treatments for substance abuse showed that all were equally effective, and the most important factor was the subjects desire to abstain.

Medications to treat addictions are helpful but not robustly effective. We are unable to restore the addicted brain to its preexisting condition. Pharmacological treatments generally fall into two categories. The first are those interventions that interfere with the reinforcing action of the drugs of abuse, for example naltrexone. The second category is those agents that replicate some of the action of the abused substance, for example methadone. Neither of these treatments cures the underlying

central nervous system (CNS) alterations, but can help in keeping a substance abuser clean.

Most problematic for the recovering addict is the intense craving that leads to relapse. Some addicts even report craving dreams during withdrawal. Efforts are underway to find medications that will decrease the thoughts and desires stimulated by memories of drug use. Much of the focus has been on agents that affect glutamate and γ-aminobutyric acid, but as yet no substantial interventions have been discovered. The challenge is to selectively eliminate the craving for drugs without affecting interest in the natural reinforcing stimuli.

Are Stimulant Medications Neurotoxic?

The diagnosis and treatment of attention deficit hyperactivity disorder (ADHD) has increased dramatically over the past decade. Psychostimulants such as methylphenidate and amphetamine remain the most effective and widespread pharmacological interventions for ADHD. These medications are potent inhibitors for the dopamine reuptake transporter and result in increased dopamine stimulation of post-synaptic neurons.

Although effective in improving attention and decreasing impulsivity, the long-term effects of these agents are not well studied. A meta-analysis of stimulant therapy and substance abuse shows that the medications did not promote substance abuse later and may even decrease the potential. However, we have seen in this review that other substances that increase dopamine at the NAc result in changes to the molecular and structural character of neurons. It is unknown if such changes occur with sustained use of the psychostimulants.

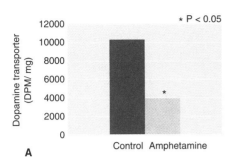
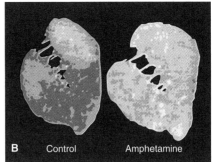

FIGURE 9.15 ● A: Significant reduction in dopamine transporter after 4 weeks of oral amphetamine treatment in nonhuman primate. B: Drawing of cross section of the basal ganglia stained for dopamine transporter. Darker brown = more dopamine transporter. (Adapted from Ricaurte GA, Mechan AO, Yuan J, et al. Amphetamine treatment similar to that used in the treatment of adult attention deficit/hyperactivity disorder damages dopaminergic nerve endings in the striatum of adult nonhuman primates. *J Pharmacol Exp Ther.* 2005;315[1]:91–98.)

Two studies with methylphenidate in rats found enduring behavioral effects after treatment during early development. As adults, these rats showed signs of reduced responsiveness to normal stimuli and increased reactions to aversive situations. These findings are similar to what we see with addicts when they are not using their drug of abuse. A compelling study by Kolb et al. found that exposure to amphetamine has enduring impairments on the development of dendritic branching and spine formation 3 months after stopping the medication. However, these studies have been criticized for using rodents, high doses of the medications, and administering the medication by injection.

A recent study by a group at Johns Hopkins Medical Institute examined the neural effects of amphetamine administered orally to nonhuman primates in equivalent doses to that used on patients with ADHD. The researchers taught a small group of baboons and squirrel monkeys to orally ingest a racemic mixture of dextro and levo amphetamine (similar to what is found in Adderall) twice a day. The plasma amphetamine levels were measured and corresponded to doses reported in humans. Treatment continued for 4 weeks. Two weeks after stopping medication, the animals were sacrificed and their brains were analyzed.

The baboons that had self-administered amphetamine showed significant reductions in striatal dopamine. Likewise, the dopamine transporter protein (the protein blocked by the amphetamine) was significantly reduced in the striatum (Figure 9.15). Similar results were found in the squirrel monkeys, a different primate species. For comparison the serotonin levels were concomitantly measured, and remained equal in the amphetamine and control groups.

While we must be cautious when we extrapolate from animal studies to humans, we also must be vigilant about avoiding harmful treatments. The history of medicine is replete with interventions that initially seemed safe, only to show problems later. Our understanding of dopamine receptor antagonism shows that supraphysiologic doses, as one gets with cocaine, can result in detrimental changes to the neurons. The long-term effects of smaller, controlled doses with stimulant medications, especially after years of continuous use, remain unknown.

Conclusion

The good news—we are designed to experience pleasure. The bad news—pleasure is supposed to wear off. We are only meant to feel satisfied for a short period. We are built to "lead lives of quiet desperation." People satisfied with their accomplishments fall behind. Some of the patients we see, particularly the chronic schizophrenic and seriously depressed, are cursed with a lack of motivation and joy. They are unable to work toward a goal that will be rewarding and bring them pleasure.

Likewise we frequently deal with patients who create havoc in their lives through their pursuit of pleasurable substances and activities. Many of these patients will say some variation of what a patient said to one of us, "Doc, I want to stop being an alcoholic, I just don't want to stop drinking." An understanding of the neuroscience of pleasure helps us conceptualize that patients, such as this, fail to find joy in alternative, natural reinforcers. Our task with such patients is to assist them in the process of developing healthy activities that will stimulate the mesolimbic cortical pathway.

QUESTIONS

1. Cocaine induces euphoria by
   a. Inhibiting GABA.
   b. Stimulating GABA.
   c. Inhibiting dopamine reuptake
   d. Stimulating dopamine reuptake

2. Heroin induces euphoria by
   a. Inhibiting GABA.
   b. Stimulating GABA.
   c. Inhibiting dopamine reuptake
   d. Stimulating dopamine reuptake

3. Microdialysis allows
   a. Pharmacologic stimulation at precise locations.
   b. The development of conditioned behaviors.
   c. Biopsy of cellular tissue.
   d. Continuous sampling of extracellular fluid.

4. Pleasurable feelings includes all of the following, except
   a. Increased dopamine at the nucleus accumbens.
   b. Dopamine receptor antagonism.
   c. Increased activity of the VTA.
   d. Receptor stimulation.

5. All of the following are involved with the development of tolerance, except
   a. Activation of the prefrontal cortex.
   b. Habituation.
   c. Down-regulation of dopamine receptors.
   d. Accumulation of inhibitor transcription factors.

6. All of the following are involved with craving, except
   a. Hypometabolism of the prefrontal cortex to natural stimuli.
   b. Hypermetabolism of the prefrontal cortex with drug cues.
   c. Enhanced GABA activation.
   d. Glutamatergic activation of the nucleus accumbens.

7. The Alpha monkey has
   a. Increased glutamatergic activation of the nucleus accumbens.
   b. Increased frontal lobe metabolism.
   c. Greater propensity to self-administer stimulants.
   d. Increased dopamine receptors.

8. Enhanced transmission of all of the following can result in relapse, except
   a. GABA.
   b. Glutamate.
   c. Dopamine.
   d. CRH.

9. All of the following result in increased spine formation in rats, except
   a. d-amphetamine.
   b. Heroin.
   c. Methylphenidate.
   d. Cocaine.

See Answers section at end of book.

Appetite

SET POINT

In spite of great fluctuation in the quantity and frequency of eating, we all maintain remarkable precision between energy expenditure and energy intake. Social factors, emotions, and time of day, as well as taste, satiety, and personal habits, influence our eating patterns, yet we maintain a reasonably stable body weight month after month. This is referred to as *energy homeostasis* or simply a metabolic "set point".

Evidence of a set point comes from a variety of sources. If a rat is deprived of food, then, when offered a normal diet it will overeat for a short period and return his body weight to its preexisting level. Likewise, after being force-fed to increase body weight, it will limit its food intake to return to normal weight (see Figure 10.1). The brain and body work in harmony to keep the body weight at a specific point.

The human corollary to this is the disturbingly low success rates with most diets. In a review of long-term efficacy of dietary treatment interventions for obesity, Ayyad and Anderson found that only 15% of the patients fulfilled at least one of the criteria for success 5 years after the study. Most people who diet will slowly return to their preexisting weight within 1 year.

Several lines of research suggest that the set point is genetically controlled. Adoption studies provide a unique way to separate the effects of genetics from environment on body weight by comparing children to their biologic parents and to the parents from the house in which they were raised. In an analysis of Danish adoptees, Stunkard

et al. found a strong relation between weight class of the adoptees and the body mass of the biologic parents. However, there was no correlation between the weight class of the adoptees and their adopted parents. These results show that genetic make-up, not environment, is the determining factor in one's body weight.

Yet, obesity was a rare condition 50 years ago. Clearly, our genes have not evolved in half a century. There must be other explanations for the significant change in body weight that is occurring in first-world nations. The Pima Indians of Mexico and Arizona can provide some insight on this issue.

The Pima Indians separated into two tribes approximately 700 to 1,000 years ago—one tribe

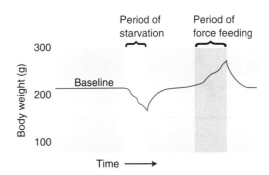

FIGURE 10.1 ● A rat will return its body weight to its preintervention weight when allowed to eat a regular diet. (Adapted from Keesey RE, Boyle PC. Effects of quinine adulteration upon body weight of LH-lesioned and intact male rats. *J Comp Physiol Psychol.* 1973;84[1]:38–46.)

that remained in Mexico and the other that settled in what is now Arizona. In spite of their similar genetic make-up, they have remarkably different average body weights. The Arizona Indians have the highest reported prevalence of obesity and non–insulin-dependent diabetes mellitus whereas their Mexican relatives are not overweight and have little diabetes. The difference can be best explained by understanding the divergent life styles these two populations developed.

The Mexican Pima Indians have remained in the mountains, continuing a traditional rural lifestyle. They exert considerable physical energy working the farms and eat a diet high in starch and fiber. The Arizona Indians on the other hand were forced to move on to reservations and abandon their former way of life. There they lead more leisurely lives and eat a diet high in fat and sugar.

The obesity problem that the Pima Indians suffer from has been attributed to a "thrifty gene"—a gene that promotes saving and storing calories. Two thousand years ago, such a genetic predisposition would enhance survival for those struggling with the fluctuations of prosperity and famine. However, with plentiful high caloric, highly palatable food, the "thrifty gene" promotes accumulation and storage beyond what is healthy. So the weight problem is genetic, but influenced by what is available in the environment.

The concept of a set point helps us understand the difficulties encountered by anyone trying to diet. One of the mechanisms the brain uses to return body weight to its baseline set point became apparent in the Minnesota Starvation Experiment.

This was an experiment conducted with conscientious objectors in Minnesota at the end of the Second World War to help clinicians understand the starving state of the civilians in Europe.

Participants were subjected to a semistarvation diet for 6 months with the goal of losing approximately 25% of their weight. From our perspective, one of the more interesting symptoms these men experienced during the experiment was obsessive thoughts about food. Not unlike the cravings discussed in the previous chapter, food became the principle topic of their thoughts, conversation, and daydreams. Reading cookbooks and collecting recipes became an intensely interesting pastime for many men. Eating, either mentioned in a book or shown in a movie, were cues that now captured and held the men's attention. The urge to eat was so powerful that the researchers established a buddy system so that participants would not be tempted to cheat when away from the dorm. Clearly, their brains were focusing on what the body needed.

In addition to regulating intake to maintain a stable body weight, the brain also has the capacity to adjust energy expenditure. Figure 10.2 shows a thermodynamic perspective of energy expenditure. Energy enters an organism as food and exits as heat or work. Energy is stored as fat or glycogen and mobilized as needed. Total energy expenditure can be subdivided into three components: obligatory energy expenditure, physical activity, and adaptive thermogenesis.

Adaptive thermogenesis is one of the mechanisms the brain uses to maintain a consistent

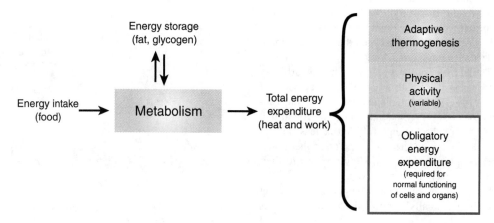

FIGURE 10.2 ● Energy accumulation and expenditure must be in balance for an organism to maintain a stable body weight. Adaptive thermogenesis is regulated by the brain and can vary in response to changes in diet or temperature. (Adapted from Lowell BB, Spiegelman BM. Towards a molecular understanding of adaptive thermogenesis. *Nature*. 2000;404[6778]:652–660.)

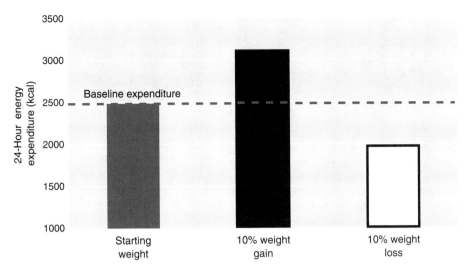

FIGURE 10.3 ● Total energy expenditure is increased in response to weight gain and decreased when weight is lost. (Adapted from Leibel RL, Rosenbaum M, Hirsch J. Changes in energy expenditure resulting from altered body weight. *N Engl J Med.* 1995;332[10]:621–628.)

weight in response to changes in diet and temperature. Activation of the sympathetic nervous system and the resulting catabolic breakdown of adipose tissue produces energy. Figure 10.3 shows the changes in energy expenditure in healthy subjects after 10% alterations in body weight. Not only does the brain increase adaptive thermogenesis when the body gains weight but also turns it down in response to weight loss—a frustration many dieters have experienced.

HOMEOSTATIC MECHANISMS

The key point is that despite large day-to-day fluctuations in food intake and energy expenditure, body weight tends to remain within a relatively narrow range. Signals from the body to the brain implement mechanisms to keep the body weight under control. Brain lesion and stimulation studies in the 1940s identified the hypothalamus as a major center controlling food intake. Although the initial studies turned out to be overly simplified, the hypothalamus remains an important command center. The best way to understand the current conceptualization of the Central nervous system (CNS) homeostatic mechanisms is to separate the short-term signals from the long-term ones.

Short-Term Signals

The short-term signals tend to effect meal size rather than overall energy storage. The signals comprise nutrients and gut hormones in the circulation as well as afferent signals sent up the

vagus nerve. These signals to the brain result in the sensation of satiety but do not produce sustained alteration in body adiposity.

Nutrients

Glucose is the primary nutrient that mediates satiety. Hypoglycemia increases hunger sensations and stimulates eating. Glucose infusions will decrease food intake. Other nutrients in the systemic circulation, such as fats and amino acids, play a real but limited role in signaling to the brain the effects of a recent meal. High levels of these nutrients tell the brain to stop eating, but these sensations will be overridden when the individual has been starving.

Mechanoreceptors

The physical presence of food in the stomach and upper small intestine activates mechanoreceptors. The stomach wall is innervated with stretch receptors that increase in activity in proportion to the volume in the stomach. The autonomic nervous system (ANS) afferents (which send information to the brain about internal organs) transmits signals about gastric distention to the hindbrain by way of the vagus nerve.

Gut Hormones

Numerous gut hormones are involved in food intake regulation. The most widely studied hormone is *cholecystokinin* (CCK). CCK is released from endocrine cells in the mucosal layer of the small intestine in response to fats and proteins.

CCK inhibits further food intake through several mechanisms, such as stimulating the vagal nerve and inhibiting gastric emptying. Additionally, there are CCK receptors in the brain. The injection of CCK directly into the ventricles will inhibit eating. CCK appears to have central and peripheral mechanisms to put the brake on a meal.

Although CCK will limit food intake, its long-term administration does not induce significant weight loss. In studies with rats the repeated administration of CCK resulted in smaller but more frequent meals. Thus, the overall energy balance was not altered. Figure 10.4 summarizes the short-term signals regulating food intake.

There are many other gut hormones that also inhibit eating: glucagon-like peptide-1 (GLP-1) and peptide tyrosine–tyrosine (PPY), just to mention two. *Ghrelin* is unique in that it is the only gut hormone that stimulates hunger. Produced in the stomach, fasting increases the levels of ghrelin, which then fall after a meal. Peripheral and central administration of ghrelin increases food intake. In contrast to CCK, there is some evidence that ghrelin has long-term effects on weight and may be a potential culprit in obesity. Some studies suggest that one of the mechanisms of successful gastric bypass surgery may be that it reduces ghrelin production.

DISORDERS: HORMONES AND WEIGHT

Pituitary disorders can be a cause of weight disturbance. Glucocorticoids stimulate appetite. Cushing's disease, as well as oral administration of such agents as prednisone, results in energy storage and adipose accumulation. Alternatively, Addison's disease and the resulting glucocorticoid deficiency cause anorexia. Thyroid hormones, on the other hand, stimulate the basal metabolic rate and cause weight loss.

Long-Term Signals

In the 1950s, it was suggested that adipose tissue releases a hormone that signals the hypothalamus about the current state of energy storage. Termed an *adiposity signal*, it must have three traits. It must circulate in blood in proportion to the amount of stored fat. It must be able to cross the blood–brain barrier and stimulate specific receptors in the brain. Lastly, changes in the level of such a signal must produce predictable changes in food intake, or energy expenditure.

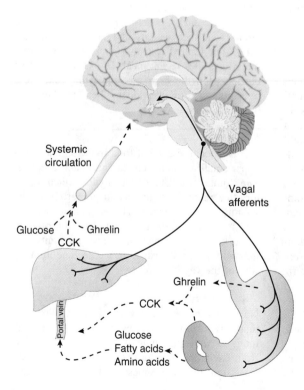

FIGURE 10.4 ● Short-term signals from the intestines (hormones in the circulation and stimulation of the vagus nerve) convey the message that the body is full. CCK, cholecystokinin. (Adapted from Havel PJ. Peripheral signals conveying metabolic information to the brain: Short-term and long-term regulation of food intake and energy homeostasis. *Exp Biol Med.* 2001;226[11]:963–977.)

Leptin

It was not until the discovery of *leptin* in 1994 that the first adiposity signal was identified. The mutant ob/ob mice (ob = obese) have an alternation in one gene, which results in hyperphagia and weight gain of three to five times the normal. Identifying the locus of the genetic defect allowed the cloning of the protein that the ob/ob mice were missing: leptin.

Leptin is primarily produced in white fat cells and circulates in direct proportion to the total fat load. The largest concentration of leptin receptors are found in the arcuate nucleus of the hypothalamus. Mice lacking leptin are obese. When given exogenous leptin they decrease food intake and lose weight (see Figure 10.5).

Other hormones have been proposed as adiposity signals, the most prominent of which is *insulin*. The role of insulin is complicated because its primary function is to enhance glucose intake into muscle and adipose tissues. Yet, insulin secretion is influenced by total body fat, and in turn it can elicit a reduction in body weight. Insulin appears to work in parallel with leptin. Figure 10.6 shows a schematic representation of the adiposity signals.

Arcuate Nucleus

The hypothalamus is at the heart of the regulation of the body's energy metabolism. So it is no wonder that the largest concentration of leptin receptors is found in the arcuate nucleus of the hypothalamus. The arcuate nucleus is located at the base of the hypothalamus next to the third ventricle (see Figure 10.7). Two groups of neurons have been identified within the arcuate nucleus that mediate the leptin signal: proopiomelanocortin (POMC) and neuropeptide Y (NPY).

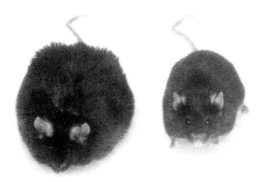

FIGURE 10.5 ● Two ob/ob mice, both of which fail to produce leptin. The mouse on the right has received daily leptin injections for 4.5 weeks and weighs about half as much as the mouse on the left. (From Amgen Inc., Thousand Oaks, California.) Photo by John Sholtis.

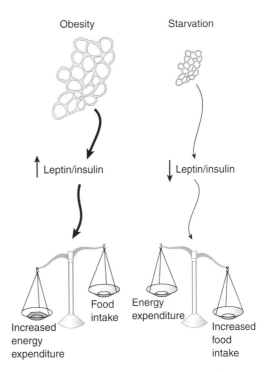

FIGURE 10.6 ● Adipose tissue secretes hormones in proportion to the total fat stored. The hormones in turn affect energy expenditure and food intake in relation to their levels in the circulation.

Proopiomelanocortin

The POMC neurons put the brakes on eating. The POMC neuropeptide is cleaved to produce α-melanocyte stimulating hormone (α-MSH), which is a potent suppressor of food intake. The effects of α-MSH are mediated through the melanocortin (MC) receptors, particularly MC3R and MC4R, which are strongly expressed in the hypothalamus.

High levels of leptin as well as other circulating hormones will stimulate the POMC neurons. Conversely, low levels of leptin inhibit the POMC neurons. Thus, POMC neurons and α-MSH are directly responsive to circulating hormones that signal an excess of adipose tissue.

Neuropeptide Y

The NPY neurons work to increase food intake and decrease energy expenditure. The NPY neurons express a peptide called *agouti-related peptide* (AGRP), which is an antagonist at the MC4 receptor. Therefore, activation of the NPY neurons blocks the effects of α-MSH and the POMC neurons. The role of NPY neurons and AGRP in the accumulation of calories has been demonstrated in many experimental situations:

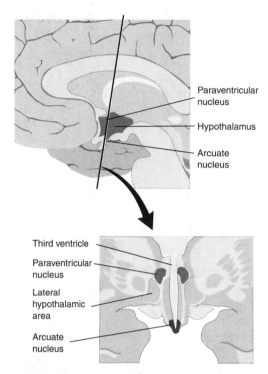

Paraventricular nucleus

Hypothalamus

Arcuate nucleus

Third ventricle

Paraventricular nucleus

Lateral hypothalamic area

Arcuate nucleus

FIGURE 10.7 ● Two sections of the brain showing the location of the arcuate nucleus within the hypothalamus along with two other important nuclei for the control of energy balance.

1. Stimulation of the NPY neurons increases food intake.
2. Increased expression of AGRP results in increased food intake.
3. During starvation there is increased activation of the NPY neurons and increased expression of AGRP.
4. Leptin inhibits the NPY neurons and AGRP expression.

Thus, there is an accelerator and brake relationship between the NPY neurons and the POMC neurons that responds to signals from the body about the long-term status of energy storage (see Figure 10.8). Of particular relevance to the current epidemic of obesity is the unequal relationship between each set of neurons. While they provide equal stimulation of the down stream effort neurons, only the NPY neurons directly inhibit the POMC neurons. The POMC neurons do not inhibit the NPY neurons. Consequently, there appears to be a slightly greater emphasis on the accumulation of calories. In other words, the accelerator is stronger than the brake, which, from an evolutionary perspective, would seem to enhance survival.

DISORDER: MC4R MUTATIONS

It is becoming increasingly apparent that the MC receptor, particularly MC4R, is the most common cause of genetic obesity. In one random study of obese individuals, 4% were found to have some MC4R mutation whereas the controls had none. Another study found a strong relationship between the severity of the mutation and the size of a test meal consumed by the patient. Clearly, an impaired MC4R means a weaker brake on meal termination and ultimately increased weight gain.

Downstream Targets

The downstream effects of the arcuate neurons are numerous and largely remain mysterious. Two important sites are the paraventricular nucleus (PVN) and the lateral hypothalamic (LH) area, also shown in Figure 10.7. The POMC and NPY neurons project in parallel to these sites with corresponding activation and deactivation, depending on the short-term and long-term signals from the periphery.

The effects of the hunger and satiety signals are carried out by three systems: the cerebral cortex (behavior), the endocrine system, and the ANS. The PVN affects the output of the endocrine system and the ANS—both of which effect energy expenditure. The LH communicates with the cerebral cortex, which in turn modulates food-seeking behavior. This simplified analysis of the downstream effects of signals from the body is shown in Figure 10.9.

POINT OF INTEREST

Smokers weigh significantly less than nonsmokers. Conversely, smoking cessation results in weight gain in 70% to 80% of people who quit. Nicotine seems to suppress appetite and enhance the basal metabolic rate; however, the exact mechanism of this action is unknown. It may be in part due to effects on the lateral hypothalamus. Lesions of the LH are known to induce anorexia. Smoking may result in weight loss due to direct and indirect inhibitory effects on the LH.

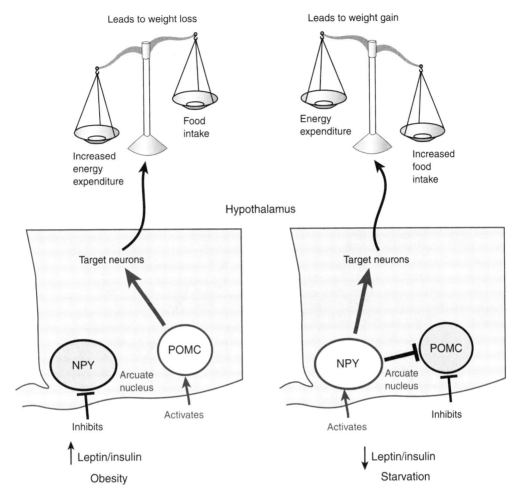

FIGURE 10.8 ● The presence or absence of adiposity signals, such as leptin and insulin, has opposite effects on the NPY and POMC neurons. In turn, the activation of the NPY and POMC neurons has different effects on energy balance and body weight. NPY, neuropeptide Y; POMC, proopiomelanocortin.

The Pleasure of Food

Eating is more than just sustenance; it is one of the great pleasures of life. The perception of pleasure that we get from some foods is most likely an adaptation that enhanced the survival of our ancestors during lean times. However, genes that favored sweet foods during times of scarcity have become a liability now, with the abundance of inexpensive highly palatable refined foods.

The hallmark of certain foods' ability to induce pleasure has been shown in studies like the one in the previous chapter (see Figure 9.8), in which chocolate was seen to increase dopamine at the nucleus accumbens. Additionally, the endogenous opioids appear to be more active during a good meal. Other evidence that eating is a highly valued pleasure that can even resemble an addiction include the following:

1. Destruction of the forebrain dopamine system leads to decreased free feeding.
2. Reduced D_2 receptors in the striatum of obese individuals are similar in magnitude to that seen with addicted subjects.
3. Activation of the orbitofrontal cortex and craving with food related stimuli.

Stress

Many patients will report that food is a source of comfort when they are "stressed-out". Several lines of evidence suggest there may be a correlation between the hypothalamic–pituitary–adrenal (HPA) axis and ability to resist the pleasures of food:

1. Childhood stress is associated with increased weight problems in adolescence and adulthood.

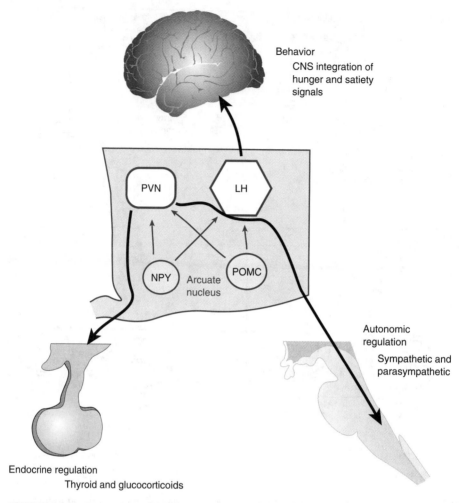

Behavior
CNS integration of
hunger and satiety
signals

PVN   LH

NPY   Arcuate   POMC
nucleus

Autonomic
regulation
Sympathetic and
parasympathetic

Endocrine regulation
Thyroid and glucocorticoids

FIGURE 10.9 ● The PVN and lateral hypothalamus (along with others) influence the three major effort pathways so that the body can maintain a stable energy balance. CNS, central nervous system; PVN, paraventricular nucleus; LH, lateral hypothalamic; NPY, neuropeptide Y; POMC, proopiomelanocortin.

2. Corticotropin-releasing hormone (CRH) and cortisol stimulate the release of dopamine at the nucleus accumbens, which makes it harder to resist temptations.
3. Glucocorticoids increase fat deposits.
4. Stressed rats given access to sweet water have lower glucocorticoid levels.

Endocannabinoids

It has been known for a long time that marijuana stimulates appetite. The naughty boys at our colleges called it *the munchies*. Stimulation of the cannabinoid receptor by the main active component of marijuana, Δ^9-THC (tetrahydrocannabinol), is believed to induce this behavior. Clinicians have successfully utilized this effect when treating anorexic conditions such as AIDS-related wasting

syndrome. With animals it has been found that the endocannabinoid system is activated with short-term fasting or the presentation of palatable food, thereby inducing appetite.

The cannabinoid (CB_1) receptor is involved with regulation of food intake at several levels. First, it enhances the motivation to seek and consume palatable food possibly by interactions with the mesolimbic pathways. Studies with rodents show that endocannabinoids enhance the release of dopamine at the nucleus accumbens and may synergize the effects of the opioids.

The endocannabinoid system also stimulates food consumption in the hypothalamus. Studies have shown that endocannabinoids are highest in the hypothalamus with fasting and lowest during food consumption. Additionally, the endocannabinoids appear to work in concert with the neurohormones such as leptin and ghrelin to control appetite. The ultimate effect may be through the CB_1 receptors at the PVN and lateral hypothalamus. One of the most exciting developments in the treatment of obesity involves blocking the CB_1 receptor (the anti-munchie pill), which seems to reduce appetite.

EATING DISORDERS
Obesity

Fifty years ago, obesity was a rare disease. Readily available palatable food accompanied by a sedentary life style has now resulted in an epidemic of obesity. Most disturbing is the rapid rise in childhood obesity. Clearly, diet and exercise are first-line interventions for this condition, but these efforts are a constant uphill battle against a genetic set point that favors rich, sweet food that historically was in short supply.

After the discovery of leptin, there was great excitement about the prospect of a treatment for obesity. Leptin was shown to reduce obesity in genetically leptin-deficient humans and rodents (Figure 10.5). Unfortunately, the magnitude of weight loss in most obese humans who received exogenous leptin in studies has been modest. In actuality, most obese people have high levels of circulating leptin, but for some reason fail to respond to the signal. This has generated speculation that obesity may be associated with, or even caused by, a resistance to leptin, as is seen with insulin resistance in type 2 diabetes.

There are several possible explanations of leptin resistance in obese individuals:

1. Down-regulation of the leptin receptors.
2. Reduced transport of leptin into the CNS.
3. The leptin signal is simply not strong enough to overcome the modern diet.

Although leptin remains of interest as a possible treatment for obesity, another area of active research is with the MC system. Enhancement of this system could induce the POMC neurons and effectively increase the brakes on eating.

Purging

It is tempting to speculate that patients with anorexia and bulimia have set-points that favor lean body mass. Some evidence suggests this might be the case. First, there is a genetic predisposition to inherit an eating disorder. Second, a single nucleotide alteration in the AGRP gene has been identified in some patients with anorexia nervosa (AN). This suggests that patients with AN may have trouble blocking the anorexic effects of the POMC neurons and the MC system. However, recent studies with rodents have shown that the affected AGRP neuropeptide is functionally as effective as the unaltered AGRP.

Other lines of reasoning suggest that AN and bulimia are conditions that arise from parts of

TREATMENT: LONGEVITY

Caloric restriction is the most reproducible intervention to extend life. Figure (Adapted from Roth, 2005.) shows the survival curves for rats whose calories were restricted by 50% compared to controls. Similar findings have been shown in primates. The biologic benefits of lean body size may include less oxygen radical damage, reduced metabolic rate, and lower temperature: in other words, less wear and tear. The brain also shows signs of slower aging with calorie restriction. Some evidence has shown an increase in brain-derived neurotrophic factor (BDNF) in rodents with restricted intake, which may promote neuronal survival. Whatever the mechanism, it is unlikely that humans will participate in such severe caloric restriction without pharmacologic intervention.

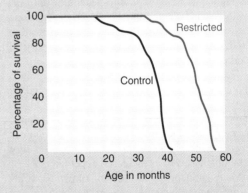

(Adapted from Roth GS. Caloric restriction and caloric restriction mimetics: Current status and promise for the future. *J Am Geriatr Soc.* 2005;53[9 Suppl]:S280–S283.)

the brain other than the hypothalamus. Specifically, the symptoms of anxiety, perfectionism, and obsessions about body image are more consistent with disorders in the prefrontal cortex and amygdala. Likewise, patients who have lost significant weight experience food cravings similar to what the men in the Minnesota Starvation Experiment experienced. Finally, the neuropeptide, and neuroendocrine alterations present when patients are restricting intake return to normal levels when the patients recover. This suggests that the hormonal disturbances are a result of starvation and not the cause.

In summary, the data suggests that the mechanisms of hunger and satiety function properly in patients with AN and bulimia. Starvation is the result of other causes that compel the patients to override the signals to eat.

PSYCHIATRIC MEDICATIONS

Weight gain is one of the most difficult side effects associated with psychiatric treatment and often a cause for patients to stop effective treatments. Surprisingly little is known about the mechanism of this problem. The new antipsychotic agents have been of particular concern. The FDA has required all manufactures to include black box warnings documenting concerns about weight gain as well as the development of diabetes and hypercholesterolemia.

The mechanism of the weight gain remains a mystery. One compelling study examined the affinity for various receptors (serotoninergic, adrenergic, dopaminergic, histaminergic, and muscarinic) compared to reports of short-term weight gain. They determined that the strongest correlation for gaining weight is with H_1 histamine receptor activity ($r = -0.72$). Table 10.1 shows the relative risk of weight gain from the second-generation antipsychotic agents, as determined by a consensus group that included the American Diabetes Association and the American Psychiatric Association (as well as others), compared to the H_1 affinity.

The histamine neurons are known to be involved with energy homeostasis—an effect enhanced by modafinil. Additionally, centrally administered histamine increases the activity of leptin in rodents. Inversely, the blocking effect of the antihistamines may result in weight gain through decreased energy metabolism as well as increased appetite.

Many antidepressants are well known for stimulating appetite and promoting weight gain, for example, tricyclic antidepressants. Unfortunately, there are few long-term placebo controlled studies examining the effect of treatment on weight. One particularly intriguing study is shown in

TABLE 10.1

The Relation Between Risk of Weight Gain with Second-Generation Antipsychotic Agents and Affinity for the H_1 Histamine Receptor

	Weight Gain	Amount of Drug Needed to Block H_1 Histamine
Clozapine	+++	1.2
Olanzapine	+++	2
Quetiapine	++	11
Risperidone	++	15
Aripiprazole	+/−	29.7
Ziprasidone	+/−	43

Greater affinity for a receptor is reflected by a smaller number.

Figure 10.10. In this study, patients with depression were put on fluoxetine in an open label trial for 12 weeks. Patients whose depression remitted were randomly and blindly assigned to placebo or stayed on fluoxetine. The groups were followed up for 1 year. Amazingly, the average weight gain was equal for those on placebo and active treatment.

The authors felt it was the resolution of the depression and not the medication that stimulated the weight gain. These results show that without good studies it can be hard to establish cause and effect. As many clinicians suspect, it is not always the medicine's fault.

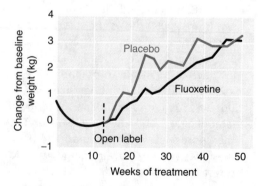

FIGURE 10.10 ● After an initial loss of weight, patients gained weight over the next 38 weeks regardless of whether they were on placebo or fluoxetine. (Adapted from Michelson D, Amsterdam JD, Quitkin FM, et al. Changes in weight during a 1-year trial of fluoxetine. *Am J Psychiatry.* 1999;156[8]:1170–1176.)

Few psychiatric medications induce weight loss. Bupropion and topiramate have demonstrated beneficial effects on weight, but results are modest and few studies exist. The stimulant medications are well known to promote weight loss, which can even be problematic for growing children being treated for attention-deficit hyperactivity disorder (ADHD). The stimulants have a long history of use as "diet pills," with the first FDA approvals being granted in the 1940s. Questions about long-term side effects have been a concern ever since. The approval and rapid removal of dexfenfluramine (Redux) in the 1990s has not helped matters.

The mechanism by which stimulants induce weight loss is not what one would expect. These medications—affectionately called "speed" and "uppers" on the street—actually reduce motor activity. This is often called *the paradoxical effect*. Figure 10.11 documents this effect in a group of boys with no behavioral or learning difficulties and an average IQ of 130. Motor activity was measured by a little sensor the children wore during a 2-hour test period. The graph shows that, with few exceptions, the boys calmed down when on amphetamine. (Some clinicians incorrectly interpret this normal response to stimulants as an indication that the subject has ADHD).

A more recent study analyzed energy expenditure for children on and off stimulants. They found a decrease in total energy expenditure, which was almost entirely explained by decreased physical activity. Basal metabolic rate was unaffected by the stimulants. Consequently, it appears that the weight loss from stimulants is due to appetite suppression. Studies with humans have consistently shown decreased caloric intake while on stimulants. In laboratory settings subjects will consume the same quantity when eating, but eat less frequently.

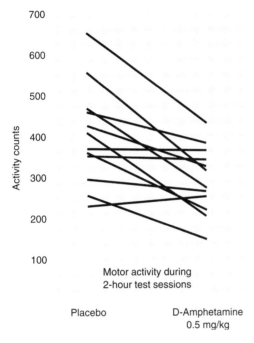

FIGURE 10.11 ● Physical activity in normal prepubertal boys decreased when they were on amphetamine compared to placebo. (Adapted from Rapoport JL, Buchsbaum MS, Zahn TP, et al. Dextroamphetamine: Cognitive and behavioral effects in normal prepubertal boys. *Science*. 1978;199[4328]:560–563.)

DISORDER: MIDDLE AGE SPREAD

The gradual accumulation of body mass is one of the more discouraging aspects of aging. Twin studies show that it is primarily genetic. Possible explanations include decreased physical activity, lower basal metabolic rate, and hormonal changes. Ultimately, it is further proof that there is no such thing as an intelligent design.

QUESTIONS

1. All of the following support the concept of a metabolic "set point," except
   a. Most diets fail.
   b. Forced feeding leads to increased energy expenditure.
   c. The "thrifty gene" promotes weight gain when high caloric food is readily available.
   d. Adaptive thermogenesis is unchanged by caloric intake.

2. Patients with anorexia nervosa and participants in the Minnesota Starvation Experiment share which of the following symptoms?
   a. Perfectionistic personality traits.
   b. Obsessive thoughts about food.
   c. Altered metabolic "set point".
   d. Increased energy expenditure.

3. Short-term signals about hunger and satiety include all of the following, except
   a. Leptin.
   b. CCK.
   c. Glucose.
   d. Ghrelin.

4. Adiposity signals must be able to do all of the following, except
   a. Cross the blood-brain barrier.
   b. Change in relation to amount of stored fat.
   c. Alter afferent signals from the Vagus nerve.
   d. Inhibit or enhance caloric intake.

5. The largest concentration of leptin receptors are in the
   a. Amygdala.
   b. Arcuate nucleus.
   c. Adrenal cortex.
   d. Anterior corticospinal tract.

6. The AGRP does which of the following?
   a. Antagonist at the MC4 receptor and stimulates eating.
   b. Antagonist at the MC4 receptor and inhibits intake.
   c. Agonist at the MC4 receptor and stimulates eating.
   d. Agonist at the MC4 receptor and inhibits intake.

7. The melanocortin system
   a. Has been implicated as cause of AN.
   b. Stimulates foraging for food.
   c. Potentiates the endocannabinoid receptor.
   d. Suppresses food intake.

8. The effects of the brain's assessment of caloric needs are carried out by all of the following, except
   a. Endocrine hormones.
   b. Changes in behavior.
   c. Modulation of the "set point".
   d. Alterations in the ANS.

See Answers section at end of book.

Anger and Aggression

DIAGNOSIS

Anger and aggression are fundamental reactions throughout the animal kingdom. Defending against intruders and hunting for the next meal are traits that were essential for the survival of our ancestors. However, some individuals are too aggressive. We all know a few dogs (and relatives for that matter) that are easily agitated and quick to bite. Animals and people with this tendency are a significant social problem.

Terms such as *road rage, spouse abuse*, and *school violence* are all too common in our daily papers. Yet, the *Diagnostic and Statistical Manual* (DSM) does not include a category for inappropriate anger. It has been suggested this is because men created DSM and they do not see anger as a problem. (PMS, on the other hand, now that is a disorder!)

The absence of a diagnostic category is clinically relevant. For example, a small Danish pharmaceutical company in the 1970s was pursuing a treatment for aggression, called *serenics*. In spite of promising results, the company shelved the medication when it became clear the U.S. Food and Drug Administration would not approve the medication because aggression is not a specific disorder. Consequently, although psychologists and other counselors provide treatment for "anger management," there is no sanctioned pharmacologic intervention for excessive anger and irritability.

Aggression is clearly influenced by one's culture and upbringing. Violence on TV and early physical abuse increase the likelihood a person will be aggressive. Alternatively, the context in which an assault occurs determines the appropriateness of the aggression. For example, fighting on the ice at hockey games is accepted, but fighting in the stands is not. These are issues beyond the scope of this text. We are interested in the processes in the brain that generate or fail to impede violence toward another.

Two Kinds of Aggression

Working with cats, Flynn at Yale, and Siegel at University of Medicine and Dentistry of New Jersey identified two types of aggressive behavior. One is more predatory—similar to hunting. The cat quietly and calmly waits to pounce on its prey. The other type of aggression is defensive. Here the cat is agitated and makes a big display of its feelings, in part to avoid a fight, but is also ready to respond if provoked. In the cat, these different responses can be elicited by electrical stimulation of different regions of the hypothalamus.

MECHANISMS IN THE BRAIN
Hypothalamus

Figure 11.1 shows the location of the hypothalamus and the two general regions (lateral and medial) that lie on either side of the third ventricle. Flynn and Siegel placed electrodes into these regions and, with stimulation, elicited the two kinds of aggressive behavior in cats. In a series of experiments over many years they located the sites that corresponded with the behavior.

Figure 11.2 shows an example of predatory aggression elicited in a cat by stimulation of the

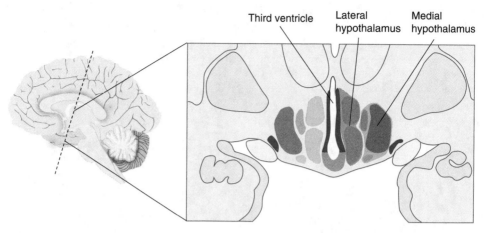

Third ventricle   Lateral hypothalamus   Medial hypothalamus

FIGURE 11.1 ● The lateral and medial regions of the hypothalamus.

lateral hypothalamus. The bite to the back of the neck is preceded by quite, stealthy circling of the rodent. It is worth noting that the researchers used cats in these experiments that would not bite the rat before the hypothalamic stimulation.

Figure 11.3 shows the defensive type of aggressive behavior, this is induced by stimulating the *medial hypothalamus.* In this case the cat becomes aroused (high sympathetic tone, increased heart rate, dilated pupils, etc.) and displays hostile behavior (hissing, growling, arching back, piloerection, etc.). The different features of each kind of aggression are summarized in Table 11.1.

These two pathways and subsequent behavior elicited in the cat also describe the two basic kinds of aggression seen in humans. Analysis of playground behavior, spousal abuse, and serial killers support the dichotomy of a reactive/impulsive/defensive type of aggression and a stealthy/premeditated/hunting type of aggression. Although a combination of the two types is a common finding in any specific aggressive act (see Treatment box, page 135).

Frontal Cortex

Various areas of the brain modify the expression of aggression by either putting on the brakes or applying the accelerator. There is substantial evidence that impairment of the frontal cortex is the equivalent of taking off the brakes on aggressive impulses. The most famous example of this is Phineas Gage. Gage was a foreman at a railroad construction company in Vermont in 1848. A tamping iron was blown through his left

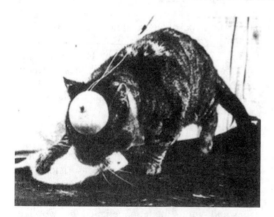

FIGURE 11.2 ● Predatory attack (quiet bite) against a rat induced by stimulating the lateral hypothalamus. (From Flynn JP. The neural basis of aggression in cats. In: Glass DC, ed. *Neurophysicology and emotion.* New York: Rockefeller University Press; 1967.)

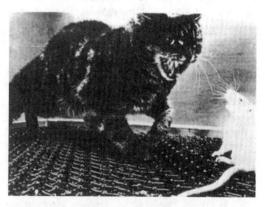

FIGURE 11.3 ● Defensive attack elicited by stimulating the medial hypothalamus. (From Flynn JP. The neural basis of aggression in cats. In: Glass DC, ed. *Neurophysicology and emotion.* New York: Rockefeller University Press; 1967.)

[4]...

TABLE 11.1

The Different Features of Predatory and Defensive Aggression

	Predatory Aggression	Defensive Aggression
CNS Location	Lateral hypothalamus	Medial hypothalamus
Sympathetic tone	Calm	Autonomic arousal
Behavior	Stealthy movement, bite to back of rat's neck	Hissing, arching back, paw swipe, piloerection
Evolutionary function	Hunting	Protection
Quality	Hidden, premeditated	Overt, reactive

CNS, central nervous system.

frontal skull when a spark inadvertently ignited explosive powder.

Gage's skull has been preserved, and Figure 11.4 shows a reconstruction of the path the tamping iron took through his skull. Remarkably, he recovered, was out of bed within a month, and lived another 12 years. However, his personality had drastically changed. While before the accident he had been efficient, balanced, and responsible, now he was fitful, impulsive, unfocused, and easily agitated.

If we imagine that the frontal cortex applies the brakes to the array of primitive impulses that arise from the subcortical brain, then we can see how taking the brakes off (due to a poorly functioning frontal cortex) allows the expression of feelings that would normally be subdued. Specifically, a poorly functioning frontal cortex allows more aggressive impulses to be expressed. Alternatively, a healthy, active frontal cortex puts the "brakes" on inappropriate aggressive behavior.

Figure 11.5 shows the results of a study from Siegel's laboratory that highlights the role of the frontal cortex in inhibiting aggression. In this study a cat has one electrode in its lateral hypothalamus and one in the lateral aspect of its frontal cortex. What is being measured is the time until the cat attacks the rat after stimulation of the electrodes. With just hypothalamic stimulation, the cat only waits approximately 12 seconds before attacking. However, with stimulation of both the hypothalamus and the frontal cortex, the time to attack is doubled.

This study was repeated with many cats with electrodes in different locations of the frontal cortex. Similar results were found. Clearly, the frontal cortex has an inhibitory effect on aggressive expressions.

One of the most consistent findings with humans and violence is frontal lobe dysfunction. With the advent of neuroimaging capabilities, many researchers have looked at activity in the prefrontal cortex (PFC) in men with violent histories. In a review of the literature on the topic, Brower and Price concluded that significant frontal lobe dysfunction is associated with aggressive dyscontrol—in particular, impulsive aggressive behavior.

A study on convicted murderers by Raine et al. provides further insight on this topic. Raine separated a group of murderers into those who

TREATMENT: PSYCHOSURGERY

There are few studies in the medical literature involving the hypothalamus and aggression in humans, with the exception of a few reports of psychosurgery. For example, in Japan, Sano, and Mayanagi performed 60 posteromedial hypothalamotomies in the 1960s for aggressive behavior. Most patients also had a history of seizures and mental retardation. In a follow-up report conducted in 1987 they reported the absence of violence and aggression in 78%, with apparently normal endocrine function. Although a drastic procedure, it accentuates the central role of the hypothalamus with aggressive behavior.

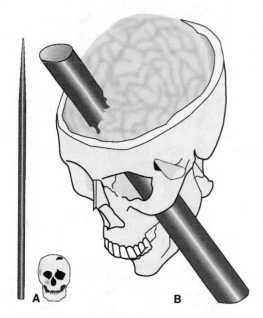

FIGURE 11.4 ● **A:** The skull of Phineas Gage and the tampering iron that exploded through his head in 1848. **B:** Drawing of a computerized reconstruction of the path the rod took through his skull and brain. The damage involved both left and right prefrontal cortices. (Adapted from Damasio H, Grabowski T, Frank R, et al. The return of Phineas Gage: Clues about the brain from the skull of a famous patient. *Science*. 1994;264:1102–1105.)

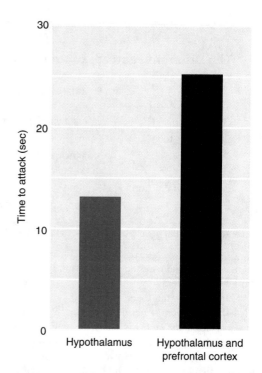

FIGURE 11.5 ● The time it takes a cat to attack a rat after the hypothalamus is stimulated is greatly increased when the frontal cortex is simultaneously stimulated. (Adapted from Siegel A, Edinger H, Dotto M. Effects of electrical stimulation of the lateral aspect of the prefrontal cortex upon attack behavior in cats. *Brain Res.* 1975;93:473–484.)

committed planned, predatory violence from those who perpetrated affective, impulsive violence. Positron emission tomography (PET) scans were conducted on these subjects along with normal controls, examining the activity in the frontal cortex. The results are shown in Figure 11.6. Both groups of murderers had less activity in the PFC compared to controls, but the impulsive, affective group had the least. This study implies that one explanation for the violent acts may be the lack of sufficient inhibition from the frontal cortex.

Amygdala

There is conflicting information about the role of the amygdala and aggressive behavior. Although better known for being activated during fearful situations, the amygdala may have a broader function in processing emotional stimuli. Early studies with monkeys showed that bilateral removal of the amygdala produced an animal that was placid—neither frightened nor aggressive. This is called the *Klüver-Bucy Syndrome*, after the two

DISORDER: VIOLENCE AND AGE

Age has a profound effect on the likelihood of being violent. The incidence of violent crime rises rapidly until the ages of 18 to 22 and then gradually declines over the next three decades. The very young and very old are the least violent. There are many sociocultural variables that contribute to this trend. However, the delay in the maturing of the brain compared to the fully developed physical body provides one explanation (see Figure 7.7). The young adult does not have enough containment by the frontal cortex of his aggressive impulses.

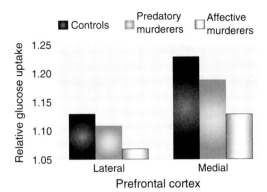

FIGURE 11.6 ● The relative activity in the lateral and medial aspect of the prefrontal cortex of predatory and affective murderers compared to normal controls. (Adapted from Raine A, Meloy JR, Bihrle S, et al. Reduced prefrontal and increased subcortical brain functioning assessed using positron emission tomography in predatory and affective murderers. *Behav Sci Law.* 1998;16[3]:319–332.)

researchers who performed the experiments. This and other research suggest that the amygdala is instrumental in recognizing whether a stimulus is threatening and that an overactive amygdala can lead to excessive defensive aggression.

There are reports in the literature of bilateral amygdalotomies for untreatable aggression in humans. Some of the reports are disturbingly optimistic. A group from India reported on 481 cases, stating that 70% showed excellent or moderate improvement after five years (see Prefrontal Lobotomy box, page 17). A report about two cases in Georgia provides a more balanced assessment of the procedure.

Two individuals who were essentially institutionalized because of aggressive behavior received amygdalotomies after years of failed medical therapies. The procedures resulted in reductions but not elimination of the assaultive behavior. Pre- and postassessments demonstrated reduced autonomic arousal as measured by skin conductance. The authors concluded that the procedure resulted in a "taming effect," which they attributed to reduced perceptions of threats. In other words, an overactive amygdala causes the individual to perceive threats where they do not exist. Removing the amygdala decreases the false perceptions.

Other research suggests that the amygdala is underactive in those with aggressive problems (see section on Psychopath in the subsequent text). Recent imaging studies have found amygdala dysfunction associated with criminal psychopaths.

One study in Finland showed decreased volume of the amygdala in a group of psychopaths. Another study used functional magnetic resonance imaging (MRI) to examine the activity of the amygdala during memory tasks involving negatively charged words. The psychopaths showed less amygdaloid activity compared to controls (see Figure 11.7). These studies suggest that an underactive amygdala may facilitate aggression.

Work by Siegel with his cats may shed light on the conflicting data about the role of the amygdala with aggressive behavior. We must remember that the amygdala is not just one organ, but made up of multiple nuclei (see Figure 2.6). Siegel found with cats that stimulating the lateral and central groups facilitates predatory attacks and suppressed defensive rage. Conversely, stimulation of the medial aspect of the basal complex has just the opposite effect. This subtle difference within the amygdala would be hard to identify in humans with current imaging technology.

In summary, the amygdala may be overactive with different subtypes of aggression and underactive with others. Alternatively, it could be that different nuclei are activated for the different types of aggression.

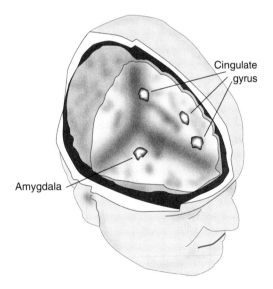

FIGURE 11.7 ● Criminal psychopaths showed less activity in the amygdala along with parts of the cingulate gyrus when recalling negative affective words compared to controls. (Adapted from Kiehl KA, Smith AM, Hare RD, et al. Limbic abnormalities in affective processing by criminal psychopaths as revealed by functional magnetic resonance imaging. *Biol Psychiatry.* 2001;50:677–684.)

HORMONES AND NEUROPEPTIDES

Testosterone

Everyone "knows" that testosterone stimulates aggression. Males fight more than females. Unfortunately, the role of testosterone and aggression is not as simple as it first seems.

In 1849, Arnold Adolph Berthold, a German physician, conducted an experiment that is considered the first formal study of endocrinology (see Figure 11.8). With this elegant little study he demonstrated the importance of a substance from the testes (later discovered to be testosterone) and aggressive behavior.

Berthold knew that male chicks grow into roosters with typical secondary sexual characteristics displaying sexual and aggressive behavior. In the experiment, Berthold removed the testes from chicks, which curtailed their normal development and eliminated sexual and aggressive behavior. In a second group he reimplanted the testes into the abdominal cavity. If the testes could establish a blood supply then the chick would develop into a normal rooster with the usual sexual and aggressive tendencies. Berthold concluded that the testes releases a substance that affected male body structures and behaviors.

Research with laboratory animals in the years since Berthold have consistently demonstrated similar correlations between testosterone and aggressive behavior. A good example by Wagner et al. shows the effect of castration on bite attacks on an inanimate target for adult male mice (see Figure 11.9). Before castration and with testosterone replacement the male mice will frequently bite the target. However, in the absence of the hormone, bite attacks drop close to the frequency seen with females.

For humans, it is not so easy to establish a direct link between plasma testosterone and magnitude of hostility. Conflicting results are found throughout the literature. In particular, it is hard to establish cause and effect. For example, testosterone levels are known to spike for the winner and to drop for the loser of a sporting event. Even in a chess match, or for men watching a sporting event, testosterone levels will drop for the loser. A better correlation may exist between a man's place in the social hierarchy and his plasma testosterone. A study of male prisoners in a Connecticut

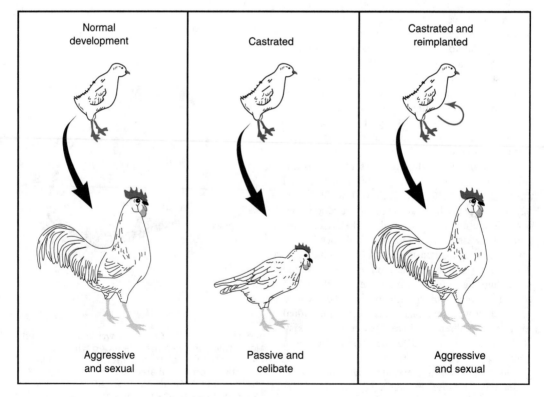

FIGURE 11.8 ● Berthold established in 1849 that a substance in the testes was necessary for the development of male behavior and body structure. (Adapted from Rosenzweig MR, Breedlove SM, Watson NV. *Biological psychology*, 4th ed. Sunderland, MA: Sinauer; 2005.)

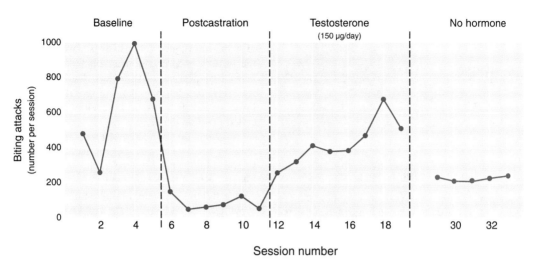

FIGURE 11.9 ● Baseline bite attacks for male mice are markedly diminished with castration. This effect can be reversed temporally with testosterone replacement. (Adapted from Wagner GC, Beuving LJ, Hutchinson RR. The effects of gonadal hormone manipulations on aggressive target-biting in mice. *Aggress Behav.* 1980;6:1–7.)

prison found that both aggressive inmates as well as those who were socially dominant but not aggressive had higher plasma testosterone than those who were non-aggressive and low on the social scale (see Figure 11.10).

Another popular belief is that exogenous steroids that some athletes take to enhance performance increases aggression in most men:

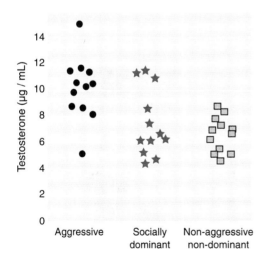

FIGURE 11.10 ● Plasma testosterone levels for prisoners organized by history of aggression and social dominance. (Adapted from Ehrenkranz J, Bliss E, Sheard MH. Plasma testosterone: Correlation with aggressive behavior and social dominance in man. *Psychosom Med.* 1974;36:469–475.)

"roid rage." This too is murky. In the best study of the effects of supraphysiologic doses of testosterone on normal men, Tricker et al. found no difference in anger for those on either testosterone or placebo, as noted by the spouse or by self-report after 10 weeks. Likewise, studies of sexual predators treated with antiandrogens have demonstrated remarkable decreases in libido but with little change in aggression.

Vasopressin

Vasopressin, better know for its role in water retention and bedwetting, is also known as an *antidiuretic hormone* (ADH). However, many neuropeptides have multiple functions in the brain and we are only beginning to understand the significance of vasopressin on aggressive behaviors. When given to hamsters, rats, and voles, for example, vasopressin will increase their aggression. Alternatively, vasopressin receptor blockers will decrease aggression.

A remarkable study by Coccaro et al. has looked at the association between cerebrospinal fluid (CSF) vasopressin and aggression in 26 subjects with personality disorders. Figure 11.11 shows the correlation between CSF vasopressin and a life-history of aggression against other people. The importance of vasopressin in social interactions goes beyond aggression. We also see this peptide involved with bonding and will discuss it further in Chapter 14, Social Attachment. In the future, this may be a neuropeptide with great interest for the mental health community.

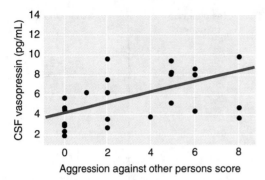

FIGURE 11.11 ● Cerebrospinal fluid vaso-pressin levels correlate with aggression in subjects with personality disorders. (Adapted from Coccaro EF, Kavoussi RJ, Hauger RL, et al. Cerebrospinal fluid vasopressin levels: Correlates with aggression and serotonin function in personality-disordered subjects. *Arch Gen Psychiatry.* 1998;55:708–714.)

Nerve Growth Factors

It is interesting to ask whether fighting changes the brain. That is, does winning or losing alter the structure of the brain in a manner that develops aggressive or submissive personalities? We know there is a strong relationship between experience and neurobiology, for example, enriched environments cause enhanced nerve cell growth (see Figure 7.4). Likewise, we know that the growth and development of neurons are enhanced by nerve growth factors (NGFs). Finally, we know that animals that are repeatedly on the losing side of fights will develop a syndrome called *conditioned defeat.*

A group in Italy has examined the effect of winning and losing on growth factors in mice. Figure 11.12(A) shows the rapid and sustained release of NGF into the bloodstream immediately after a fighting episode. Further studies looked at growth factors in areas that are known for the proliferation of new nerve cells, for example, the subventricular zone (SVZ) (see Figure 7.3). In this area the researchers found enhanced levels of NGF as well as brain derived neurotropic factor (BDNF). However, the levels depended on who was the winner or loser.

Figure 11.12(B) shows the results of NGFs in the SVZ after 3 consecutive days of fighting episodes. It was only the subordinate mouse that had increases in NGF. The dominant mouse had increased levels of BDNF. These results suggest that being the winner or loser may have different effects on the proliferation of new nerve cells. If

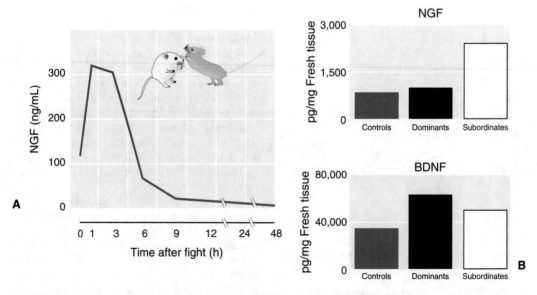

FIGURE 11.12 ● **A:** Fighting results in an increase in nerve growth factor (NGF). **B:** In the subventricular zone, NGF only increases for the subordinate mouse whereas brain derived neurotropic factor (BDNF) increases for the dominant mouse. (Adapted from Fiore M, Amendola T Triaca V, et al. Fighting in the aged male mouse increases the expression of TrkA and TrkB in the subventricular zone and in the hippocampus. *Behav Brain Res.* 2005;157[2]:351–362 and Branchi I, Francia N, Alleva E. Epigenetic control of neurobehavioural plasticity: The role of neurotrophins. *Behav Pharmacol.* 2004;15(5–6):353–362.)

this is true, it may explain why winners and losers behave differently.

TREATMENT: LITHIUM

One of the most unique treatment studies for aggressive behavior was conducted in a prison in Connecticut in the 1970s. They randomly assigned volunteers with a history of violence to receive lithium or placebo. The exclusion of inmates with psychosis was the only psychiatric criteria applied to this study. The number of infractions reported by the institutional staff that was blind to the treatment administered served as the measure of response. Figure shows the results.

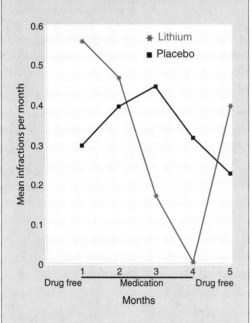

Although the study has methodological problems (small n, high drop out for those on lithium), it nonetheless demonstrates the powerful effect that lithium has on violent behavior. This is consistent with lithium's well-documented ability to decrease suicide—which can be considered violence against oneself. Exactly how lithium accomplishes this remains a mystery.

SEROTONIN

There is actually a more robust association between low serotonin and aggression than between low serotonin and depression. Because there is no feasible way to directly measure serotonin in humans or animals, most studies examine the correlation between violence and CSF 5-hydroxyindoleacetic acid (5-HIAA), a metabolite of serotonin.

Studies with monkeys have found high rates of wounding, violence, and inappropriate aggression in subjects with low CSF 5-HIAA. Analysis of these monkeys has shown that they are not necessarily uniformly more aggressive. However, they are more likely to engage in rough interactions that escalate into unrestrained aggression with a high probability of injury. This behavioral trait can be viewed as poor impulse control, which could underlie the aggressive tendency.

A group has studied the relationship between 5-HIAA and violence in a longitudinal study of free-ranging rhesus monkeys secluded on a small island on the coast of South Carolina. The researchers captured 49 two-year-old males and measured their CSF 5-HIAA. They were then followed up for 4 years. Two years is an age in monkeys that corresponds to middle to late childhood in humans, and is a particularly dangerous age for male monkeys. This is a phase of life when males move from their group of origin to a new social group.

By the time most of the subjects had reached young adulthood, 11 had died. Figure 11.13 shows the percentage of subjects that died and the percentage that had survived, separated by their CSF 5-HIAA concentrations at the start. Note that

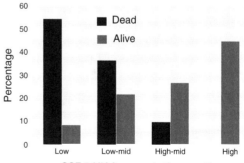

FIGURE 11.13 ● The percentage of 2-year-old monkeys who are still alive after 4 years, separated by the metabolite of serotonin (5-HIAA) in the CSF. (Adapted from Higley JD, Mehlman PT, Higley SB, et al. Excessive mortality in young free-ranging male nonhuman primates with low CSF 5-hydroxyindoleacetic acid concentrations. *Arch Gen Psychiatry.* 1996;53[6]:537–543.)

all those in the high concentration group were still alive. The researchers observed that those monkeys with the lowest levels of 5-HIAA were much more likely to engage in risky behavior, including aggressive acts directed at older, larger males. They would pick fights they could not win. They were not only aggressive but also impulsive.

Studies with humans are equally impressive. A variety of researchers from many different sites have shown the following results:

1. Lower 5-HIAA correlates with greater suicide intent and higher lethality in those who have attempted suicide.
2. 5-HIAA levels show an inverse correlation with lifetime histories of aggression.
3. Low 5-HIAA levels predict recidivism for violent offenders.
4. Acute tryptophan depletion, which causes a transient decline in brain serotonin, will result in increased irritability and aggression.

Most relevant for the practicing clinician are the studies with selective serotonin reuptake inhibitor (SSRIs) and aggression. Several double-blind, placebo-controlled studies have found reduced aggression with SSRIs in patients with personality disorders, autism, schizophrenia, and dementia.

THE PSYCHOPATH

Being violent is not the same as being cruel or mean. Violence in defense of oneself or one's family is not even considered a crime. Alternatively, there are many examples of violence that seems to have no purpose other than being mean and inflicting emotional or physical pain.

Psychopathy is the closest definition we have in psychiatry to describing cruel or mean behavior. It is not included in the DSM. The Psychopathy Checklist-Revised (PCL-R) created by Robert Hare defines psychopathy and is made up of two factors. Impulsive aggression and a wide variety of offenses defines one factor, which correlates closely with antisocial personality disorder in the DSM.

The other factor defines the emotional shallowness of the psychopath: superficial, egotistical, lack of remorse, lack of empathy, and manipulative. This factor has a smaller correlation with antisocial personality disorder and more closely resembles what we would consider cruel and mean. It tends to persist as the subject ages, although the impulsive, aggressive factor decreases with maturity. The older psychopath is no more empathetic or remorseful, but less likely to be violent.

Hare has suggested that the psychopath lacks some internal control. From the viewpoint of the neuroscientist the specific neural systems that are lacking are starting to come into focus.

Raine has shown that men with antisocial personality disorders have decreased prefrontal gray matter when compared to normal controls or substance abusers. This suggests a lack of containment from the frontal cortex, similar to what has been discussed earlier. Unique to the psychopath are findings showing low autonomic arousal and less activity in the amygdala.

Resting Heart Rate

One of the most consistent physiologic findings in psychiatry is the correlation between low resting heart rate and aggressive behavior in children. Furthermore, a low heart rate in a child is predictive of future criminal behavior independent of all other psychological variables. Some people speculate that the low heart rate reflects a fearless, stimulus-seeking temperament. A fascinating study from Europe supports this conclusion.

The study is based on Pavlovian (classical) conditioning. When presented repeatedly with a neutral stimulus followed by an aversive stimulus, most people will show some anxiety when seeing the neutral stimulus in anticipation of what will follow. Birbaumer et al. set up such a paradigm for 10 criminal psychopaths out on bail and 10 healthy controls while their brains were being scanned. Figure 11.14 shows that the controls showed increased activity in areas underlying conditioned fear response: amygdala, orbitofrontal cortex, insula, and anterior cingulate. Remarkably, the psychopaths showed almost no activity in these areas. This may help us understand the lack of emotion that is an essential aspect of being a psychopath.

The Pleasure of Violence

The lack of fear alone does not seem sufficient for some of the cruel actions perpetrated by psychopaths. For example, decorated bomb-disposal operators have been shown to have unusually low heart rates during experimental simulations. We can imagine that other high-stress professions are overly represented with individuals who are innately calm: firefighters, air-traffic controllers, trauma surgeons, etc. However, these are people trying to help society, not inflict pain. Something else is needed to understand the behavior of the psychopath. A study with rats suggests a possible neurologic mechanism to explain what else may be aberrant with psychopaths.

First, we must acknowledge that many people enjoy violence. One has to only look at what is

Healthy controls   Psychopaths

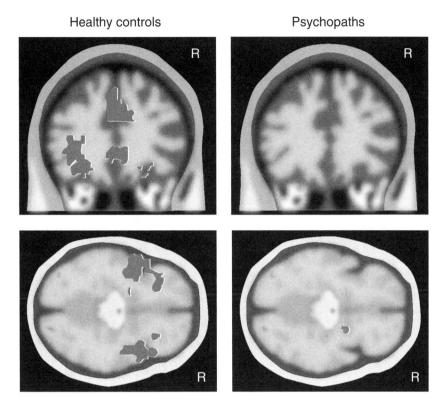

FIGURE 11.14 ● Healthy controls show a robust fear response in anticipation of an adverse stimulus. Psychopaths fail to develop a similar fear. (Adapted from Birbaumer N, Veit R, Lotze M, et al. Deficient fear conditioning in psychopathy: A functional magnetic resonance imaging study. *Arch Gen Psychiatry.* 2005;62[7]:799–805.)

popular at the movies, in video games, and on the news to see that blood sells. Second, as we described in Chapter 9, Pleasure, the nucleus accumbens lights up with dopamine during pleasurable activities: cocaine, sex, gambling, and so on.

The missing link is shown in Figure 11.15. In this study, male rats were implanted with micropipettes that sampled the extracellular concentration of dopamine at the nucleus accumbens every 10 minutes. The sampling was done during an aggressive encounter with a naive male intruder in which two to six bites and at least 140 seconds of aggressive behavior were displayed by the rat under study. The graph shows that dopamine

DISORDER: TEMPORAL LOBE EPILEPSY

There is a subgroup of patients with temporal lobe epilepsy who have aggressive outbursts between seizures. Some have attributed this to an interictal syndrome often called *episodic dyscontrol.* However, many of these patients have alternative explanations for their aggression, for example, low IQ, antisocial personality disorder, etc. The concept remains controversial but may apply to a few patients with seizure disorder.

More appealing is the prospect that patients with aggressive outbursts may be having unrecognized subclinical temporal lobe seizures. Unfortunately, this has been difficult to substantiate. However, the anticonvulsants do show some positive effects as treatment for aggression, although the benefits are primarily limited to those with impulsive aggressive acts rather than premeditated acts.

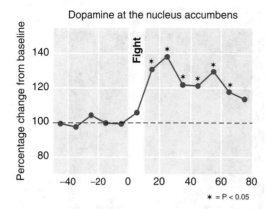

Dopamine at the nucleus accumbens

FIGURE 11.15 ● Increase in dopamine at the nucleus accumbens following an aggressive encounter with another rat. (Adapted from van Erp AM, Miczek KA. Aggressive behavior, increased accumbal dopamine, and decreased cortical serotonin in rats. *J Neurosci*. 2000;20:9320–9325.)

significantly rose above baseline for up to 60 minutes after the encounter.

Imaging studies of humans suggest similar neural mechanisms. Researchers in Switzerland set up an elaborate study to examine the activity in the brain when a subject is playing a game with an untrustworthy partner. In instances when the subject wants to retaliate after the partner keeps all the money, there was increased activity in the dorsal striatum—an area that contains the nucleus accumbens. Furthermore, the stronger the activity in the striatum the more willing the subject was to incur a deficit to inflict the punishment.

Using this data, we can conceptualize in an overly simplified manner that violence and aggression give a squirt of pleasure to the aggressor. This could explain why some people seem to enjoy aggression, either watching or participating.

In summary, the neurobiology of the psychopath may be a constellation of problems: not enough constraint from the frontal cortex, lack of fear, and too much activation of the nucleus accumbens. It could be that psychopathy, like alcoholism or cocaine dependence, is an addiction. Although in this case the addiction is to violence. This could explain why psychopathy, like the addictions, is so difficult to treat and does not respond to traditional interventions.

QUESTIONS

1. When dealing with a patient with an anger problem and trying to make the right diagnosis, which of the following do you not do?
   a. Refuse to treat him because there is no DSM diagnosis for anger.
   b. Call it a variation of bipolar disorder.
   c. Call it a wastebasket term, such as depression not otherwise specified (NOS) or anxiety not otherwise specified (NOS).
   d. Call it Intermittent Explosive Disorder because it sounds good, even although you know it does not actually apply.

2. Which of the following is not associated with predatory aggression?
   a. Activation of the lateral hypothalamus.
   b. Stealthy movement.
   c. Autonomic arousal.
   d. Premeditated.

3. In simple terms, the frontal cortex plays what role with anger?
   a. Activates the autonomic neurons system.
   b. Applies the brakes on the impulses.
   c. Modulates the nucleus accumbens.
   d. Activates the lateral hypothalamus.

4. All of the following apply to the amygdala and aggression, except
   a. Klüver-Bucy Syndrome.
   b. Shows less activity with criminal psychopaths.
   c. Different nuclei could be activated with different subtypes of aggression.
   d. Facilitates the expression of the serotonin receptor.

5. Testosterone
   a. Is the primary cause of fighting.
   b. Increases plasma levels for the loser.
   c. May show a better correlation with social dominance.
   d. Stimulates overt hostility in weight lifters.

6. After a fight, the dominant mouse has which of the following?
   a. Decreased testosterone and decreased NGF.
   b. Decreased testosterone and increased BDNF.
   c. Increased testosterone and decreased NGF.
   d. Increased testosterone and increased BDNF.

7. All of the following statements about low CSF concentration of the serotonin metabolite 5-HIAA are true, except
   a. Common with major depression.
   b. Correlates with greater lifetime history of aggression.
   c. Predicts relapse for criminal offenders.
   d. Associated with Greater suicide intent.

8. The psychopath can be conceptualized as having all of the following, except
   a. Low resting heart rate.
   b. Activated frontal cortex.
   c. Hypofunctioning amygdala.
   d. Increased activity at the nucleus accumbens.

See Answers section at end of book.

Sleep

NORMAL SLEEP

Sleep remains a mystery. We spend roughly a third of our lives in this suspended state. All mammals sleep, as does most of the animal kingdom. Even the fruit fly sleeps—although not enough. Most people look forward to sleeping, especially if they have been deprived of sleep. Without enough sleep, people function as poorly as if they are drunk. Significant sleep deprivation will cause psychosis and physical problems. What is it that happens to us when we sleep?

The average length of sleep is approximately 7.5 hours per night (see Figure 12.1). Remarkably, some people require much less—who have been called *nonsomniacs*. Meddis studied a retired nurse who was happily functioning on an hour of sleep a night. She reported she had needed little sleep all her life. When studied in Meddis's sleep laboratory, she did not sleep the first night and then slept, on average, only 67 minutes for each of the remaining four nights. She did not complain of being tired or wanting more sleep. (As an aside, some in the psychiatric community might diagnose this woman with a bipolar spectrum disorder, although her condition may simply be a variant of sleep need.)

Most people show deterioration in performance when deprived of sleep. Figure 12.2 shows the results of changes on neurobehavioral tasks as subjects were increasingly sleep deprived. The study looked at the effects of four different sleep conditions on various tasks of psychomotor skill and cognitive functioning. One group was totally sleep deprived for 3 days, two other groups were restricted to 6 or 4 hours of sleep per night for

14 days, and the control group got 8 hours of sleep per night. Figure 12.2(A) shows the effects of sleep restriction on a sustained attention task whereas Figure 12.2(B) shows the effects on a test of memory. Note how chronic sleep deprivation takes a toll on the subjects' performance as the study progresses. Of interest, the subjects were largely unaware of their impairments—a finding that is not uncommon when cognition declines.

A recent intervention with medical interns working in an intensive care unit (ICU) in a Boston hospital demonstrated a practical application of this

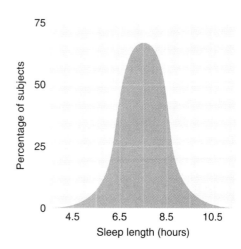

FIGURE 12.1 ● The duration of sleep for adults is normally distributed around a mean of 7.5 hours per night. (Adapted from Hobson JA. *Sleep*. New York: Scientific American Library; 1989.)

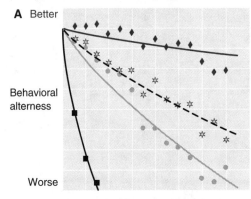

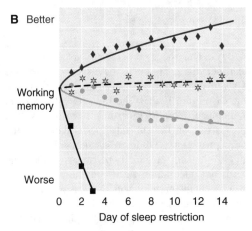

- ■ Total sleep deprivation
- ● 4 hrs sleep/night
- ✳ 6 hrs sleep/night
- ♦ 8 hrs sleep/night

A Better

Behavioral alterness

Worse

B Better

Working memory

Worse

0   2   4   6   8   10   12   14

Day of sleep restriction

FIGURE 12.2 ● The effects of total sleep deprivation for 3 days and chronic sleep restriction for 14 days are measured with neurobehavioral tasks. The Psychomotor Vigilance Task (**A**) measures alertness and attention. The Digit Symbol Substitution Task (**B**) measures working memory. (Adapted from Van Dongen HP, Maislin G, Mullington JM, et al. The cumulative cost of additional wakefulness: Dose-response effects on neurobehavioral functions and sleep physiology from chronic sleep restriction and total sleep deprivation. *Sleep.* 2003;26[2]:117–126.)

knowledge. Interns who had their workday limited to 16 hours (compared with the traditional 24+ hours) got more sleep each week and made half the attentional errors during on-call nights compared with the interns following the traditional schedule.

Stages of Sleep

For centuries sleep had been considered a passive, uniform process that simply restored the body. That changed in 1953 when Nathaniel Kleitman

and Eugene Aserinksy examined electroencephalographic (EEG) recordings from sleeping healthy subjects. They discovered that sleep comprises different stages that repeat in characteristic patterns throughout the night. They identified the three states of consciousness: awake, non-rapid eye movement (non-REM) sleep, and rapid eye movement (REM) sleep. Non-REM sleep has been further subdivided into four stages.

Electroencephalographic Patterns

Figure 12.3 shows the characteristic EEG patterns during the different stages of sleep. From an awake state to the deepest sleep of stage 4 there is a progression of decreasing frequency and increasing amplitude of the EEG activity. Stage 1 sleep, also called the *drowsy period*, is so light that most people when awoken from this stage will say that they were not asleep. Stage 2 sleep shows the development of sleep spindles, which are periodic bursts of activity resulting from interactions between the thalamus and the cortex. Stage 3 and 4 sleep, also called *slow wave sleep* (SWS), are the deepest

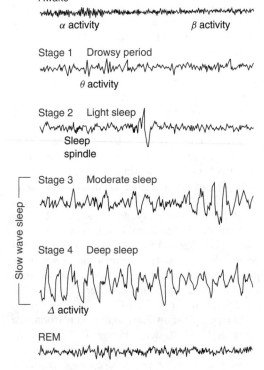

FIGURE 12.3 ● Characteristic electroencephalographic rhythms during the stages of consciousness. REM, rapid eye movement. (Adapted from Horne JA. *Why we sleep: the functions of sleep in humans and other mammals.* Oxford: Oxford University Press; 1988.)

stages of sleep characterized by the development of delta waves. REM sleep is the most unusual finding that Kleitman and Aserinksy discovered. In REM sleep the EEG activity is remarkably similar to the awake state.

In a typical night, a person cycles through five episodes of non-REM/REM activity (see Figure 12.4(A)). The first REM episode occurs after approximately 90 minutes of sleep. This period is called *REM latency* and is usually reduced in patients who are exhausted as well as those with depression, narcolepsy, and sleep apnea. The deepest stage of sleep occurs only in the early phases of the night. The REM episodes increase in length as the night unfolds.

Figure 12.4(B) shows some of the other physiologic changes that take place during the stages of sleep. The most remarkable findings are the differences in physiologic activity between non-REM and REM sleep. Non-REM sleep is characterized by limited eye movement and decrease in muscle tone, heart rate, and respirations. Metabolic rate and body temperature are also decreased

in these stages. They reach their lowest levels during stage 4 sleep. REM sleep, as the name implies, is characterized by rapid, darting movements of the eyes along with paralysis of most major muscle groups. Heart rate and respirations increase almost to the level found when awake. Penile/clitoral erections also occur during REM sleep—a finding that helps rule out physiologic impotence.

Muscle Tone
Muscle activity varies depending on the phase of sleep. During non-REM sleep, the muscles are capable of movement, but rarely do. On the other hand, REM sleep is characterized by a loss of skeletal muscle tone. Respiratory muscles along with the muscles of the eyes and the tiny muscles of the ear remain active in REM sleep.

Brain Imaging
Brain imaging studies during sleep reveal a pattern that is consistent with EEG findings. During non-REM sleep, positron emission tomography (PET)

POINT OF INTEREST

All mammals sleep. Mammals living in the water are able to sleep, but still regularly surface for air. Additionally, from the day they are born until they die, dolphins are continuously moving and avoiding obstacles. They do not have a period of immobility that in terrestrial mammals marks the state of sleep. How do they do all this and still sleep?

Studies of EEG tracings of the bottlenose dolphin show that they rest one hemisphere at a time (see Figure). Note how the large amplitude waves of SWS are only present in one hemisphere at a time. The eye contralateral to the brain hemisphere showing slow waves is usually closed while the other eye is almost always open. Lastly, these dolphins do not display REM activity, which may be an adaptation so they can keep moving.

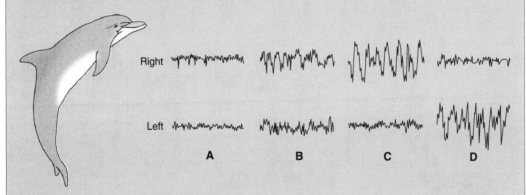

Electroencephalographic tracings from bottlenose dolphins. (Adapted from Mujhametov LM. Sleep in marine mammals. In: Borbely AA, ed. 1984 and Purves D, Augustine GJ, Fitzpatrick D, et al. *Neuroscience*, 3rd ed. Sunderland, MA: Sinauer; 2004.)

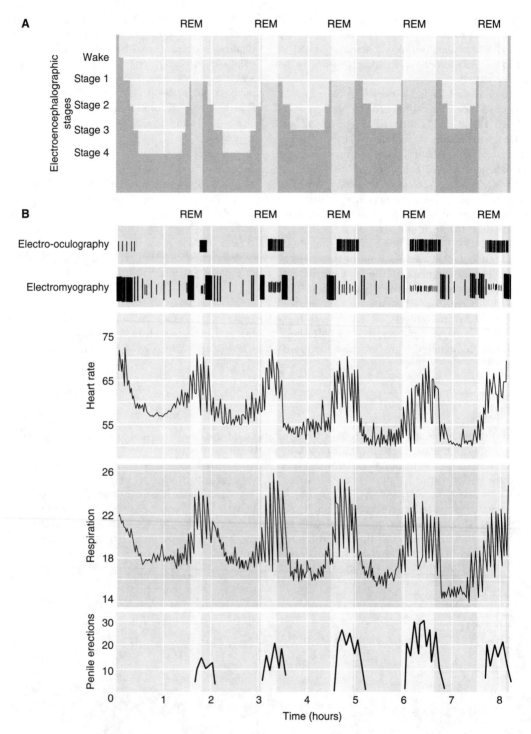

FIGURE 12.4 ● Physiologic changes in a healthy volunteer during 8 hours of sleep. REM, rapid eye movement. (Adapted from Purves D, Augustine GJ, Fitzpatrick D, et al. *Neuroscience*, 3rd ed. Sunderland, MA: Sinauer; 2004.)

studies show decreased cerebral blood flow, and energy metabolism. The greatest decreases correlate with greater depth of sleep. Alternatively, REM sleep shows a cerebral energy metabolism, which is equal to that occurring during awakening.

William Dement, a prominent sleep researcher from Stanford, has eloquently summarized the difference between the phases of sleep. He has characterized non-REM sleep as an idling brain in a movable body. In contrast, REM sleep is an active, hallucinating brain in a paralyzed body.

DISORDERS: SLEEPWALKING AND NIGHT TERRORS

Approximately 40% of the people are *sleepwalkers* as children, although few are sleepwalkers as adults. This behavior usually occurs in the first stage-4 non-REM period of the night. In a typical episode, the child's eyes will be open and the child will avoid obstacles when moving about the room or house. The cognition is clouded and the child will usually have no memory of the event. The best intervention is to gently guide the sleepwalker back to bed.

Night terrors are characterized by extreme terror and an inability to be awakened. Typically occurring in children between the ages of 4 and 7, this condition only affects approximately 3% of the population. As with sleep walking, it develops in the deep stages of non-REM sleep. Night terrors are not to be confused with nightmares, which are vivid dreams during REM sleep.

The child appears in a state of panic, may even scream, and cry. Fortunately they usually return to sleep in 10 to 20 minutes and little is remembered the next day. The greatest toll may be on the parents who have to comfort the frightened child. The best intervention is support.

Changes with Aging

Total sleep duration and the proportions of time spent in various stages change as people age. Figure 12.5 shows the duration of sleep across the life span. Neonates (on the left of the figure) spend most of their time sleeping, with a large percentage of that time in REM sleep. Some have suggested that REM serves a developmental purpose and this is why neonates and young children require so much time in this phase.

On the right side of Figure 12.5 is a meta-analysis of sleep duration from childhood to old age. Note the gradual reduction in the deepest stages of sleep and the increase in awakening after sleep onset as people age. Dissatisfaction with sleep is a common complaint in the elderly, and the origins of those complaints can be seen in this figure.

Dreaming

Historically it has been believed that dreaming is limited to REM sleep. A thorough analysis of what people are experiencing at different stages of consciousness reveals that dreams occur in all stages of sleep, but the content varies. Researchers gave college students a pager and instructed them to sleep with a special nightcap that recorded eye and head movement (see Figure 12.6(A)). The students were considered to be in non-REM sleep when there was an absence of eye movement. REM sleep was defined as rapid eye movements without head movement. The students dictated what they were doing, thinking, and feeling when they were paged or spontaneously awoke.

The results showed that the subjects had dreams at all stages of sleep; however, the nature of dreams was different. In non-REM sleep the dreams were more thoughts—as though the person is solving a problem. In REM sleep the dreams are illogical, bizarre, and even hallucinatory. Figure 12.6(B) shows the decrease in thoughts as the subject goes from an awake state to REM sleep and the corresponding marked increase in hallucinations.

NEURONAL CIRCUITS

Until the 1940s, sleep was generally conceptualized as the body's reaction to the lack of stimulation, that is, the brain passively turns "off" when there is no input. We now know that sleep is an active process initiated and terminated by different regions of the brain.

Suprachiasmatic Nucleus

The master clock of the brain is the suprachiasmatic nucleus (SCN) located in the anterior hypothalamus (see Figure 12.7). The SCN orchestrates circadian rhythms throughout the brain and body. The SCN is synchronized (entrained) by signals from the retina, which are activated by inputs from the sun. When humans are prevented

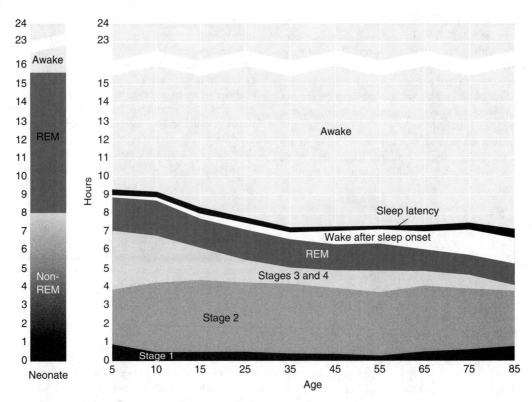

FIGURE 12.5 ● Sleep duration across the lifespan. Neonates are shown on the left and on the right is a meta-analysis of sleep parameters in healthy individuals across the life span. REM, rapid eye movement. (Adapted from Ohayon MM, Carskadon MA, Guilleminault C, et al. Meta-analysis of quantitative sleep parameters from childhood to old age in healthy individuals: Developing normative sleep values across the human lifespan. *Sleep.* 2004;27[7]:1255–1273.)

from receiving cues about the solar day (such as living in a cave for weeks), the 24-hour sleep–wake cycle will gradually increase to approximately 26 hours—a condition that is called *free-running.*

The SCN is made up of some of the smallest neurons in the brain and has a volume that is >0.3 mm^3. Output from the SCN synchronizes other cellular oscillators throughout the brain and body. Studies with hamsters have established the crucial roll this tiny collection of neurons play in the regulation of sleep–wake cycles. Figure 12.8(A) shows how recordings of the time a hamster spends on the running wheel can be used to establish their circadian rhythm. When the SCN is ablated, the 24-hour rhythm is lost and no regular pattern can be identified. If the hamster receives a transplant from a strain of mutant hamsters with a 22-hour circadian rhythm, the foreign rhythm becomes established.

TREATMENT: MELATONIN

Under normal circumstances, the SCN is reset each day by signals of light from the retina. However melatonin secreted during the dark cycle from the pineal gland can also entrain the SCN. This justifies the use of melatonin to promote sleep in those with delayed sleep onset or to reset the internal clock that occur with jet lag. Studies with melatonin agents have been effective although less robust than we might hope. An important part of melatonin dosing is the time of taking it. Taking a dose at the wrong time will not only be ineffective, but can make things worse!

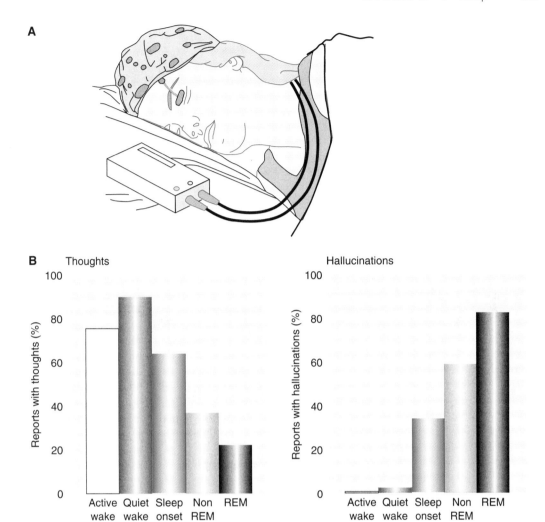

FIGURE 12.6 ● A special home-based sleep-monitoring system (A) allows researchers to correlate dream content with stage of consciousness (B). REM, rapid eye movement. (Adapted from Fosse R, Stickgold R, Hobson JA. Brain-mind states: Reciprocal variation in thoughts and hallucinations. *Psychol Sci.* 2001;12[1]:30–36.)

Molecular Mechanisms

Recent work with fruit flies and mice has begun to tease out the molecular mechanisms that control circadian rhythm. Although all the details remain to be worked out, the basic mechanism is becoming clear. The cell (is this in the SCN only?) produces two proteins: CLOCK and BMAL1. These proteins bind together to form a dimer, which then activates the transcription of other proteins, called *PER (Period)* and *CRY (Cryptochrome)*. PER and CRY form a dimer that inhibits the transcription of CLOCK and BMAL1, providing a negative feedback loop.

The buildup and breakdown of these proteins takes 24 hours. Figure 12.9 shows the daily fluctuation in the proteins PER and CRY from a mouse SCN. Note the 6-hour lag between the buildup of the messenger RNA and the production of the proteins. Although the functions of PER and CRY remain to be elucidated, this molecular mechanism is believed to drive the 24-hour cycling of the SCN.

An area of great interest involves the genes that control these proteins in humans and their role with sleep disorders. For example, mutations of CLOCK and PER have been found in some individuals with delayed or advanced sleep phase

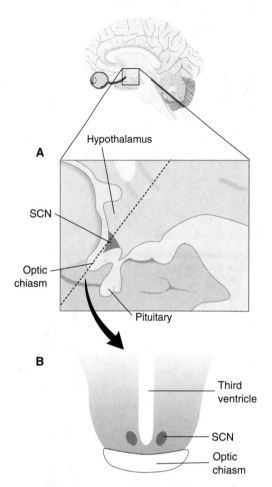

FIGURE 12.7 ● A sagittal view (**A**) and frontal view (**B**) of the human suprachiasmatic nucleus (SCN). (Adapted from Bear MF, Connors BW, Paradiso MA, eds. *Neuroscience: exploring the brain*, 3rd ed. Baltimore: Lippincott Williams & Wilkins; 2007.)

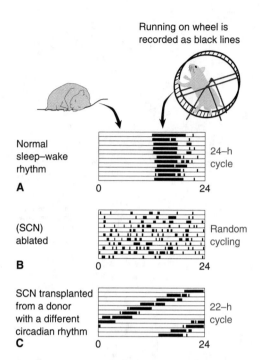

FIGURE 12.8 ● Usual 24-hour circadian rhythm (**A**). Lack of rhythm after the suprachiasmatic nucleus (SCN) is destroyed (**B**). New 22-hour rhythm after transplantation of SCN from hamster with genetically different rhythms (**C**). (Adapted from Ralph MR, Lehman MN. Transplantation: A new tool in the analysis of the mammalian hypothalamic circadian pacemaker. *Trends Neurosci.* 1991;14[8]:362–366.)

syndromes. Additionally, of great interest to us, is the question of damaged *clock* genes and psychiatric disorders. Clearly, sleep impairments have a strong correlation with psychiatric disorders, but as yet there is only limited evidence implicating *clock* genes as the culprits.

Ascending Arousal Systems

In 1949, the Italian neurophysiologists Horace Magoun and Giuseppe Moruzzi discovered the first circuits governing sleep and wakefulness. They found that stimulating a group of neurons in the midline of the brain stem aroused a sleeping animal. Likewise, lesions of this region resulted in persistent sleep. They called this region the *reticular activating system*.

It is likely that Magoun and Moruzzi were stimulating many different sets of ascending arousal neurons during their experiments. Further study in the intervening years has identified several of the important nuclei and neurotransmitters. One group is the cholinergic neurons with cell bodies located near the pons–midbrain junction. These neurons project to the thalamus and activate the thalamic relay neurons that are crucial for transmission of information to the cerebral cortex. Stimulation of these nuclei causes high frequency, low amplitude EEG activity.

The second group comprises four neuronal systems: the noradrenergic neurons of the locus coeruleus, the serotoninergic neurons of the raphe nuclei, the dopaminergic neurons from the periaqueductal gray matter, and the histaminergic neurons in the tuberomammillary nucleus (see Chapter 4, Neurotransmitters, for further details). These neurons project to the hypothalamus and throughout the cerebral cortex.

All five neuronal systems are active during arousal and quiescent during non-REM sleep.

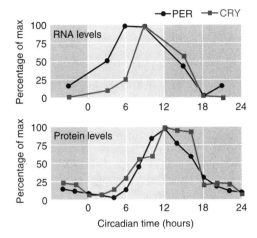

FIGURE 12.9 ● Fluctuations of gene expression and protein levels in the mouse suprachiasmatic nucleus (SCN). These proteins are believed to be the molecular signal of circadian rhythm. (Adapted from Pace-Schott EF, Hobson JA. The neurobiology of sleep: Genetics, cellular physiology and subcortical networks. *Nat Rev Neurosci.* 2002;3[8]:591–605.)

However, the cholinergic neurons resume their activity during REM sleep while the monoaminergic neurons slow down even further. This is another example of how wakefulness and REM sleep (conditions that seem so similar) are different. A summary of these arousal networks is given in Table 12.1.

The Sleep Switch

In general, most people experience a relatively rapid transition from arousal to asleep or vice versa. This transition can be conceptualized as the flipping of a switch. The closest approximation to a "sleep switch" in the brain is the ventrolateral preoptic nuclei (VLPO). The VLPO has projections to the main components of the ascending arousal system shown in Table 12.1. The VLPO is inhibitory and primarily active during sleep. In other words, an active VLPO induces sleep by putting the brakes on the arousal nuclei. Likewise, people with damage to their VLPO have chronic insomnia.

Conversely, the VLPO must be inhibited so that people can wake up. Indeed, the VLPO receives inputs from the monoaminergic neurons—the very neurons that it inhibits. So the "sleep switch" has mutually inhibitory elements in which activity from one slide shuts down the other side and disinhibits its own actions. This helps explain the relatively abrupt change from awake to asleep that occurs in most mammals (see Figure 12.10).

A problem with such a switch is that rapid, unwanted transitions from one state to another can occur when it is unstable. One such condition is *narcolepsy*. Attacks of irresistible sleepiness as well as episodes of physical collapse and loss of muscle tone during emotional situations (*cataplexy*) characterize narcolepsy. In 2000 it was discovered that patients with narcolepsy have few orexin neurons in the hypothalamus (see Figure 12.11). Orexin neurons (also called *hypocretin*) are mainly active during wakefulness and reinforce the arousal system.

It appears that patients with narcolepsy have lost the stabilizing influence of the orexin neurons and can abruptly switch from one state of consciousness to another. In other words they have a floppy "sleep switch". Patients with narcolepsy do not sleep more than normal individuals, they just take more naps during the day and awaken more frequently during the night.

TABLE 12.1

A Summary of the Major Neuronal Systems that Mediate Arousal and Comprise the Ascending Reticular Activating System

Neurotransmitter	Cell Bodies	Projections	Active During
Cholinergic	Nuclei of pons–midbrain junction	Thalamus	Awake and rapid eye movement
Noradrenergic	Locus coeruleus	Hypothalamus and cerebral cortex	Awake
Dopaminergic	Periaqueductal gray matter		
Serotoninergic	Raphe nuclei		
Histaminergic	Tuberomammillary nucleus		

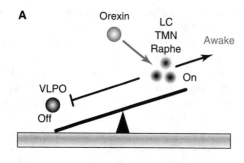

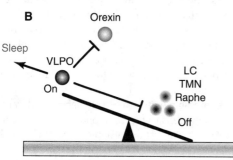

FIGURE 12.10 ● A schematic diagram of the "sleep switch". **(A)** locus coeruleus (LC), tubero-mammillary nucleus (TMN), and Raphe nuclei in the awake state are stabilized by the orexin neurons. They also inhibit the VLPO. **(B)** In the sleep state, the VLPO inhibits the orexin neurons as well as the LC, TMN and raphe nuclei. VLPO, ventrolateral preoptic nuclei. (Adapted from Saper CB, Scammell TE, Lu J. Hypothalamic regulation of sleep and circadian rhythms. *Nature.* 2005;437[7063]:1257–1263.)

TREATMENT: NARCOLEPSY

Amphetamines were first used in 1937 as a treatment for narcolepsy and remain popular. More recently, modafinil, an agent with minimal potential for abuse and a different mechanism of action, has become the first-line treatment for patients with the disorder. Modafinil works by indirectly activating the histamine network—the opposite effect of an antihistamine. Although effective for excessive daytime sleepiness, modafinil has limited benefits for cataplexy. Some clinicians add a tricyclic antidepressant or a newer antidepressant with dual-action to decrease cataplectic attacks. Such a combination will affect histamine, serotonin, and norepinephrine—all components of the "sleep switch".

DISORDER: OBESITY

A recent analysis of more than a thousand volunteers found a U-shaped curvilinear association between sleep duration and body mass. Subjects who slept, on average, 7.7 hours per night had the lowest weight whereas those sleeping for more or less time were heavier. The authors suggest the cause may be due to changes in hormones regulating appetite, such as leptin and ghrelin.

The link between SCN and the "sleep switch" is more confusing than one might expect. SCN actually has few direct projections to the VLPO and orexin neurons. There appears to be a third system: the dorsomedial nucleus of the hypothalamus (DMH). Why might the brain have evolved a three-stage pathway for control of sleep? Well, the SCN is always active during the light cycle and the VLPO is always active during sleep. Without an intermediate step, nocturnal animals could not sleep during the day.

The DMH receives projections from the SCN and sends projections to the VLPO. However, the DMH appears to do more than just relay signals from one nucleus to another. There are many factors that influence the sleep–wake cycle: hunger, stress, and sleep debt—not just the cycle of the sun. In turn, many physiologic functions are affected by the DMH: eating, temperature, and corticosteroid cycles, as well as sleep and arousal. The three-stage pathway allows greater integration of multiple factors and greater flexibility in behavioral response.

WHY DO WE SLEEP?

Life is competitive. However, when we sleep, we can neither advance our position nor protect ourselves or our families. From this perspective, sleep is a costly process. So it must be important for us to pay such a high price. As one researcher puts it, "If sleep doesn't serve an absolutely vital function, it is the biggest mistake evolution even made."

A rat deprived of sleep will die faster than if deprived of food. Humans with fatal familial insomnia, an inherited disease that develops in middle age and results in degeneration of the thalamus, usually die within 24 months (although there may be other reasons for death). Humans forced to remain awake will pursue sleep with a

Normal   Narcoleptic

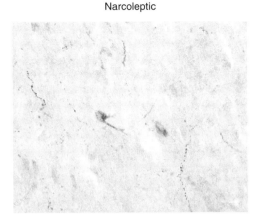

FIGURE 12.11 • Neuronal degeneration of orexin neurons in lateral hypothalamus of a patient with narcolepsy compared with a control. (Courtesy of Jerome Siegel.)

vigor that rivals sex and food. When allowed to sleep, they will make up for the loss by sleeping deeper and longer—called *sleep rebound*. Clearly, something essential happens when we sleep, but what is it?

Development

Some have speculated that sleep serves to establish brain connections during the critical periods of development. For example, all the twitching that infants exhibit during sleep may serve to help babies get control of their muscles. If this theory is true, then it would explain why we sleep most when young and less as we age. Additionally, species that are more mature at birth (e.g., those that can thermoregulate and ambulate) have sleep durations close to adult levels.

Frank and his group have conducted studies that suggest sleep enhances the plasticity of the developing cortex. We discussed the devastating effects that occluding an eye at critical periods has on normal development in Chapter 7, Adult Development and Plasticity. Frank and his group took this research one step further. They occluded an eye of one-month-old cats for 6 hours. Then one group was allowed to sleep for 6 hours and the other group was kept awake in darkness for an equal amount of time. Both groups were anesthetized and their visual cortex was probed. Electrodes inserted almost parallel to the visual cortex recorded activity from different locations while a light shone in the cats eyes.

The results are shown in Figure 12.12. Compare these results with the studies shown in Figure 7.11. Note that the cats that were allowed to sleep developed the typical pattern of ocular dominance. That is, the opened eye dominates the neurons in the visual cortex. The cats that did not

DISORDER: DREAM ENACTMENT

The muscle atonia that accompanies REM sleep is one of the most interesting developments of normal sleep. Unfortunately, some people lose the ability to induce muscle paralysis—a condition called *REM sleep behavior disorder*. The most common patients are men older than 50. Often this condition precedes by many years the emergence of a neurodegenerative disorder such as Parkinson's disease.

Patients who fail to suppress muscle tone during REM sleep are condemned to act out their dreams. Such patients thrash about in bed and frequently hurt themselves or their partners. In some cases it even gets violent. In cats a similar condition has been elicited with small lesions of the pons just above the locus ceruleus. In humans it has been harder to find a specific lesion. It is presumed that some subtle disruption of the balance between atonic and motor generation may be occurring in the spinal cord, brain stem, or even higher cortical areas.

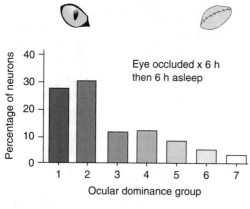

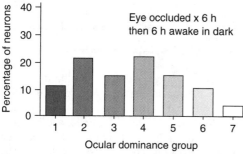

FIGURE 12.12 ● The effects of sleep and sleep deprivation on ocular dominance plasticity during the critical period of visual development in 1-month-old cats. (Adapted from Frank MG, Issa NP, Stryker MP. Sleep enhances plasticity in the developing visual cortex. *Neuron.* 2001;30[1]:275–287.)

sleep maintained a more even distribution of ocular dominance. This research suggests that the effects of occluding an eye are not fully processed until the animal is asleep; to put this in another way, the changes in the brain that develop with experience are imprinted during sleep.

Taken together, these observations suggest that sleep is instrumental to normal development. However, Siegel has noted an almost complete absence of sleep for dolphin mothers and their newborns after birth. The calf will gradually increase its sleep to adult amounts over a period of months. This is the opposite of what is seen with terrestrial mammals, which suggests that sleep is either not essential for normal development or dolphins have adapted alternative mechanisms.

Neurogenesis
A group at university of California, Los Angeles (UCLA) examined the effects of sleep deprivation on neurogenesis. Adult rats were deprived of sleep for 4 days and then examined for new cells in the dentate gyrus of the hippocampus. There

was a 68% reduction in new cells in the sleep-deprived group compared with the controls. Stress hormones did not mediate the change, as the serum corticosterone levels were not significantly different in the two groups.

Energy Conservation
Sleep may be a form of energy conservation across the 24-hour day, the way hibernation conserves energy through a winter. An animal that is protected in a warm location minimizes the energy expenditure that will later need to be replaced. However, conserving energy does not explain the drive to sleep or sleep rebound.

Restoration
Comparing sleep amounts across species sheds some light on the function of sleep. One established relationship in biology is the inverse correlation between body mass and metabolic rate; that is, smaller animals have higher metabolic rates and a higher metabolic rate means greater metabolic activity in the brain. Greater activity in the brain means greater metabolic by-products. Small animals with higher metabolic rates tend to sleep longer. For example, bats and opossums sleep approximately 18 to 20 hours per day whereas elephants and giraffes sleep as little as 3 to 4 hours a day.

A high metabolic rate results in increased oxidative stress produced from the mitochondria. Higher rates of oxidative stress have been linked to aging, arthritis, and dementia in the mouse. Sleep may be the time that the brain "cleans up" and repairs the damage that accumulated during the day.

Siegel et al. have shown that sleep deprivation in the rat results in increased oxidative stress, which can be reversed with sleep. Additionally, they have shown tissue damage in the brain stem, hippocampus, and hypothalamus with sleep deprivation. The greatest area of disruption was in the supraoptic nucleus of the hypothalamus. Siegel believes that wakefulness produces a gradual toxic state that is corrected with sufficient sleep. Animals with a higher metabolic rate require greater sleep amounts to repair the more extensive wear and tear on their neurons during arousal.

Memory Consolidation
The idea that sleep improves the consolidation of memories has been debated and studied for more than 80 years. There is still no consensus. The underlying hypothesis proposes that information acquired during the day is reviewed and strengthened during sleep. Many different experimental designs have shown that memory for procedures

or the ability to recognize patterns improve after sleeping—or even just napping during the day. However, memories for facts (declarative memory) do not seem to improve with sleep. So, the relationship between sleep and memory depends on the material learned.

It was discovered in the 1970s that some neurons in the rat hippocampus fire when the animal is in a specific location or moving toward that location. These cells were called *place cells*. It was subsequently shown that specific patterns of activity by the place cells during the day were reactivated during non-REM sleep that night. Furthermore it has been shown that there are correlations between hippocampal cells and cortical neurons during the behavior and again when asleep. This suggests that the hippocampus revisits the events of the day "off line" and possibly orchestrates the consolidation of memories to long-term cortical stores.

Pierre Maquet et al. in Belgium has taken this one step further and used functional imaging studies to look at the activity in the human hippocampus the night after learning a new task. Participants were instructed to learn their way through a complicated virtual town. It was observed that regions of the hippocampus that were active during the task were reactivated during subsequent non-REM sleep. Of particular interest, everyone improved on the task the following day. However, those with the greatest activity expressed during SWS also showed the greatest improvement navigating the virtual town the following day (see Figure 12.13).

In summary, it is not entirely clear what happens during sleep. It is likely that sleep serves many functions simultaneously.

MOOD DISORDERS

There is a long-standing suspicion that mood disorders are initiated or at least maintained by circadian dysfunction. Several lines of evidence suggest this to be true for depression. For example:

1. Depression has a diurnal variation—worse in the morning.
2. Insomnia is one of the most common complaints.
3. Insomnia resolves with effective treatment.
4. Sleep deprivation is an effective, although short-lived, antidepressant.

Seasonal Affective Disorder

Seasonal affective disorder (SAD), also called *winter depression*, is most suggestive of circadian changes affecting mood. Many mammals display seasonal fluctuations in behavior that is regulated by the change in day length. Hibernation may be the extreme form of this seasonal change. Humans

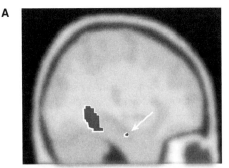
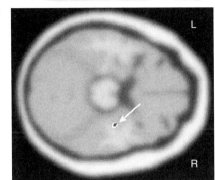
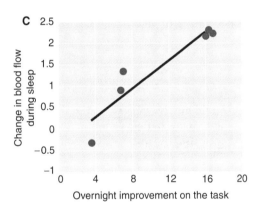

FIGURE 12.13 ● Hippocampal reactivation during non-REM sleep and memory consolidation. The sagittal (**A**) and horizontal (**B**) sections show the areas of the right hippocampus that were reactivated during sleep and correlated with improved scores on the task. (Adapted from Peigneux P, Laureys S, Fuchs S, et al. Are spatial memories strengthened in the human hippocampus during slow wave sleep? *Neuron.* 2004;44[3]:535–545.)

with SAD develop symptoms of depression in the winter, along with weight gain, increased sleep, and decreased activity. This array of symptoms resembles changes seen in animals preparing to hibernate.

The changes in daylight hours are transmitted from the retina to the SCN. The SCN activates the paraventricular nucleus of the hypothalamus, which indirectly (by way of the sympathetic nervous system) inhibits the pineal gland. When the SCN is inactive during darkness, the inhibition is removed, and the pineal gland secretes melatonin. In other words, melatonin is secreted during the night when the "brakes" are off. The duration of elevated nightly melatonin provides every tissue with information about the time of day and time of year. Some have called the pineal gland both a *clock* and a *calendar*. For example, animals that hibernate, such as the Syrian hamster, produce more melatonin in winter, and less in summer.

Recent research has examined melatonin secretion in 55 patients with SAD in summer and winter. They found that for patients with SAD the nocturnal duration of melatonin secretion was longer in winter than in summer, but there was no change in duration for the healthy volunteers. Other research has found that early morning light therapy for patients with SAD improved their mood and produced phase advances of the melatonin rhythm. In total these results suggest that the neural circuits that mediate season change in mammals may be impaired in patients with SAD.

DISORDER: HYPERAROUSAL

Trouble in sleeping is a common complaint. Some patients cannot turn off the arousal networks at bedtime. Patients with anxiety disorders, attention deficit hyperactivity disorder (ADHD), and hyperthymic temperament will often complain that they cannot stop thinking when trying to sleep. Patients who abuse alcohol, opioids, and marijuana often use the substance as a hypnotic and frequently show rebound insomnia when substance free. Furthermore, insomnia is a risk factor for relapse with recovered alcoholics.

A recent neuroimaging study of patients with insomnia showed greater global cerebral metabolism while awake and asleep compared with controls. Additionally, the patients showed a smaller decline in relative metabolism from waking to sleep states in some of the structures discussed earlier, for example, ascending reticular activating system and hypothalamus.

TREATMENT: INSOMNIA

Insomnia is generally a long-term problem. Hypnotic medications are not without risk. Nonpharmacologic interventions, such as cognitive behavior therapy and stimulus control, are as effective as medications, show enduring benefits, and have no side effects. Such treatments should be the first-line interventions, particularly for the young and middle aged.

The evolution of sleep medications is a story of searching for agents with shorter duration, more specific mechanisms of action, and less potential for abuse. Alcohol is perhaps the oldest sleep medicine. Chloral hydrate, first synthesized in 1832, was the first medication specifically indicated for insomnia. The development of barbiturates in the early 1900s brought a new class of agents that were widely used for 50 years. The introduction of benzodiazepines in the 1960s provided a treatment that was effective and safer.

As shown in Figure 5.3, benzodiazepines work by sensitizing the γ-aminobutyric acid (GABA) receptor, which in turn increases the movement of negatively charged chloride ions into the cell and ultimately enhances the activity of the GABA neurons. More GABA activity means more inhibition of the central nervous system (CNS).

There are two benzodiazepine receptor subtypes on the GABA receptor. The traditional benzodiazepines bind to both, but the newer agents (zolpidem, zaleplon, and eszopiclone) bind to just one subunit. This subunit mediates the sedating and amnesic effects, but not the anxiolytic, or myorelaxation. Whether this selective binding translates into fewer side effects remains to be determined.

Bipolar Disorder

Bipolar disorder is another condition associated with circadian dysfunction. The delay in sleep onset and reduction in sleep duration accompanying a manic episode are clear examples of disrupted circadian rhythm. Additionally, the mood stabilizer lithium is known to lengthen the circadian period, which may be one of its mechanisms of action.

Of particular interest is the predictive value of sleep disruption and mania. It is well known that a decreasing need to sleep can precede a manic episode. There is some evidence that the prevalence of bipolar disorder, particularly the rapid cycling subgroup, is increasing. Although the increased use of antidepressants and/or illicit drugs are possible causes, another explanation may be sleep disruption due to the modern lifestyle.

Wehr et al. believe that individuals with bipolar disorder are predisposed to exacerbations of the illness when sleep deprived. Because manic behavior interferes with sleep and sleep deprivation makes mania worse, a vicious downward cycle can be established. They describe a highly educated, successful individual who developed bipolar disorder in his mid-40s. Despite aggressive

pharmacologic management, he cycled between depression and mania every 6 to 8 weeks. He also showed great fluctuations in his sleep–wake phases across these cycles.

The group intervened by getting the subject to remain at bed-rest in a dark room for 14 hours each night. This was later tapered to 10 hours per night. Remarkably, his mood and sleep stabilized. Periods of hyperactivity and hypoactivity were greatly reduced. The effects were still present after 1 year. It is worth noting that he remained on divalproex sodium and sertraline. The authors believe that enforced bed-rest synchronized and stabilized the circadian rhythms, which were so easily disrupted by his modern lifestyle. If nothing else, this case highlights the importance of good sleep hygiene for any patient.

QUESTIONS

1. Which do you typically see in Stage 2 of sleep?
   a. Sleep spindles.
   b. α-waves.
   c. δ-activity.
   d. SWS.

2. REM latency is decreased in all of the following, except
   a. Depression.
   b. Generalized Anxiety.
   c. Narcolepsy.
   d. Sleep Apnea.

3. Which of the following is true?
   a. The average length of sleep is 8 hours/night.
   b. The deepest sleep occurs in the latter third of the night.
   c. Muscle tone increases during REM sleep.
   d. PET scans show decreased cerebral blood flow during SWS.

4. Which of the following is true about dolphin sleep?
   a. They never show REM sleep.
   b. New born calfs sleep the most during the neonatal period.
   c. They close their eyes and navigate by echolocation.
   d. They sleep on the surface so they can breath.

5. All of the following are true regarding sleep and aging, except
   a. We sleep less as we age.
   b. Arousal after sleep onset increases with age.
   c. REM sleep increases in the latter part of life.
   d. SWS decreases with aging.

6. Which of the following is active during the night in humans?
   a. The SCN.
   b. Orexin neurons.
   c. The ventrolateral preoptic nucleus.
   d. Tuberomammillary nucleus.

7. Which of the following systems is active during arousal and REM sleep?
   a. Noradrenergic.
   b. Dopaminergic.
   c. Histaminergic.
   d. Cholinergic.

8. Possible functions for sleep include all of the following, expect
   a. Memory consolidation.
   b. Energy conversation.
   c. Neurotransmitter reaccumulation.
   d. Metabolic restoration.

See Answers section at end of book.

Sex and the Brain

SEXUAL DIMORPHISM

Humans are sexually dimorphic (*di*, "two"; *morph*, "type"). That is, they come in two styles. How one conceptualizes these differences depends on one's perspective. Table 13.1 summarizes the major categories of sexual dimorphism. In this chapter we will focus on how the hormones change the morphology of the brain and how this affects behavior and sexuality.

Pink and Blue

On average, men and women behave differently and enjoy different activities. The etiology of this difference remains a hotly debated topic. Is it nature or nurture—innate or learned? With humans it is almost impossible to tease out these opposing causes. The signals a baby receives about its sexual identity starts early—in the nursery. Typically, boys favor construction and transportation toys. Girls show less rough physical play and prefer toys such as dolls. Is this a product of learned gender social roles or something more innately wired in the brain?

A study with vervet monkeys suggests that the choice of toys children make to play with are more ingrained than some might think. Monkeys in large cages at the university of California, Los Angeles (UCLA) Primate Laboratory were allowed 5 minutes of exposure to individual toys classified as "masculine" (police car and ball) or "feminine" (doll and pot). The amount of time they were in direct contact with each of the toys was recorded. Figure 13.1 shows a male and female monkey playing with the toys and the percent time that each gender spent in contact with the toys. These results

shows that even nonhuman primates who are not exposed to social pressure regarding toy preference, will choose gender-specific toys.

If we remember the important role of pleasure in determining behavioral preferences, we can speculate that the monkeys spend more time with the toys they enjoy. Likewise we can speculate that the association between an object and pleasure is hard wired in the brain. Furthermore, some of this "wiring" must have arisen early in human evolution before the emergence of our hominid ancestors.

The Boy Who was Raised as a Girl

One of the more remarkable stories of sexually dimorphic behavior involves a tragic story of a

TABLE 13.1

Different Ways of Conceptualizing Sexual Dimorphism

Perspective	Example
Chromosomal	XX, XY
Gonadal	Ovaries, testes
Hormonal	Estrogen, androgens
Morphological	Genitalia, body size, body shape
Behavioral	Nurturing, aggressive, hunter, gatherer, etc.
Sexual	Identity, orientation, preference

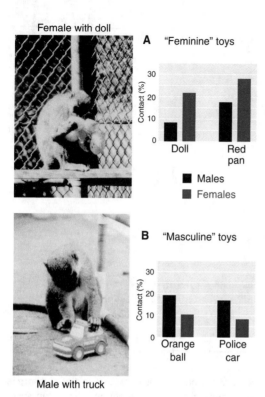

Female with doll

A "Feminine" toys

Doll   Red pan

■ Males
■ Females

B "Masculine" toys

Orange ball   Police car

Male with truck

FIGURE 13.1 ● Male vervet monkeys spent more time in contact with "masculine" toys while females spent more time with "feminine" toys. (From Alexander GM, Hines M. Sex differences in response to children's toys in nonhuman primates (Cercopithecus aethiops sabaeus). *Evol Hum Behav.* 2002;23:467–479.)

boy raised as a girl. David was 8 months old in 1966 when his entire penis was accidentally burned beyond repair during a routine circumcision. Dr. John Money, a psychologist at Johns Hopkins Hospital with an expertise in sexual reassignment, convinced the family to proceed with surgical sex change and raise the boy as a girl. Dr. Money believed that sexual identity/orientation developed after 18 months of age and children could adapt to a new sexual identity if the procedure was started soon enough. David provided an ideal case study as he had a twin brother with a normal penis.

Amazingly, Dr. Money reported in the medical literature that the reassignment was a success, but it was in actuality a disaster. David, whose name was changed to Brenda, did not want to wear dresses, or play with dolls. She preferred to play with guns and cars. She would beat up her brother and threw a ball like a boy. Worst of all, this unusual behavior was not well received

at school. Brenda was relentlessly teased for her masculine traits and was shunned by the girls and the boys.

By the time Brenda was 14 years old she was still unaware of the sexual reassignment, and remained distressed. A local psychiatrist who was treating Brenda convinced the parents to reveal the truth. Brenda recalls her reaction, "Suddenly it all made sense why I felt the way I did. I wasn't some sort of weirdo."

David immediately decided to revert to his genetic sex. Within several months he began going out in public as a boy. He stopped estrogen and started testosterone. He had bilateral mastectomies and several operations to rebuild male genitalia. He eventually married in his twenties although he could not have children. However, he battled with depression and the demons from this childhood experience. In May 2005 at the age of 38 he killed himself.

The significant point about this case is that in spite of being raised as a girl, estrogen hormones, and the absence of testosterone, David continued to have male pattern psychosocial and psychosexual development. Larger case studies are consistent with David's experience. One analysis of XY individuals assigned female roles at birth due to a severe pelvic defect (cloacal exstrophy) found that all showed masculine tendencies. Slightly more than half chose to declare themselves male when older. These studies suggest that something permanent happens *in utero* that determines sexual identity/orientation.

Environment

It would be naive to dismiss the significance of environment on sexually stereotypical behaviors. History is replete with examples of men and women showing varying amounts of masculine and feminine behavior that are clearly molded by shifts in social norms. Kim Wallen reviewed 30 years of research with rhesus monkeys and attempted to separate hormonal and social influences. For example, rough and tumble play is one of the most robust sexually dimorphic behaviors. Juvenile males wrestle more frequently than females in almost every rearing condition. However, if reared in a group with only males, they actually engage in less rough play. Likewise, mounting behavior is seen more with males than females. However, when reared in isolated, same-sex environments, males display less mounting while females display more.

Rust et al. looked at gender development in preschool children and the effect of an older sibling. They found that having an older brother was

associated with greater masculine and less feminine behavior in boys and girls. However, boys
with older sisters were more feminine but not less
masculine whereas girls with older sisters were
less masculine but not more feminine.

Together, these studies suggest interplay between hormones and environment. That is, biologic factors predispose individuals to engage in
specific behaviors, which can be modified by social experience.

HORMONES

Figure 11.8 showed the classic experiment by
Berthold who was the first to establish that the
testes contain a substance that controls the development of male secondary sexual characteristics. In Chapter 6, Hormones and the Brain,
we discussed the relationship between the cortex, hypothalamus, pituitary gland, and end organ.
Briefly, with input from the cortex, the hypothalamus produces gonadotrophin-releasing hormone
(GnRH), which in turn stimulates the anterior pituitary gland to produce luteinizing hormone (LH)
and follicle-stimulating hormone (FSH). LH and
FSH stimulate the gonads to produce the sex
hormones.

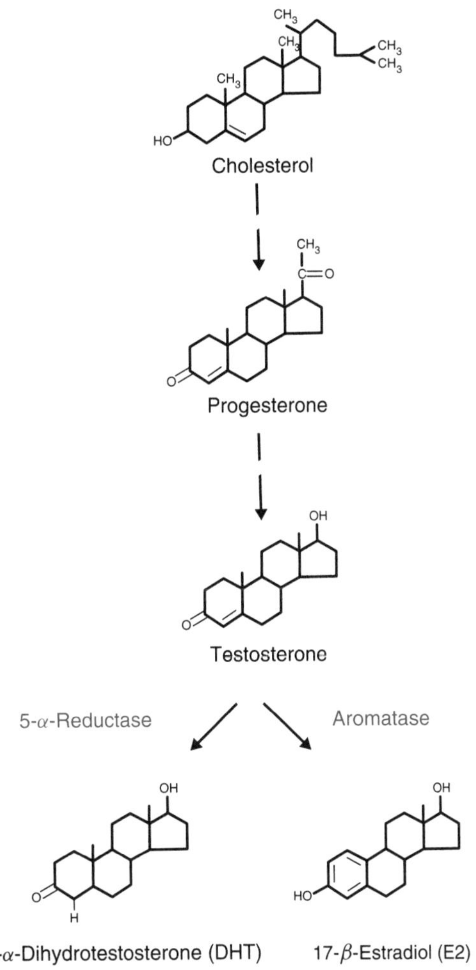

FIGURE 13.2 ● The sex hormones are synthesized from cholesterol. Testosterone serves as a
prohormone for 17-β-estradiol.

GONADS

The gonads (ovaries and testes) serve two
major functions. Firstly, they produce
eggs or sperm to pass on DNA to the
next generation. Secondly, they produce
the sex hormones that not only promote
the development of secondary sexual
characteristics but also drive the behavior
that increases the chances of an egg and
sperm meeting.

Cholesterol is the precursor of all steroid hormones. Figure 6.7 shows the three major steroids
synthesized from cholesterol: glucocorticoids, mineralocorticoids, and the sex steroids. The sex
steroids are synthesized in the adrenals or gonads.
Because the steroid hormones are lipid soluble and
easily pass through the cell walls, they are released
as they are synthesized.

Testosterone, as shown in Figure 13.2, is converted into 17-β-estradiol (E2) and an androgen,
5-α-dihydrotestosterone (DHT). Amazingly, much
of the androgen effects in the brain are actually
implemented by 17-β-estradiol. For example, an

injection of estrogen to a newborn rat is more mas-
culinizing than an injection of testosterone.

Why do the maternal estrogens not masculinize
all fetuses? One of the functions of α-fetoprotein
is to bind with maternal estrogens, which are then
cleared through the placenta. This protein, which
does not bind testosterone effectively, prevents
estrogens from reaching the brain.

We have discussed in other chapters how the
sex steroids can work directly on synaptic receptors or indirectly through gene transcription (see
Figures 5.3, 6.1, and 6.3). These different effects
are summarized in Figure 13.3. The direct effects
are fast while the indirect effects take longer to
transpire.

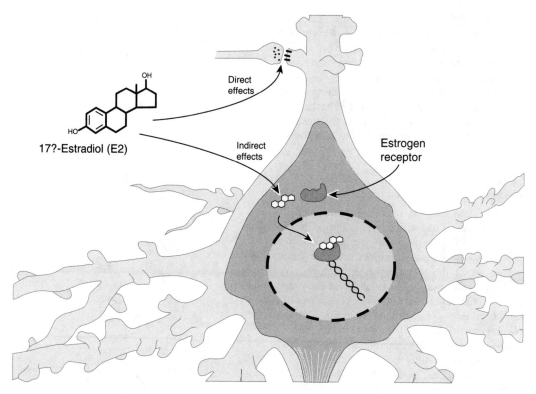

17?-Estradiol (E2)

Direct effects

Indirect effects

Estrogen receptor

FIGURE 13.3 ● Steroids can directly affect transmitter synthesis/release or postsynaptic transmitter receptors. They can also indirectly influence gene transcription. (Adapted from Bear MF, Connors BW, Paradiso MA, eds. *Neuroscience: exploring the brain*, 3rd ed. Baltimore: Lippincott Williams & Wilkins; 2007.)

Differentiation and Activation

The development of sexual dimorphism is dependent on the sex hormones. The presence of testosterone at critical periods of time both masculinizes and defeminizes the brain. Likewise, the absence of testosterone feminizes and demasculinizes the brain. William C. Young et al. published in 1959 a classic paper that rivals Berthold's work with roosters in helping us understand the fundamental principles of hormones and behavior.

To understand Young's study it is important to be aware of the different sexual postures males and females display at appropriate times. Female rodents will stand immobile and arch their backs: *lordosis*. Males will *mount* such a receptive female. Females and males rarely (although not completely) exhibit the opposite behavior. Researchers use the presence or absence of lordosis and mounting as expressions of sexual behavior. For example, castration of a male stops his mounting behavior. But this can be reinstated with injections of testosterone.

Young's group sought to understand the effects of early and late exposure to sex hormones on sexual

behavior. Their experiment, which is shown in Figure 13.4, started with injecting testosterone in a pregnant female guinea pig. Their first observation (not shown in the figure) was that female pups exposed to high doses of androgens *in utero* were born with masculinized external genitalia.

The rest of the study focused on the female pups that were allowed to mature and then spayed. Later they were all given estrogen and progesterone to stimulate female sexual behavior. Each was paired with a normal male guinea pig. Some time later, the procedure was reversed. All were injected with testosterone and paired with a receptive female. The results were striking. The females exposed to testosterone *in utero* failed to display lordosis when given estrogen and progesterone. However, they would mount other females when given testosterone. The control group displayed the opposite behavior.

This elegant experiment established a clear distinction between the differentiating effects of sex hormones during development and the activating effects during adulthood. The females exposed to testosterone *in utero* had alterations in

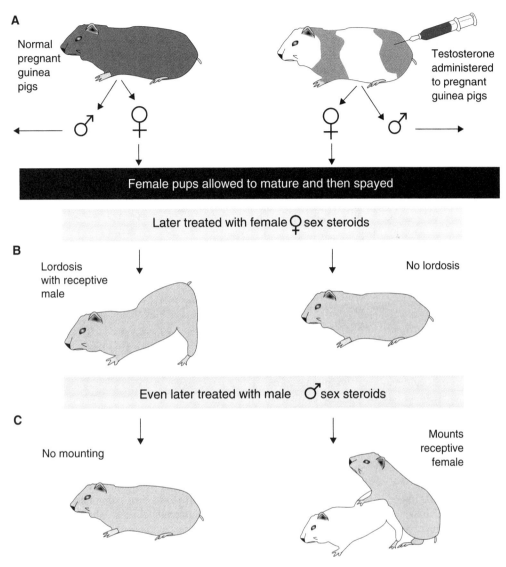

FIGURE 13.4 ● Guinea pigs exposed to testosterone *in utero* (A) fail to show feminine sexual behavior (B) when given female sex hormones and instead act like males (C) when given testosterone.

the organization of their brains that prevented the normal activation by female sex hormones as an adult.

Human Congenital Anomalies

Occasionally people are born with genetic alterations that give us insight into the differentiation and activation of human sexual dimorphism. One such condition is *congenital adrenal hyperplasia* (CAH). Children with this condition are exposed to excessive androgens due to overactive fetal adrenal glands. Paradoxically, the condition is caused by an impaired ability of the fetal adrenal gland to produce cortisol. Because the pituitary fails to receive the appropriate negative feedback, it continues to secrete adenocorticotropic hormone (ACTH), which in turn induces hyperplasia of the steroid-producing cells of the adrenal cortex.

As we might predict from Young's studies with guinea pigs, human males are unaffected by the exposure to adrenal androgens *in utero*. Females, on the other hand, are born with masculinized external genitalia. Additionally, the females tend to exhibit more rough and tumble play as children. As adults, they have an increased tendency to prefer other females as partners.

An extraordinary condition in men provides a different example of anomalous sexual development. *Androgen insensitivity syndrome* (AIS) is a condition in which XY (male) individuals are born as normal appearing females. The problem is caused by a mutation in the androgen receptor. These individuals produce testosterone, but the cells are unable to recognize it. Consequently there is no activation of the genes necessary for male characteristics.

These individuals are born looking like normal little girls and are raised as such (see Figure 13.5). Typically, they only come for a medical evaluation when they fail to menstruate in adolescence. Unfortunately, they are unable to conceive as they have failed to develop uteri, fallopian tubes, and ovaries. However, their behavior is unequivocally feminine. Hines et al. examined the psychological development of 22 XY individuals with complete AIS compared with 22 XX normal controls and found no differences on any measure of psychological outcome. They concluded that these results argue against the need for ovaries and two X chromosomes in the development of traditional feminine behavior. Likewise, it reinforces the importance of the androgen receptor in masculine development. It is an interesting thought that all humans (both men and women) would develop into women unless other hormones intervene. The default model for mankind, is a woman!

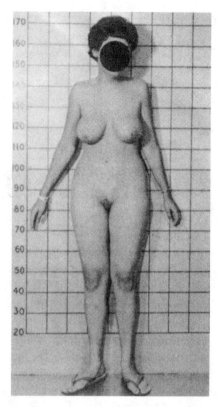

FIGURE 13.5 ● This person with complete androgen insensitivity syndrome has an XY genotype, but has developed unambiguous feminine characteristics. (Courtesy of John Money.)

NEURONAL CIRCUITRY
Nerve Growth

Gonadal steroids grow more than just testes and breasts—they also cause selective neuronal growth. As shown in Figure 13.3, gonadal steroids stimulate gene expression through the androgen and estrogen receptors. These receptors are also transcription factors, which, in turn, stimulate gene transcription and protein synthesis. Ultimately the gonadal steroids can affect nerve volume, dendritic length, spine density, and synaptic connectivity.

TREATMENT: REVEALING THE DIAGNOSIS

In the 1950s the standard practice was to withhold the actual diagnosis from individuals with AIS. They were told that childbearing was impossible, but not told they were genetically male. It was believed that such information would produce psychiatric disorders and possibly even thoughts of suicide. In the 1990s the prevailing attitude shifted to greater disclosure, and now it is the standard practice to reveal all the details to patients with this disorder. However, there remains a small cohort of women whose management was started in the era of less autonomy and who are still unaware of their diagnosis.

Many patients can sense when a secret is being kept. In this age of the Internet it is possible for curious patients to discover their own diagnosis. Some patients have avoided further medical care or even committed suicide when finally discovering their true condition. When confronted with such a patient, clinicians struggle with the appropriate manner and timing of sharing the diagnosis, particularly with a patient who has been kept in the dark for so long.

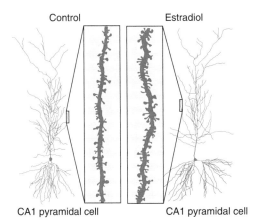

Control   Estradiol

CA1 pyramidal cell   CA1 pyramidal cell

FIGURE 13.6 ● Ovariectomized rats treated with estradiol display greater spine formation on CA1 pyramidal cells from the hippocampus. (Adapted from Woolley CS, Weiland NG, McEwen BS, et al. Estradiol increases the sensitivity of hippocampal CA1 pyramidal cells to NMDA receptor-mediated synaptic input: Correlation with dendritic spine density. *J Neurosci.* 1997;17[5]:1848–1859.)

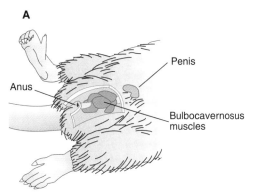

A

Penis

Anus

Bulbocavernosus muscles

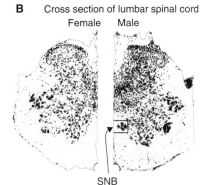

B   Cross section of lumbar spinal cord
Female   Male

SNB

FIGURE 13.7 ● **A:** The male rat has bulbocavernosus muscles that are needed to control the penis for copulation. **B:** Cross sections of the female and male lumbar spinal cord show the presence of the spinal nucleus of the bulbocavernosus for the male, but not the female (A: Adapted from Breedlove SM, Arnold AP. Hormonal control of a developing neuromuscular system. II. Sensitive periods for the androgen-induced masculinization of the rat SNB. *J Neurosci.* 1983;3[2]:424–432.)

Woolley et al. demonstrated this effect by administering estradiol or placebo to ovariectomized rats and examining the structure and function of the hippocampal cells. Figure 13.6 shows two CA1 pyramidal cells and a closer examination of their dendritic spines. The estradiol-exposed neurons had 22% more spines than the controls. Additionally, the N-methyl-D-aspartate (NMDA) glutamate receptors were also increased by 30% in the estradiol-treated neurons. Furthermore, the treated neurons exhibited less electrical resistance to cellular input. So not only did the estrogen change the structure of the neuron, but also the function.

Growth Factor Proteins

The astute reader might wonder about the role of growth factor proteins with sex hormones and nerve plasticity. Indeed there is considerable evidence linking gonadal steroids with growth factors such as brain-derived neurotrophic factor (BDNF). However, it is unclear if the sex hormones stimulate the production of the growth factor protein, or work synergistically with them, or both. A study looking at the rat motoneuron sheds some light on this issue.

The motoneurons projecting from the spinal cord to the skeletal muscles in rodents are generally similar for males and females. However, the male requires innervation of the *bulbocavernosus* muscles around the penis, which are necessary for erections and copulation (see Figure 13.7). Consequently, the motoneurons in the lumbar region of the spinal cord of the male rat (collectively called the *spinal nucleus of the bulbocavernosus* [SNB]) are approximately four times larger than in the female. These motoneurons regress in the female shortly after birth. Similar regression occurs with castrated males. Androgen treatment will preserve the motor neurons.

The dendrites of the motoneurons have extensive branchings that make connections spanning several spinal segments. Cutting the SNB motoneurons results in regression of the dendrites. Previous research has shown that testosterone or BDNF can limit the dendritic regression.

Yang et al. took this a step further. They cut the SNB motoneurons in castrated males. Then they put BDNF over the cut axons or administered testosterone, or both, in different groups of rats. A month later the motoneurons were injected

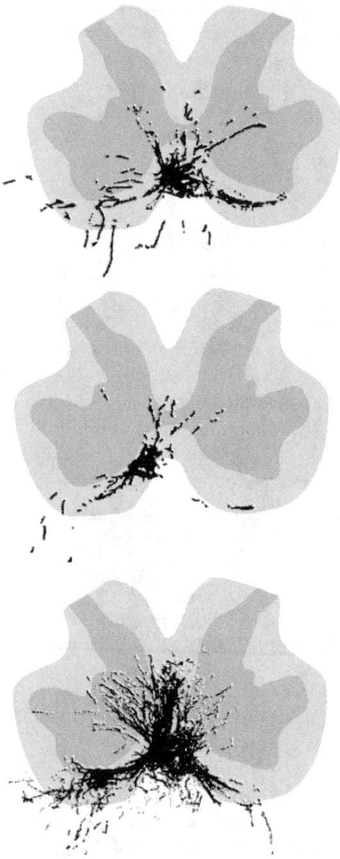

Testosterone

BDNF

Testosterone
and BDNF

FIGURE 13.8 ● Composite lumbar cross
sections showing the extent of spinal nucleus of
the bulbocavernosus motoneurons that remain
1 month after surgical excision. Testosterone
plus brain-derived neurotrophic factor preserved
more of the motoneurons than either alone.
(Adapted from Yang LY, Verhovshek T, Sengelaub
DR. BDNF and androgen interact in the maintenance of dendritic morphology in a sexually
dimorphic rat spinal nucleus. *Endocrinology*.
2004;145[1]:161–168.)

with a marker that allows visualization of the dendrites and axons after the animal is sacrificed.
Figure 13.8 are computer-generated composite
sections marking the presence of the SNB motoneurons for the three groups of rats. The BDNF
plus testosterone group preserved substantially
more dendritic branching than seen with either
alone (similar to what would be seen in a normal control). This suggests that BDNF and testosterone act synergistically to maintain the SNB
motoneuron morphology.

Songbirds

The study of the sexually dimorphic brain structures of the songbirds is one of the great stories of

neuroscience—one that helped transform the way
we think about the brain. The leader in this research is Fernando Nottebohm at the Rockefeller
University in New York. He and others wanted to
understand why male songbirds sing and females
seldom do.

They initially looked at the syrinx (vocal cords)
trying to find differences, without success. Later
they focused on the neuronal mechanisms that
control singing: the high vocal center (HVC),
robust nucleus (RA), and area X. These nuclei
send projections to the XII cranial nerve which
controls the syrinx. Lesions of the HVC bilaterally
will silence a bird.

The big discovery came when they realized
that the song nuclei are approximately three times
larger in males (see Figure 13.9). This was the
first discovery of sexual dimorphism in the brain.
Furthermore, they showed that the size of the HVC
correlates with the number of song syllables a
male canary sings.

Their next discovery has fundamentally altered
the way we think about the brain. Adult canaries
change their songs every year. This is accomplished by adding new syllable types and discarding others. Remarkably, this is accomplished
through the birth and death of neurons in the song
nuclei. Nottebohm et al. were the first to show that
working neurons develop in adult warm-blooded
vertebrates—an idea that received a cool recep-
tion when first presented in 1984.

The reason to discuss this topic in the current
chapter is the fact that much of the differences
in the male canaries' nuclei and song production
are controlled by testosterone. Evidence to support
this include the following:

1. The nuclei of the adult song system have high
   concentrations of testosterone.
2. Adult males with higher testosterone sing more
   than adults with less testosterone.
3. Females given testosterone will sing more and
   show increased volume of their HVC and RA.
4. Drops in testosterone levels at the end of the
   breeding season correspond with the death of
   HVC neurons.

Hypothalamus

The hypothalamus is instrumental in regulating
gonadotrophin secretion. Specifically, the anterior
aspect of the hypothalamus is known to control a
wide variety of mating behaviors: desire, sexual
behavior, and parenting. Lesions in this area can
lead to alterations in sexual behavior. The *preoptic
area* (POA) in the rat is an area where significant differences between the sexes are found (see

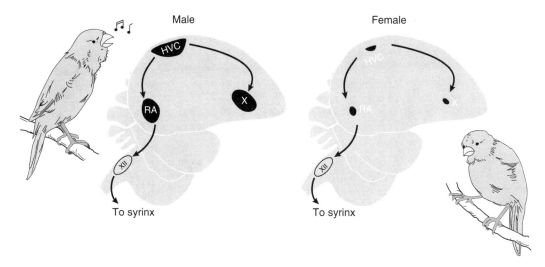

Male

Female

To syrinx

To syrinx

FIGURE 13.9 ● Male canaries sing but females seldom do. The song nuclei are approximately three times larger in the male. HVC, high vocal center; RA, robust nucleus. (Adapted from Nottebohm F. The road we travelled: Discovery, choreography, and significance of brain replaceable neurons. *Ann N Y Acad Sci.* 2004;1016:628–658.)

Figure 2.7). In the male rat the POA is five to seven times larger than in the female. The difference is so prominent that it can be accurately identified with the naked eye. This region of the POA is called the *sexually dimorphic nucleus of the preoptic area* (SDN-POA). Female rats given androgens will develop an SDN-POA approximately the size of a male's. As with the SNB motoneurons, it appears that the androgens preserve the nerve cells, which otherwise waste away.

Humans

Allen et al. examined the anterior aspect of the hypothalamus in a postmortem analysis of 22 human brains: half of each sex. They focused their attention on an area that is the human equivalent of the rat SDN-POA. They identified four cell groupings within the anterior hypothalamus, which they called the *interstitial nuclei of the anterior hypothalamus* (INAH). They numbered the INAH from 1 to 4 and reported that INAH-2 and INAH-3 are approximately twice as large in males compared with females. Figure 13.10 shows actual comparative micrographs through the INAH of males and females.

Sexual Orientation

Simon LeVay took this work one step further and compared the INAH for females, heterosexual males, and homosexual males. He confirmed the work by Allen et al., that is, two of the four interstitial nuclei are sexually dimorphic. However, even more interesting, he found that INAH-3 was

twice as large in heterosexual men as it was in homosexual men (see Figure 13.11). Although this provides compelling evidence that sexual orientation is "hardwired," we must be cautious for there could be other explanations. For example, almost all of the homosexual men died of AIDS, whereas only approximately one third of the heterosexual men did. Likewise, there was considerable overlap in the size of the nuclei between groups, implying that it is impossible to predict the sexual orientation of any individual based on the measurement of his INAH-3.

More recently, research on this issue has returned to animals. Approximately 8% of the domestic male sheep display sexual preference for other males. A group in Oregon identified a cluster of cells within the POA of the anterior hypothalamus (analogs to the INAH) that is significantly larger in rams than ewes. They compared these nuclei for rams with different sexual preferences and found it was twice as large in heterosexual rams as it was in homosexual rams. These results provide an animal model that is consistent with the work by LeVay.

Taken together, the above studies suggest a possible explanation for the continuum of human sexual behavior. Small differences in nuclei in the anterior hypothalamus produce significant differences in sexual identity and behavior. Early exposure to sexual hormones during critical periods of development determines the development of these relevant nuclei. Full expression of the

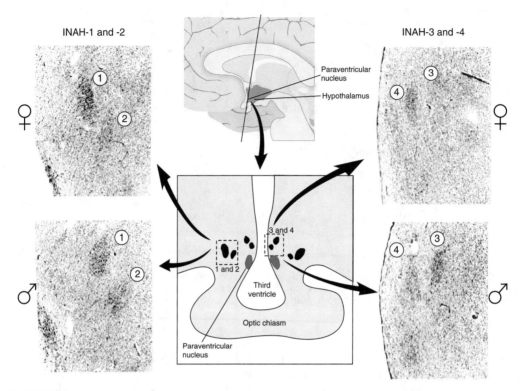

FIGURE 13.10 ● Representative micrographs showing the interstitial nuclei of the anterior hypothalamus for women (top) and men (bottom). Note that INAH numbers two and three are less distinct in the women. Micrographs (From Allen LS, Hines M, Shryne JE, et al. Two sexually dimorphic cell groups in the human brain. *J Neurosci.* 1989;9[2]:497–506.)

sexual behavior in adulthood requires activation by the sexual hormones.

TREATMENT: HOMOSEXUALITY

A few mental health professionals across the country offer treatment for individuals who want to be heterosexual rather than homosexual. Hardly any studies exist that establish the effectiveness of such treatment. However, Robert Spitzer has published a survey of 200 individuals who claim to have changed their sexual orientation. Many reported changing from predominantly or exclusively homosexual to predominantly heterosexual. Few reported complete changes. Is it possible that some motivated individuals were able to change their brain or were they not actually homosexual at the start? Only prospective studies will answer this controversial question.

PSYCHIATRIC DISORDERS
Cognitive Decline

There is considerable evidence that estrogens (and presumably testosterone) are neuroprotective. Figure 13.6 shows the robust increase in spine formation that can be induced by estrogen in hippocampal neurons. Presumably, such an

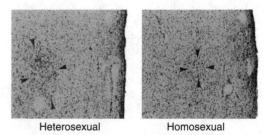

Heterosexual   Homosexual

FIGURE 13.11 ● Micrograph of interstitial nuclei of the anterior hypothalamus (*arrows*) of a heterosexual man on the left and a homosexual man on the right. (From LeVay S. A difference in hypothalamic structure between heterosexual and homosexual men. *Science.* 1991;253:1034–1037.) Reprinted with permission from AAAS.

arborization of the neurons enhances memory. Research with rodents and nonhuman primates demonstrates beneficial effects of estrogen on cognition. Multiple observational studies in humans have found that hormone replacement protects against the development of Alzheimer's disease, although there are other risks of continued hormone replacement.

Figure 13.12 is an example of one such observational study with humans. This was a study of more than 3,000 elderly people from one county in Utah. The objective was to test for the development of Alzheimer's disease and see if a history of hormone replacement therapy (HRT) was protective. Note that the men (who presumably maintain adequate levels of sex hormones) fare better than the women in terms of developing Alzheimer's disease. Likewise, the women who took HRT displayed a dose–response effect. That is, the longer a woman took HRT the less likely she was to develop Alzheimer's disease.

Unfortunately, the only large double-blind placebo-controlled trial of HRT for women (the Women's Health Initiative [WHI]) failed to find any beneficial effect from the hormones and actually showed some cognitive decline for those women taking estrogen and progestin. How can this be?

One intriguing explanation for the failure of the WHI to demonstrate neuroprotective benefits revolves around the age of the women in the study. The average age of the women in the study was 72, a full 20 years past the average age of menopause. Some speculate that HRT must be started within a critical period of time after the initiation of menopause, or the benefits are lost. Indeed, studies with animals have demonstrated preserved cognition when HRT was started shortly after ovariectomy, but not if delayed. Certainly,

a pattern we have seen with the brain and sex hormones is the importance of having the correct hormone available at the correct time.

Sexual Dysfunction

A survey of adults between the ages of 18 and 59 in the United States found a high prevalence of sexual dysfunction: 31% for men and 43% for women. The most common complaint for men was premature ejaculation whereas for women it was lack of interest. There are pharmacologic interventions available for premature ejaculation. For example, the selective serotonin reuptake inhibitors (SSRIs) make it harder to have an orgasm, although they are not U.S. Food and Drug Administration (FDA) approved for this indication.

Lack of interest in sex, on the other hand, is difficult to treat. Certainly the qualities of the relationship, secondary medical conditions, and the presence of other psychiatric disorders have strong influences on the joy of sex. Likewise loss of interest in sex is a feature of depression. However,

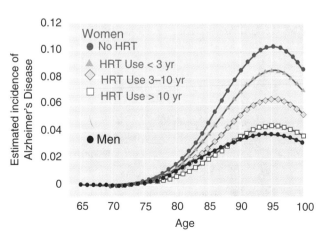

FIGURE 13.12 ● A prediction of the incidence of Alzheimer's disease calculated from data collected about men and women over 3 years shows the beneficial effects of sex hormones. HRT, hormone replacement therapy. (Adapted from Zandi PP, Carlson MC, Plassman BL, et al. HRT and incidence of Alzheimer's disease in older women: The Cache County Study. *JAMA.* 2002;288[17]:2123–2129.)

the prospect of giving a patient something legally sanctioned to enhance their sexual interest is currently not an option. The phosphodiesterase-5 inhibitors (e.g., Viagra) have been tested in large trials for female sexual dysfunction and failed to enhance interest any more than placebo. The testosterone patch, although effective for some patients, failed to win FDA approval owing to safety concerns.

Recent research suggests that α-melanocyte-stimulating hormone (α-MSH) may be, what some call, a genuine aphrodisiac. We mentioned in Chapter 8, Pain, that a large precursor neuropeptide in the pituitary gland, pro-opiomelanocortin (POMC), is cleaved to form active neuropeptides, which include ACTH, β-endorphin, and α-MSH (see Figure 13.13). α-MSH is the peptide that also causes the skin to darken in patients with Addison's disease and also suppresses appetite (see Chapter 10, Appetite). The story is told that a company was testing a melanocortin product as a possible tanning agent that did not require sun exposure. While it was being tested, it triggered erections in most of the men. Eureka! Subsequently, a peptide analog of α-MSH, called *bremelanotide*, was developed for study.

Recent research has shown that bremelanotide enhances female sexual solicitation in rats. The female rats displayed behavior one might call flirtatious—even climbing through little holes in the walls to get to the males. FDA studies of this product administered to humans as a nasal spray are under way. Anecdotal reports include men and women experiencing a rapid onset, with a warm feeling in the groin and a desire for sex.

It is not clear why the pituitary neuropeptide α-MSH enhances sexual interest. Studies in

which the medication was injected directly into a female rat's lateral ventricles increased solicitations establishing that its effects are mediated centrally. Additionally, α-MSH activated the Fos proteins (markers of gene expression) in the POA of the hypothalamus as well as the nucleus accumbens—areas that would be consistent with sexual pleasure.

Mood Disorders

The lifetime prevalence of mood disorders in women is approximately twice that of men. Although the cause of this difference remains undetermined, one possible explanation is the sex hormones—or more specifically, the fluctuation in sex hormones. Figure 13.14 shows the alterations in estrogen levels for a hypothetical woman across her lifespan. The times of greatest risk for mood disturbances are during times of fluctuating estrogen levels: menarche, premenstrual syndrome (PMS), postpartum, and perimenopausal.

The correlation between dropping sex hormones and depressive symptoms are not limited to women. The difference is that men typically have a stable testosterone level, so to find an effect we must look at times of dropping hormone levels. In one veterans administration (VA) study the researchers followed up the testosterone level and emergence of depressive illness in men older than 45 for 2 years. They found that 22% of the hypogonadal men (total testosterone <200 ng/dL) developed depression whereas only 7% of the eugonadal men did. Another group looked at the emergence of psychiatric symptoms in men treated for prostate cancer with reversible chemical castration. They found significant increases in anxiety and depression during the time when the testosterone levels dropped almost to zero.

Some of the most convincing data regarding the effects of sex hormones on mood have been treatment studies. Both with men and women, positive results have been shown for elevating depression when sex hormones were administered. Figure 13.15 shows two representative studies. These studies have many differences, but they both reveal improved mood with sex hormones.

The study on the left is on perimenopausal women who have mild or moderate depressive symptoms. One group was given placebo and the other estradiol. No antidepressants were used. The graph on the right was a study on men. This group of men had failed antidepressant therapy and had low or borderline testosterone levels. All participants remained on their antidepressant while one group received supplemental testosterone gel.

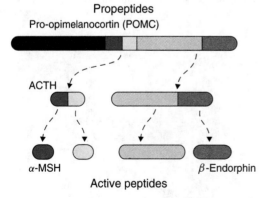

Propeptides
Pro-opimelanocortin (POMC)

ACTH

α-MSH β-Endorphin

Active peptides

FIGURE 13.13 ● The propeptide POMC is produced in the pituitary gland where it is cleaved to smaller active peptides such as ACTH, α-MSH, and β-endorphin.

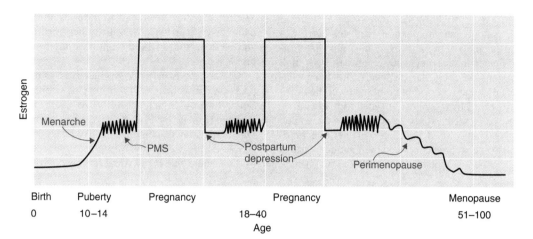

FIGURE 13.14 ● Estrogen levels fluctuate for women from puberty to menopause. The times of greatest vulnerability for depression occur when estrogen levels are changing. (Adapted from Stahl SM. *Essential psychopharmacology. Neuroscientific basis of practical applications*, 2nd ed. New York: Cambridge University Press; 2000.)

These are both small studies and need to be repeated with larger numbers. Likewise, it is important to remember that hormone replacement is not without significant risks. However, the studies demonstrate the powerful effects sex hormones can have on mood.

Throughout this chapter we have discussed the capacity of sex steroids to alter the brain and how this influences behavior. Traditionally, the prescription of hormone replacement has been for physical symptoms, and administered by medical physicians. In the future, mental health professionals may find themselves working closer with their medical colleagues to optimally treat a spectrum of emotional problems.

HOT FLASHES AND ANTIDEPRESSANTS

Some women want treatment for the hot flashes associated with menopause, but do not want HRT. The newer antidepressants have been shown to have some benefit. In the best study, the researchers felt that venlafaxine was clearly superior to placebo, but not as effective as estrogen. Their study stands as further evidence that mood and gonadal steroids are linked in ways that we are only beginning to understand.

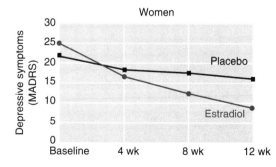

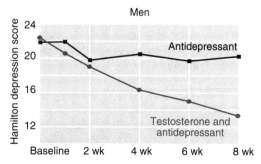

FIGURE 13.15 ● Two studies highlighting the mood-altering effects of sex hormones for women and men with sluggish gonads. (Left: Adapted from Soares CN, Almeida OP, Joffe H, et al. Efficacy of estradiol for the treatment of depressive disorders in perimenopausal women: A double-blind, randomized, placebo-controlled trial. *Arch Gen Psychiatry*. 2001;58[6]:529–534. Right: Adapted from Pope HG Jr, Cohane GH, Kanayama G, et al. Testosterone gel supplementation for men with refractory depression: A randomized, placebo-controlled trial. *Am J Psychiatry*. 2003;160[1]:105–111.)

Pregnancy and Depression

One can get the impression that sex hormones keep people happy. However, it is not that simple. For example, pregnancy, a time of very high estrogen and progesterone levels, has been conceptualized as a period of emotional well being—even protective against psychiatric disorders. However, a recent study was conducted on women with a history of depression who became pregnant. Some women continued their antidepressants while others stopped them during the pregnancy.

The relapse rates for depression during the pregnancy were 26% for those still on their medication and 68% for those who discontinued their antidepressants.

Clearly, pregnancy is not protective against depression for women with a history of depression. Some think the high levels of progesterone during pregnancy may have negative effects on mood. Others speculated about the negative effects of low BDNF during pregnancy. More research is needed to understand this paradoxical finding.

QUESTIONS

1. Female gonadal steroids include all of the following, except
   a. Testosterone.
   b. Estradiol.
   c. Progesterone.
   d. GnRH.

2. Many of the androgen effects in the brain are triggered by
   a. 17-β-Estradiol.
   b. 5-α-Dihydrotestosterone.
   c. Aromatase.
   d. α-Fetoprotein.

3. Which rat will display lordosis when primed with estrogens and progesterones and paired with a sexually active male?
   a. Males of normal pregnancies.
   b. Males exposed to androgens *in utero*.
   c. Females of normal pregnancies.
   d. Females exposed to androgens *in utero*.

4. Known effects of female sex hormones include all of the following, except
   a. Increased spine formation.
   b. Decreased risk of stroke.
   c. Increase γ-aminobutyric acid (GABA) inhibition.
   d. Gene transcription.

5. Evidence of sexual dimorphism in the vertebrate central nervous system (CNS) include all of the following, except
   a. SNB.
   b. The robust nucleus.

   c. SDN-POA.
   d. Paraventricular nucleus.

6. As suggested by some research, which area is smaller in homosexual men compared with heterosexual men?
   a. Interstitial nuclei of the anterior hypothalamus-1.
   b. Interstitial nuclei of the anterior hypothalamus-2.
   c. Interstitial nuclei of the anterior hypothalamus-3.
   d. Interstitial nuclei of the anterior hypothalamus-4.

7. The propeptide POMC is cleaved into all the following active peptides, except
   a. Δ-Fos.
   b. ACTH.
   c. α-MSH.
   d. β-Endorphin.

8. Evidence of the importance of sex hormones and mood includes all of the following except,
   a. PMS
   b. Athletes on anabolic steroids.
   c. Chemical castration for prostate cancer.
   d. Randomized controlled trials.

See Answers section at end of book.

Social Attachment

PARENTAL BEHAVIOR

The goal of reproduction is successful offspring. Parents want offspring who can survive the rigors of the world and produce their own descendents. Many animals produce offspring that require sustained assistance to successfully reach maturity. The particular actions that parents undertake to ensure the growth and survival of their offspring constitute *parental behavior.*

The extent of parental behavior in the animal kingdom occurs along a spectrum ranging from none to the extreme. Female salmons lay hundreds of eggs to be fertilized and then swim away. Humans are at the other end of the spectrum—investing many years of enormous resources, and perhaps hoping to be surrounded by their children until the very end.

Females in the animal kingdom do most of the parenting, although there are some exceptions. It is generally believed that males seek to fertilize as many eggs as possible whereas females seek to successfully raise the few they sire. Parental behavior constitutes any behavior that the parent does for the offspring. For example, a pregnant dog will build a nest a day or two before giving birth. After the delivery, she will lick them clean, eat the placentas, feed them, and keep them warm. Additionally, she will aggressively defend the pups against any suspicious intruders.

The onset of maternal behavior is remarkably precise. An inexperienced mother must immediately perform a full range of new behaviors without much room for error. How does this happen? Terkel and Rosenblatt established that there must be something in the blood that induces maternal

behavior. They transfused blood from a female rat that had just delivered to a virgin rat (see Figure 14.1). Within 24 hours, she was displaying maternal behavior.

Hormones

Biologic endocrinologists have spent considerable time and energy trying to tease this out. Although they have gotten close, there is still no definitive concoction of hormones that will immediately trigger maternal behavior in a nulliparous (virgin) rat. The leading culprits are estrogen, progesterone, and prolactin. An important ingredient appears to be the changing levels of the hormones. In Figure 14.2, note how the progesterone is seen to drop while the estrogen and prolactin raise in a rat just before delivery.

Oxytocin also plays some important role. Traditionally we conceptualize oxytocin as the neuropeptide released from the posterior pituitary into general circulation, which leads to uterine contractions and milk ejection (see Figure 6.4). Recent research has found receptors for oxytocin within the brain, establishing central actions for this neuropeptide. Indeed, injecting oxytocin directly into the lateral ventricles in a rat will induce maternal behavior in a hormone-primed virgin rat. More recently, it has been shown that oxytocin levels in the paraventricular nucleus (PVN) increase with maternal aggression. Likewise, infusion of synthetic oxytocin into the PVN also increases maternal aggression toward an intruder.

Further complicating this picture is the fact that hormones facilitate maternal behavior but are not required for it. Nulliparous rats will initially

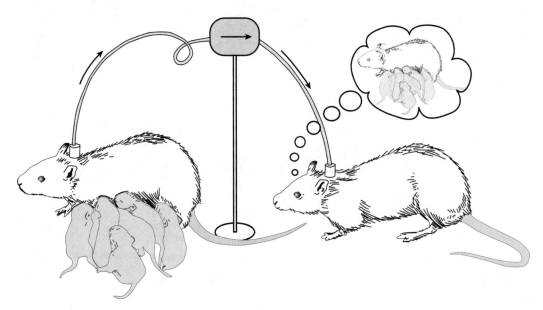

FIGURE 14.1 ● When nulliparous rats are transfused with blood from a new mother, they will display maternal behavior within 24 hours. (Adapted from Nelson RJ. *An introduction to behavioral endocrinology*, 3rd ed. Sunderland, MA: Sinauer; 2005.)

avoid new pups put into their cage. However, if exposed over a series of days (1 hour each day), they will respond maternally to the pups within 5 to 6 days. Pregnant rats will show similar avoidance until they have delivered. Once they have delivered, they will quickly display maternal behavior to any pup for the rest of their lives, proving that "once a mother, always a mother" (see Figure 14.3).

The Brain

Taken together, these studies suggest that the hormonal fluctuations late in pregnancy act on the brain to decrease fear or aversion and increase attraction or approach toward infants. Because maternal behavior persists once it is established, it is likely that the experience permanently changes some regions in the brain. An area that has been intensely studied is the one that we discussed in the last chapter (Chapter 13, Sex and the Brain): the preoptic area (POA) located in the anterior hypothalamus.

The POA is rich in estrogen, progesterone, prolactin, and oxytocin receptors, all of which increase during gestation. Lesions of the POA will disrupt maternal behavior. The POA appears

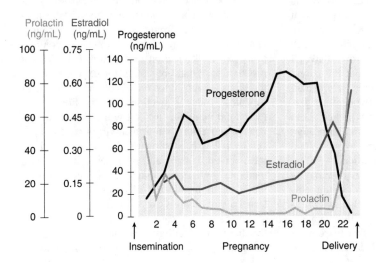

FIGURE 14.2 ● Blood levels of progesterone, estradiol, and prolactin in the pregnant rat. (Adapted from Rosenblatt JS, Siegel HI, Mayer AD. Blood levels of progesterone, estradiol and prolactin in pregnant rats. *Adv Study Behavior*. 1979;10:225–311.)

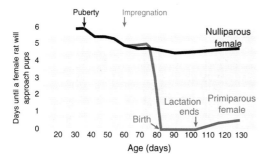

FIGURE 14.3 ● Female rats initially avoid pups. Several days of exposure are required for a nulliparous rat to display maternal behavior. Pregnant rats act similarly until after they deliver. (Adapted from Bridges RS. Endocrine regulation of parental behavior in rodents. In: Krasnegor NA, Bridges RS, eds. *Mammalian parenting: biochemical, neurobiological and behavioral determinants.* New York: Oxford University Press; 1990.)

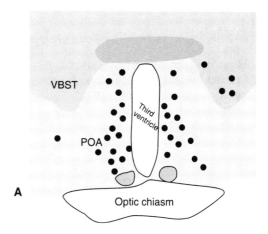

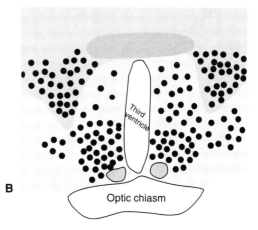

FIGURE 14.4 ● Hypothalamic region of post-partum rats exposed to candy (**A**) or newborn pups (**B**). Each dot represents five cells labeled with Fos activity. VBST, ventral bed nucleus of the terminalis; POA, preoptic area. (Adapted from Numan M, Sheehan TP. Neuroanatomical circuitry for mammalian maternal behavior. *Ann N Y Acad Sci.* 1997;807:101–125.)

to be a region that receives olfactory and somatosensory input and has projections to midbrain and brain stem nuclei. Numan and Sheehan describe an elegant experiment that demonstrates the central role of the POA with maternal behavior. Postpartum rats were exposed to either pups or candy for 2 hours. Then their brains were analyzed for the presence of the transcription factor Fos. (Fos is used as a general marker of brain cell activation.)

Figure 14.4 shows the results of the study. This is a slice through the forebrain which includes the anterior hypothalamus on either side of the ventricle. (For a human comparison, see Figure 13.10.) Note the increased activation in the POA as well as other regions of the rat exhibiting maternal behavior.

Dopamine

Up to this point, we have stressed the importance of gonadal steroids and neuropeptides in the development of maternal behavior, but the neurotransmitter dopamine also appears to play an important role. We discussed in Chapter 9, Pleasure, the activation of the orbitofrontal cortex (OFC) and the ventral tegmental/nucleus accumbens area (see Figure 9.3) in the experience of pleasure. Indeed, these areas are active in mothers.

One study scanned new mothers while they were looking at pictures of their own child and pictures of unfamiliar children. The mothers showed greater activation of the OFC when viewing their own child. With rats, researchers have found that mother rats will press a bar for access to pups the way they will press a bar for amphetamines or electrical stimulation. Additionally, pup exposure increases

the release of dopamine at the nucleus accumbens. Alternatively, dopamine blockers will impair maternal behavior (see box page 180). These studies give some neurobiologic explanations for the "joys of motherhood".

Licking and Grooming

This brings us to a series of studies from Michael Meaney's laboratory in McGill University, which may be some of the most important neuroscience studies for mental health professionals. Their studies tie together maternal behavior with lasting effects on the offspring's behavior, hypothalamic-pituitary-adrenal (HPA) axis, and even their DNA.

The story starts in the 1960s when researchers noted that pups "handled" once a day during the first

SCHIZOPHRENIA AND DOPAMINE BLOCKERS

Mothers who suffer from schizophrenia are known to be less involved with their children. They are generally more remote and less responsive during mother–infant play. This could be another example of the negative symptoms of the disorder. Worse yet, the problem can be exacerbated by the medications used to treat the patients.

In a recent study, Li et al. looked at the effect of injections of haloperidol, risperidone, and quetiapine on maternal behavior in rats. The antipsychotic medications inhibited maternal behaviors, such as nest building, pup licking, and pup retrieval. Figure shows the results for pup retrieval. Shortly after the injections, mothers failed to retrieve their own pups. Such studies suggest caution when treating human mothers with antipsychotic agents.

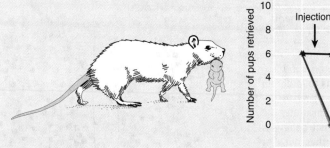
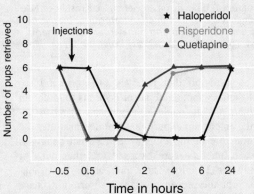

Antipsychotic medications disrupt a mother rat's tendency to retrieve her pups. (Adapted from Nelson RJ. *An introduction to behavioral endocrinology*, 3rd ed. Sunderland, MA: Sinauer; 2005 and Li M, Davidson P, Budin R, et al. Effects of typical and atypical antipsychotic drugs on maternal behavior in postpartum female rats. *Schizophr Res.* 2004;70[1]:69–80.)

weeks of life showed a reduced adenocorticotropic hormone (ACTH) and corticosterone response to stress. Later it was established that it was not the "handling" *per se* that produced this effect, but the mother's increased licking of the pups when they were returned to the nest. The mothers were simply trying to get the human odor off their pups and this extra attention to the pups resulted in their improved response to stress when they grew up to be adults.

Meaney discovered naturally occurring strains of rats that licked and groomed their pups at different rates. This particular behavior occurs when the mother rat enters the nest and gathers her pups around her for nursing. She will intermittently lick and groom the pups as they nurse. Meaney named one group the high lick and groom (high L and G) mothers and the other the low lick and groom (low L and G) mothers.

In a flurry of experiments in Meaney's laboratory, it was established that high L and G mothers produced offspring with subtle but significantly different brains. After 20 minutes of restraint (very stressful for a rodent), the rats from high L and G mothers secrete less corticosterone (see Figure 14.5A). They also produce less corticotrophin-releasing hormone messenger RNA (CRH-mRNA) in the hypothalamus (Figure 14.5B). Additionally, the amount of maternal licking and grooming correlates with the number of glucocorticoid receptors in the hippocampus (Figure 14.5C). Perhaps most significantly, the pups from a high L and G mother show a great willingness to explore novel environments as adults.

In summary, the mothers, increased attention somehow enhances the sensitivity of the HPA axis. Offspring of attentive high licking mothers demonstrate greater negative feedback to the hypothalamus by way of the increased glucocorticoid receptors, which inhibits CRH production and corticosterone release. Ultimately these offspring show greater resilience and less fear.

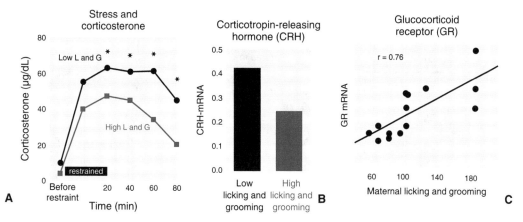

FIGURE 14.5 ● Rats raised by a mother with a high frequency of licking and grooming behavior show a more modest corticosterone release in response to stress (**A**), less corticotrophin-releasing hormone messenger RNA (CRH-mRNA) (**B**), and greater glucocorticoid receptors (GR) in the hippocampus. (**C**) The correlation between glucocorticoid receptors and licking and grooming by the mother. (Adapted from Liu D, Diorio J, Tannenbaum B, et al. Maternal care, hippocampal glucocorticoid receptors, and hypothalamic-pituitary-adrenal responses to stress. *Science*. 1997;277[5332]:1659–1662.)

Trading places

In a follow-up study, Meaney et al. switched some of the mothers and pups. That is, pups from high L and G mothers were raised by low L and G mothers and vice versa. The results were stunning and show how behaviors and patterns emerge from combinations of genetic predisposition and environment. Figure 14.6 shows the behavior of the female rats once they matured. They were more inclined to explore an open area and provided greater licking and grooming to their own pups. Note how the determining factor is not the genetic make-up, but the nurturing behavior of the mother that raised them. In other words, a low L and G female will become a high L and G mother if she is raised by a high L and G mother. So the behavior can be passed from generation to generation, but does not come from the DNA.

Effect on the DNA

Meaney and his group have taken this knowledge to the next level by searching for the mechanisms that sustain the effects of the maternal behavior over the lifespan of the pup. To understand what they have

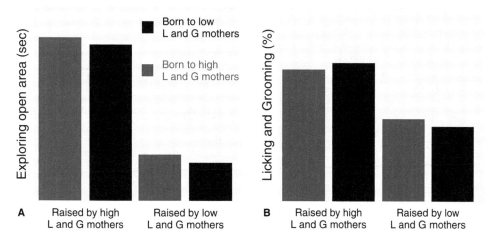

FIGURE 14.6 ● Female rats raised by mothers who were high lickers and groomers are less anxious in an open area (**A**) and are more likely to be high lickers and groomers when raising their own pups (**B**)—regardless of their genetic lineage. L and G, lick and groom. (Adapted from Francis D, Diorio J, Liu D, et al. Nongenomic transmission across generations of maternal behavior and stress responses in the rat. *Science*. 1999;286[5442]:1155–1158.)

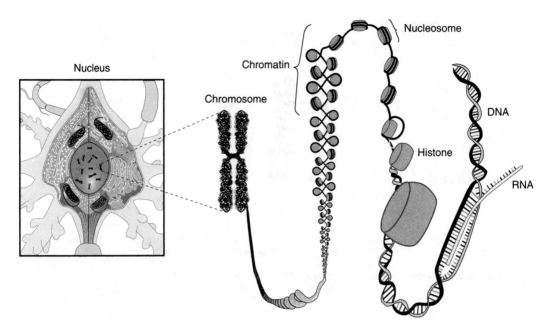

FIGURE 14.7 ● Packaging of the DNA involves wrapping around histones and folding into structures called *chromatin*. Unfolding of the packaging is required for gene expression.

discovered, we must first review some aspects of how the DNA is managed in the nucleus.

The DNA from each of our 46 chromosomes is actually one long strand of a double-helix fiber that would measure approximately a meter if laid end to end. The cell must package these strands into the nucleus of the cell (see Figure 14.7). This is accomplished by the addition of dense proteins called *histones*. The DNA, which is negatively charged, wraps around a series of histones that which are positively charged. These "beads on a string" are then folded into a compact structure called *chromatin*. The chromatin is further coiled and folded to form the chromosome.

The histones do more than just package the DNA. They also regulate gene expression. DNA is inaccessible to regulatory signals when it is folded in its chromatin structure. The activation of the gene and the transcription of RNA require the unfolding of the chromatin and the unwrapping of the histone. Transcription factors cannot transcribe RNA from the DNA they cannot get to.

Another mechanism that alters the chromatin structure and consequently limits gene expression is DNA methylation. *DNA methylation* involves the addition of a methyl group to the cytosine nucleotide (see Figure 14.8A). Genes that contain high frequencies of methylation are silenced. The methyl groups appear to limit the ability of the transcriptional factors to lock on to the DNA (Figure 14.8B).

One can think of this as "gumming-up" the machinery, thereby closing up the book. You can't read the information on the pages when the DNA has been methylated.

Meaney's group identified a section of the rat DNA that encodes for hippocampal glucocorticoid receptor. Looking specifically at the promoter region of the DNA—the region where the transcription starts—they analyzed methylation of the cytosine nucleotide at this site. Figure 14.9(A) shows that almost all of the low L and G group had methylation at this promoter region whereas the high L and G group had almost none.

The next step is almost unbelievable. The researchers administered directly into the cerebral ventricles an inhibitor (trichostatin A) that results in demethylation of the DNA (Figure 14.9B). When analyzed, these rats displayed less methylation of their DNA and greater numbers of glucocorticoid receptors. Furthermore, when stressed, these animals showed a modest HPA response (Figure 14.9C); that is, their corticosterone levels become indistinguishable from those of rats raised by a high L and G mother.

The implications from these studies are profound. We can now trace from a mother's behavior all the way to the offspring's DNA. If we can find ways to cleanse the DNA, we might be able to correct the problem, not just treat symptoms. However, it is important to note that although demethylation may be the treatment of the future,

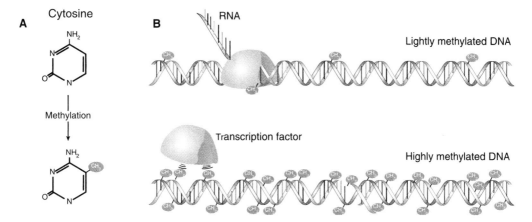

FIGURE 14.8 ● DNA methylation entails the addition of a methyl group to the nucleotide cytosine (A). A high frequency of methylation prevents the transcription of the DNA and silences the gene (B).

it is not without risks. Some cancers are believed to result from demethylation of gene sequences that are better left silenced.

The topic of methylated DNA will come up again in Chapter 18, Depression, but the recently published findings from the Star*D trials are worth mentioning. They found that successfully treating mothers with depression affected the psychiatric condition of their children. That is, the children of mothers who achieved remission had decreases in anxiety, depression, and behavioral disorders. Conversely, the psychiatric status worsened in the children with mothers who failed to achieve remission. Does treating a depressed mother affect the DNA of her children? To the degree that we

are similar to rats (and we are both mammals), the answer is probably yes.

PAIR BONDING

The attraction between men and women is a special form of social attachment. Not only is it required for sexual reproduction, but also for the formation of a lasting pair bond that is advantageous for reproductive success. Surprisingly, monogamous pair bonds are rare among mammals: approximately 5%. Monogamy is much more common among birds. The unusual bonding and rebonding that is common with humans might be best described as serial monogamy. What parts of the brain drive the affiliation of males and females?

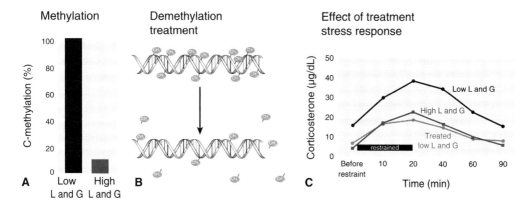

FIGURE 14.9 ● Pups raised by low lick and groom (L and G) mothers have greater methylation of the DNA on the promoter region that transcribes glucocorticoid receptors (A). The inhibitor removes the methyl groups (B). Rats from low L and G mothers who have been treated with the inhibitor display a normal hypothalamic-pituitary-adrenal response to stress (C). ((A) and (C) Adapted from Weaver IC, Cervoni N, Champagne FA, et al. Epigenetic programming by maternal behavior. *Nat Neurosci.* 2004;7[8]:847–854.)

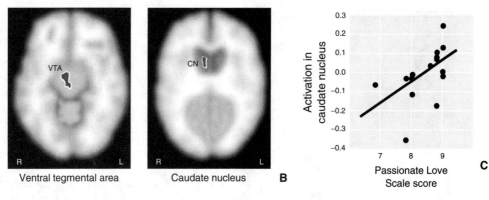

FIGURE 14.10 ● Subjects intensely in love show activity in the ventral tegmental area (VTA) and caudate nucleus (CN) when looking at pictures of their lover **(A and B)**. Activity in the CN correlated with scores on the Passionate Love Scale **(C)**. (Adapted from Aron A, Fisher H, Mashek DJ, et al. Reward, motivation, and emotion systems associated with early-stage intense romantic love. *J Neurophysiol.* 2005;94[1]:327–337.)

Romantic Love and Dopamine

Romantic love is a universal human experience. The feeling of attraction that one person may feel for another can be intense, all-consuming, and difficult to control. A person in love feels euphoric. A spurned lover is despondent and even violent. The obsessional thinking and the willingness to "cross mountains" to be with a lover suggest the activation of the brains reward system (see Figure 9.6) when one is in love.

Anthropologist Helen Fisher at Rutgers University has spent her career studying the science of love. Recently, she and her colleagues completed imaging the brains of people who were "intensely in love". The researchers alternatively showed pictures of their beloved one or a neutral individual to the subjects while they were being scanned, and compared the difference. As expected, the images of the beloved lit up the ventral tegmental area (VTA) (see Figure 14.10A). As we discussed in Chapter 9, Pleasure, the VTA is a dopamine-rich area with projections to the nucleus accumbens. These are the subcortical regions that mediate motivation and reward.

Another area activated in the study was the caudate nucleus (CN) (Figure 14.10B). This is the area that is also active in obsessive-compulsive disorder. Furthermore, activity in the CN correlated with the total score from a test of the subject's feelings: the Passionate Love Scale. Consequently, in simple terms we can conceptualize love as both an addiction and an obsession.

Growth Factors

A group in Italy—a country that knows a thing or two about romance—studied growth factors in subjects who had recently fallen in love. They

speculated that nerve growth factors (NGFs) might be activated when people experience romantic feelings. They drew blood from subjects who fell recently "in love" and couples in long-lasting relationships. They measured the values of four growth factors. Only one—NGF—was significantly higher in the subjects recently in love. Moreover, there was a positive correlation between the level of NGF and the subject's score on the Passionate Love Scale.

Of particular interest, the researchers re-examined the levels of NGF a year or two later in the subjects in love. They found that the levels of NGF had dropped back to the levels seen in the control group (see Figure 14.11). This is a neuroendocrine example of what we all know: the honeymoon does not last. It is another example that the brain does not tolerate euphoria for too long. However, if the pleasure wanes, why do we stay in a relationship? In addition to psychological and practical answers, it may be that other neuropeptides kick-in. Work with voles (discussed next) may shed some light on this.

Vasopressin

The vole is a rodent that looks like a plump mouse, but is related to the lemming. They are common in the grassy fields of North America. Voles are relevant to our discussion because of their diversity in forming pair bonds. For example, the *prairie vole* will form enduring pair bonds and mutually care for the offspring. In nature, most prairie voles which lose a mate never take on another partner. The closely related *meadow vole,* on the other hand, is socially promiscuous and does not display biparental care.

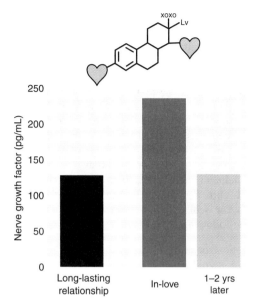

FIGURE 14.11 ● Nerve growth factor (NGF) in subjects in long-lasting relationships, subjects actively "in love," and these same subjects a year or two later. The hearts on the NGF molecule are the authors' license.

In the laboratory, researchers have observed that prairie vole males prefer to spend time next to their partners: called *huddling* (see Figure 14.12A). The meadow vole, on the other hand, is more independent. With the proper arrangements, this behavior can be measured and quantitated (Figure 14.12B).

Vasopressin has emerged as a critical neuropeptide mediating the pair bond formation in male voles. Infusion of vasopressin into the male cerebral ventricles accelerated pair bond formation. Likewise, infusion of a vasopressin antagonist prevents pair bond formation. Furthermore, differences in expressions of the vasopressin receptor can be demonstrated in the two species of voles (Figure 14.12C). The prairie vole has significantly more receptors in the ventral pallidum (VP).

In a study that seems like something out of a science fiction novel, Young et al. have increased partner preference in meadow voles. They used a viral vector to transplant into the VP of meadow voles the segment of DNA that encodes for the vasopressin receptor. This resulted in increased expression of vasopressin receptors. The usually solitary meadow voles now were huddling with their partners. In essence, they changed a male from being promiscuous into being monogamous. (Won't the social conservatives be thrilled?)

Oxytocin

Female vole partner preference, on the other hand, is mediated by *oxytocin*. Infusion of oxytocin directly into the cerebral ventricles will accelerate pair bonding formation. Conversely, infusion of an oxytocin antagonist will block the development of this behavior.

The relevance of oxytocin in humans is of great interest, but little about it is known. One recent study measured the level of oxytocin in

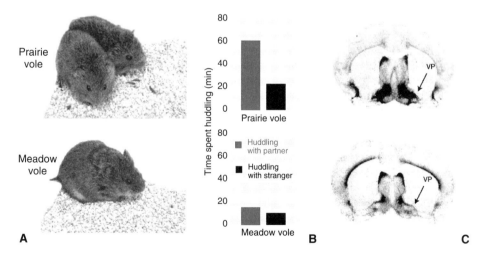

FIGURE 14.12 ● The male prairie vole will spend more time huddling with his partner than will the meadow vole **(A and B)**. The difference in vasopressin receptors (dark areas in **(C)**) in the ventral pallidum (VP) may explain the difference in this behavior. (From Lim MM, Wang Z, Olazabal DE, et al. Enhanced partner preference in a promiscuous species by manipulating the expression of a single gene. *Nature.* 2004;429:754–757.)

couples after a brief period of warm contact. Oxytocin levels increased in women after the contact, but not in men. Furthermore, women with greater partner support showed greater increases in oxytocin levels. In another experiment the researchers gave one group of students intranasal oxytocin and the other group placebo. The group that got oxytocin displayed more trust and readiness to tolerate social risk when playing an investment game with real monetary exchange. These studies suggest that we are just beginning to understand the important role of oxytocin with affiliative behavior.

Enduring Bonds

A simple explanation of human male–female affiliation is that it starts with dopamine and the pleasure centers of the brain. We speculate that other neuroendocrine systems such as oxytocin and vasopressin may then take over to ensure enduring pair bond formation once "the thrill is gone." While there is no data to support this as yet, data from twin studies suggest that the propensity to divorce is more biologically determined than traditionally thought. For monozygotic twins, when one is divorced the odds ratio for the other twin also divorcing is 5.6. With dizygotic twins the same odds ratio is 1.6—a three-fold difference. We wonder if those individuals who are prone to jumping from one relationship to another are genetically less endowed with the neuropeptides of attachment.

DISCONNECTED

Affiliation and pair bonding are on one end of the social attachment spectrum. On the other end are those individuals who are isolated and disconnected—individuals who are aloof, distant, and fail to derive pleasure from social interactions. The Unabomber is an extreme example of this sort of person. A graduate of Harvard, with a Ph.D. in mathematics, he lived alone for 16 years in a 10 foot by 12 foot cabin in the woods of Montana without electricity or plumbing. A psychiatrist conducting a court evaluation of the Unabomber gave him a provisional diagnosis of schizophrenia.

The schizophrenic spectrum disorders include the following:

- Schizotypal personality disorder
- Schizoid personality disorder
- Delusional disorder
- Schizoaffective disorder
- Schizophrenia

These comprise a large percentage of the cases of severely disconnected individuals seen in most clinical practices. Impairment in social interaction can be seen as being part of the negative signs of the schizophrenic spectrum (more on this in Chapter 20, Schizophrenia.) The behavioral similarities between the schizophrenia spectrum disorders and animal models of impaired bonding are apparent. Despite this, there is very little known about the neuroanatomic deficits, if any, in these systems in schizoid patients.

TEND-AND-BEFRIEND

Fight-or-flight has been the prevailing model to describe the mammalian response to stress. That is, stress causes a hormonal cascade that produces secretion of catecholamines and the organism either fights or retreats. Taylor has proposed that this model is male centric and does not describe how females cope in difficult times. Taylor believes females respond to stress by nurturing others and enhancing their social network. What she calls "tend-and-befriend". Although the neuroendocrine mechanisms are the same, the behavior is different. In fact, the gender difference in affiliation is one of the most robust findings in human behavioral research.

Engh et al., provide an example from a free ranging troop of baboons in Africa that they have been following. They have observed and recorded grooming behavior among the females. More recently they have also been measuring glucocorticoid levels from the feces. They found that females who lost a close relative experienced a significant increase in glucocorticoid levels after the death. However, they did not experience a decrease in their grooming although they had lost their close partner. Instead, other associations were established and the rate of grooming remained stable. The authors speculated that this social networking might modulate the stress response.

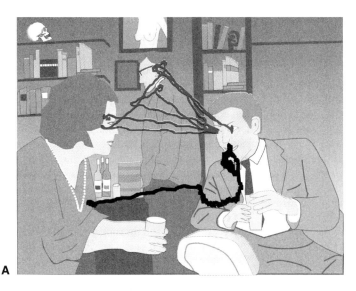

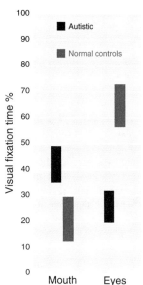

FIGURE 14.13 ● A drawing of a scene from "Who's Afraid of Virginia Woolf" shows the different aspects of the movie that subjects with autism (black) and normal controls (brown) track with their eyes (**A**). A study comparing 15 patients with autism and 15 controls demonstrated significant differences in time spent observing the eyes and mouths from similar film clips (**B**). (Adapted from Klin A, Jones W, Schultz R, et al. Visual fixation patterns during viewing of naturalistic social situations as predictors of social competence in individuals with autism. *Arch Gen Psychiatry.* 2002;59[9]:809–816. and Klin A, Jones W, Schultz R, et al. Defining and quantifying the social phenotype in autism. *Am J Psychiatry.* 2002;159[6]:895–908.)

Autism Spectrum

Kanner first described autism in 1943 at Johns Hopkins University. We now envision autism as anchoring the more extreme end of a spectrum of disorders characterized by the following:

- Severe social dysfunctions
- Early communication failure
- Presence of repetitive, rigid, and stereotypic behaviors

Asperger's disorder and childhood disintegrative disorder are other conditions in the autism spectrum which are believed to share common biologic foundations. These conditions may simply be a less severe form of the underlying disorder.

The social dysfunctions constitute the core deficits of the disorders. The inability to understand other people's feelings and a failure to establish reciprocal relationships emerge early in those with autism. Robert Schultz et al. at Yale have developed techniques to study this aspect of autism. They used eye-tracking technology to study spontaneous viewing patterns while watching video clips of complex social situations. They showed clips from the 1967 movie "Who's Afraid of Virginia Woolf?" to subjects with autism and to age- and IQ-matched normal controls.

Figure 14.13 shows a drawing of one scene from the movie. In the foreground, two adults lean toward each other in a flirtatious interchange. The woman's husband is in the background, silent, but irritated by his wife's behavior. The eye movements from a control (brown) and an autistic subject (black) are collapsed onto this one still scene. Note how the control subject focuses on the eyes of the actors. Additionally, the control's focus moves from face to face, literally outlining the charged social triangle.

The autistic subject, on the other hand, attends to less relevant aspects of the scene. This subject displays the following three findings commonly seen in subjects with autism:

- Avoidance of the eyes
- Focus on the mouth
- Preferential attention to objects rather than people

Clearly, this method of observation fails to gather the subtle social cues that are essential to understand the thoughts and feelings of other people. A quantitative assessment of the subject's visual fixation on the eyes and mouths is shown in the graph on the right side of Figure 14.13. Note the dramatic separation between the groups with regard to eye fixation. A finding this large is seldom found in behavioral studies.

Brain Size

The underlying neuroanatomic abnormalities of autism remain unknown. One consistent finding has been enlarged brain volume. In a recent meta-analysis, Redcay and Courchesne collected studies measuring head circumference and brain size with magnetic resonance imaging (MRI). They calculated the percent difference from the normal for each study so that the measurements could be compared. The results are plotted by age in Figure 14.14. The authors noted that for autism the brain size is initially reduced, dramatically increases within the first year of life, but then returns to the normal range by adulthood. These findings show a period of pathologic brain growth in autism that is largely restricted to the first year of life.

The phenomenon of abnormal growth in the first years of life mirrors what some parents have reported about their children. Namely, that they appeared to be developing normally for the first 15 to 24 months and then showed a regression in social and/or communication skills. In a clever use of technology, Werner and Dawson got blinded observers to review home video tapes of autistic children who were reported to have regressed. Indeed, they noted normal social attention and word babble at 12 months of age, but displayed significant impairment by 24 months. This was in contrast to the group of children with early onset autism who showed impairment at 12 and 24 months of age.

Mirror Neurons

Mirror neurons were discovered in one of those serendipitous scientific moments. Researchers in Italy placed an electrode in a neuron in a monkey's motor cortex and noted that it was active when he grabbed an object. Much to their amazement it also became active when the monkey watched someone else grabbing the same object. With further work, they discovered that neurons have a variety of specific functions. The ones that responded to an action and when observing the same action were termed *mirror neurons* by them. Figure 14.15 shows an example of a mirror neuron. Note that the neuron is active both when a human (a) grasps the object and when the monkey grasps the same object. However, the mirroring does not translate to all actions. If the object is grasped with pliers, the neuron does not become active.

Functional imaging studies on humans have also demonstrated mirroring. For example, a person moving a finger or observing a finger move will show similar activity in the same region of the motor cortex. Another study looked for mirroring with facial expressions. In this study, subjects were shown pictures of people displaying emotional expressions (happy, sad, angry, etc.). The subjects were instructed to either imitate the expression or just observe the picture. Figure 14.16 shows that imitating the expression and just observing it generated similar activity in the premotor region of the cortex, as measured by the functional MRI.

Additional research by this same group has identified a network of neurons connecting the frontal, parietal, and temporal lobes (see Figure 14.17). Furthermore, they found that imitating emotional facial expressions not only activated this network, but

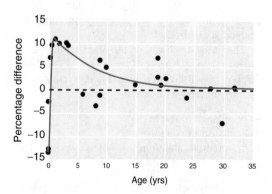

FIGURE 14.14 ● A meta-analysis of brain measurements including head circumference and MRI scans are plotted by percent difference from norm and age. (Adapted from Redcay E, Courchesne E. When is the brain enlarged in autism? A meta-analysis of all brain size reports. *Biol Psychiatry*. 2005;58[1]:1–9.)

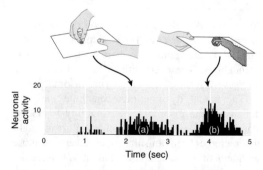

FIGURE 14.15 ● A neuron in the premotor cortex of a monkey is active when it observes a food morsel grasped by a human (A). The same neuron is active when the monkey grasps the morsel (B) (Adapted from Rizzolatti G, Fogassi L, Gallese V. Neurophysiological mechanisms underlying the understanding and imitation of action. *Nat Rev Neurosci*. 2001;2[9]:661–670.)

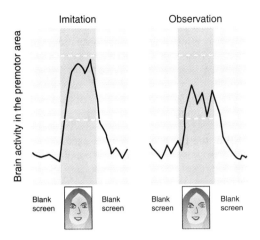

FIGURE 14.16 ● Activity in the facial region of the motor cortex is similar, as measured by functional MRI (fMRI), when subjects are imitating a facial expression or just observing it. (Adapted from Carr L, Iacoboni M, Dubeau MC, et al. Neural mechanisms of empathy in humans: A relay from neural systems for imitation to limbic areas. *Proc Natl Acad Sci USA*. 2003;100[9]:5497–5502.)

also activated the emotional centers of the brain, such as the insula and amygdala. The capacity to reflect another person's emotions may be the neuronal mechanism facilitating empathy.

Dysfunction of the mirror neuronal network may underlie the lack of empathy in patients with autism. To test this hypothesis, researchers conducted similar facial imitation and observation studies with high functioning autistic children and normally developing children matched for age and IQ. Their results showed a marked decrease in activation of the mirror neuronal network in the children with autism, particularly in the frontal cortex (see Figure 14.18A, B). Additional analysis

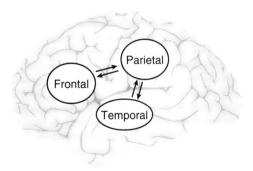

FIGURE 14.17 ● A schematic diagram of the neuronal network of imitation. (Adapted from Iacoboni M. Neural mechanisms of imitation. *Curr Opin Neurobiol*. 2005;15[6]:632–637.)

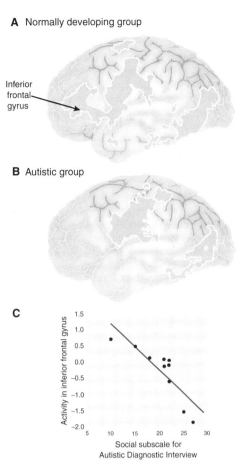

FIGURE 14.18 ● Functional magnetic resonance imaging studies for normally developing preteens compared to high functioning age/IQ-matched subjects with autism while imitating emotional facial expressions. The subjects with autism show less activity of the mirror neuronal network, particularly in the frontal cortex. (Adapted from Dapretto M, Davies MS, Pfeifer JH, et al. Understanding emotions in others: Mirror neuron dysfunction in children with autism spectrum disorders. *Nat Neurosci*. 2006;9[1]:28–30.)

showed that activity in the frontal cortex during the study correlated with the score on the social subscale of the Autistic Diagnostic Interview (Figure 14.18C).

The propensity to empathize with other's feelings is one of the central features of human social interactions. Individuals with autism are impaired in this ability. Failing to understand the emotions in others may be a result of deficient mirror neurons in patients with autism spectrum disorders. Whether this neuronal failure is the central deficit of the disorder, a downstream effect of some other problem, or just one of a host of deficits, remains to be determined.

QUESTIONS

1. Which combination of hormones is believed to trigger maternal behavior in rats just before delivery?
   a. Rising progesterone and rising estradiol.
   b. Rising progesterone and falling estradiol.
   c. Falling progesterone and rising estradiol.
   d. Falling progesterone and falling estradiol.

2. Oxytocin receptors are found in all of the following, except
   a. Uterus.
   b. PVN.
   c. POA.
   d. Optic chiasm.

3. Pups born to mothers who are high lickers and groomers show
   a. Increased reluctance to explore a novel environment.
   b. Increased glucocorticoid receptors in the hippocampus.
   c. Increased CRH during stress.
   d. Increased corticosterone when restrained.

4. Lightly methylated DNA
   a. Allows greater access to transcription factors.
   b. Results in greater glucocorticoid response to stress.
   c. Decreases gene expression.
   d. Is induced by mothers with low licking and grooming behavior.

5. Romantic love has a strong correlation with activity in the
   a. VTA.
   b. CN.
   c. Nucleus accumbens.
   d. Amygdala.

6. All of the following are false, except
   a. Vasopressin promotes pair bonding in male voles.
   b. Meadow voles have more vasopressin.
   c. Transplanting oxytocin receptors induces monogamous behavior in male voles.
   d. Tend-and-befriend behavior modulates dips in oxytocin.

7. Eye-tracking studies have shown that autistic subjects
   a. Focus on the eyes.
   b. Avoid looking at objects.
   c. Attend to the subtle social cues.
   d. Prefer to look at the lower face.

8. All of the following are true about mirror neurons, except
   a. They play a role in empathy.
   b. They are impaired in autism.
   c. The fronto-subcortical network is the most active.
   d. Frontal mirror neurons inactivity correlates with social impairment in autism.

See Answers section at end of book.

Memory

The next three chapters will review important aspects of cognition. *Cognition* is loosely defined as the ability to do the following:

- Attend to external or internal stimuli
- Identify the significance of the stimuli
- Respond appropriately

This complex processing takes place in the cortices of the brain. It occurs between the arrival of sensory input and the behavioral reaction. In the next two chapters we will discuss intelligence and attention. Here we will start with memory.

The ability to store information and retrieve it later is one of the most fascinating aspects of the brain. Indeed, research into learning and memory were some of the first experiments in psychology and continue to be aggressively studied in modern neuroscience. *Learning* is defined as new information acquired by the nervous system and observed through behavioral changes. *Memory* describes encoding, storage, and retrieval of learned information.

TYPES OF MEMORY

Experts in memory have identified different types and subtypes of memory. Many of these subtle distinctions are not relevant for our purposes. One important distinction is separating memory of details from learning procedures. The facts we learn in school or historic events from our lives are called *declarative memory* (also called *explicit memory*). This is usually what people are referring to when they speak of memory.

Another type of memory is *nondeclarative memory* (also called *implicit memory*). It describes the process of learning a skill or making associations. Examples include learning to ride a bike or playing an instrument. This type of memory is outside the conscious thought and actually can deteriorate if one concentrates too hard. Another example includes the exaggerated startle response seen with post-traumatic stress disorder (PTSD). This reaction is immediate and takes place before the subject is consciously aware of the stimulus.

The importance of separating declarative from nondeclarative memory is that these two types of memory are encoded through different mechanisms in the brain. Likewise, they are disrupted by different central nervous system (CNS) lesions or disorders—more on this later.

Immediate, Short, and Long

Memories begin to decay as soon as they are formed. The temporal stages of retention are divided into immediate, short-term, and long-term (see Figure 15.1). These are the stages we test in a comprehensive mental status examination. *Immediate memory* describes the ability to hold a few new facts in mind for a matter of seconds. Looking up a new phone number and successfully dialing the number within seconds is an example of this. We test this function when we ask a person to repeat three objects immediately. Another test of immediate memory is asking a patient to repeat a series of numbers. Surprisingly, the maximum "digit span" successfully repeated is seven plus or minus two.

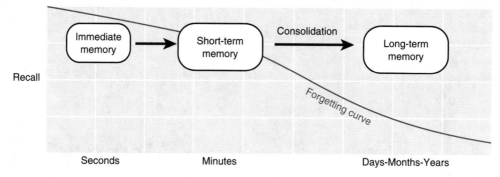

FIGURE 15.1 ● The temporal stages of memory superimposed on a hypothetical curve of memory retention.

Short-term memory describes those memories that exist from seconds to minutes. An example of this process is searching the house for a lost item and remembering where you have looked. We test this process when we ask a patient to repeat three objects at 5 minutes. Both immediate and short-term memories are vulnerable to disruption.

Long-term memories are enduring representations that last for days, months, and years: the historic events and facts of our lives. This requires the development of a more permanent form of storage. The process of moving information from immediate and short-term into long-term memories is called *consolidation*. The physical representation of memories and the areas of the brain dedicated to this function are the focus of the rest of this chapter.

Amnesia

There are two types of amnesia: retrograde and antegrade. *Retrograde amnesia* describes the loss of memory before the event. *Antegrade amnesia* is the inability to store memories after the event. Diagnostic and Statistical Manual (DSM) Mental Disorder has a specific category called *Amnestic*

Disorder. Although commonly occurring in the movies, it is almost impossible to find a true case of idiopathic global amnesia, as depicted by Hollywood, in a mental health setting. Alcohol and Alzheimer's disease are the most common causes of amnesia and are excluded as a cause in amnestic disorder.

CELLULAR MECHANISMS

The Canadian psychologist Donald O. Hebb proposed in 1949 that some changes must take place between two neurons for memories to develop. He wrote as follows:

> When an axon of cell A is near enough to excite a cell B and repeatedly or persistently takes part in firing it, some growth process or metabolic change takes place in one or both cells such that A's efficacy, as one of the cells firing B is increased.

This has come to be called *Hebb's Postulate* and can be more easily stated like this: neurons that fire together, wire together. Almost 60 years of research has affirmed that the brain changes with learning and experience.

ALCOHOLIC BLACKOUTS

Alcoholic blackouts occur when someone has consumed too much alcohol and awakens without memories of what happened the night before. It is believed that the high blood level of alcohol disrupts the consolidation of short-term memories into long-term memories. The drinker failed to preserve lasting images of the party because long-term memories were never formed. This can happen with short-acting hypnotics and benzodiazepines as well.

Amazingly, memories formed before drinking are actually enhanced by alcohol. That is, drinking after learning actually improves recall compared to not drinking. It is possible that memories already consolidated are stored in a more pristine state, because there is less interference from new memories during intoxication.

Long-Term Potentiation

In Chapter 5, Receptors and Signaling the Nucleus, we have discussed long-term potentiation (LTP), which serves as a model for memory formation. In summary, they are as follows:

- A series of rapid signals between two neurons results in a greater stimulus in the postsynaptic neuron when normal activity resumes (see Figure 5.6).
- Increased activity between two glutamate neurons will open the N-methyl-D-aspartate (NMDA) receptor, which results in molecular signals to the nucleus that induce gene expression (see Figure 5.7).
- Gene expression results in structural changes on the neuron such as spine formation on the dendrites (see Figure 5.8).

Protein Synthesis

LTP is simply a laboratory mechanism to study memory, but it appears to follow the same principles that occur with actual memories. Specifically, it has been shown that gene expression and protein synthesis are required for long-term memory formation in mammals. For example, a rat can be taught to quickly find a submerged platform to stand on in a tub of water—called a *water maze* (see Figure 15.2A, B). However, if one group of rats is given intraventricular injections of the protein synthesis inhibitor *anisomycin* 20 minutes before each test, they cannot remember the location of the submerged platform from one session to the next. These rats spend about the same amount of time each day trying to find the submerged platform (Figure 15.2C). Anisomycin inhibits the production of proteins that are needed to consolidate short-term memories into long-term memories.

Extinction

Extinction is the gradual reduction in the response to a feared stimulus when the stimulus is repeatedly encountered without an adverse experience. For example, a person who is afraid of bridges will have a reduction in fear if they repeatedly cross the bridge without falling off or the bridge collapsing. Extinction is the bedrock of behavioral therapy and one of the most effective treatments for anxiety disorders.

Several lines of evidence suggest that extinction is accomplished through the development of new memories rather than erasing the old memories. Studies have established this by looking at the effect of anisomycin on extinction. Rats given intraventricular injections of anisomycin before repeated exposure to a stimulus (without the negative consequences) fail to show extinction the following day. In other words, they did not remember what they had learned the previous day.

Faster Extinction?

Would faster learning during extinction therapy improve the effectiveness of exposure and response prevention therapy? A group at Emory University is studying just this possibility. Using the understanding of how memories are formed, they proposed that an NMDA agonist might increase the signal to the nucleus, increase gene expression, and increase learning. The reader should remember that the glutamate neurons (the most common neurons in the brain) have several different types of receptors. Opening the NMDA receptor as well as the α-amino-3-hydroxy-5-methyl-4-isoxazole propionate (AMPA) receptor increases the excitatory postsynaptic potential and the signal to the nucleus (see Figure 5.2).

Researchers at Emory developed a virtual reality simulator that gives participants the sensation

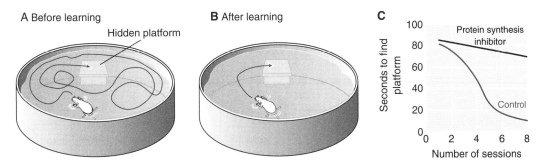

A Before learning — Hidden platform

B After learning

C Seconds to find platform / Number of sessions — Protein synthesis inhibitor; Control

FIGURE 15.2 ● A rat will learn the location of a hidden platform after several sessions in a pool of water. However, rats given a protein synthesis inhibitor fail to learn (C). (Adapted from Bear MF, Connors BW, Paradiso MA, eds. *Neuroscience: exploring the brain*, 3rd ed. Baltimore: Lippincott Williams & Wilkins; 2007 and Meiri N, Rosenblum K. Lateral ventricle injection of the protein synthesis inhibitor anisomycin impairs long-term memory in a spatial memory task. *Brain Res.* 1998;789[1]:48–55.)

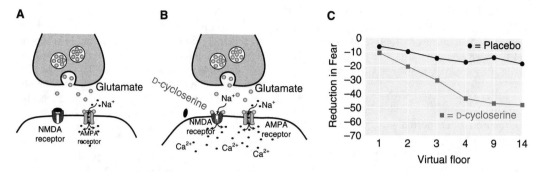

FIGURE 15.3 ● A: Activity at the AMPA receptor is insufficient to generate gene expression. **B:** D-CYCLOSERINE OPENS THE NMDA RECEPTOR AND CAN GENERATE A STRONG SIGNAL TO THE NUCLEUS. **C:** A STUDY USING D-CYCLOSERINE AND JUST TWO SESSIONS OF VIRTUAL EXPOSURE THERAPY SHOWED A MARKED REDUCTION IN FEAR OF HEIGHTS. NMDA, N-METHYL-D-ASPARTATE (**C**). (ADAPTED FROM RESSLER KJ, ROTHBAUM BO, TANNENBAUM L, et al. COGNITIVE ENHANCERS AS ADJUNCTS TO PSYCHOTHERAPY: USE OF D-CYCLOSERINE IN PHOBIC INDIVIDUALS TO FACILITATE EXTINCTION OF FEAR. *Arch Gen Psychiatry.* 2004;61[11]:1136–1144.)

of riding an elevator with a glass floor. Patients with fear of heights can extinguish much of their anxiety with many sessions in this device. D-cycloserine, an antibiotic used to treat tuberculosis, is also a partial agonist at the NMDA receptor. D-cycloserine will open the NMDA receptor and the postsynaptic nucleus will receive a heightened signal (see Figure 15.3). The Emory group gave patients D-cycloserine or placebo before just two sessions in the virtual elevator and found a 50% reduction in fear with those on the active medication (Figure 15.3C).

These results suggest that medications targeting the mechanisms of memory can work in conjunction with techniques of psychotherapy. This may lead to a whole new approach to treating mental illness.

Structural Plasticity

Some memories last an entire lifetime. These long-term memories persist despite surgical anaesthesia, epileptic seizures, and drug abuse. Protein molecules are not stable enough to survive these insults. Therefore, long-term memories must be the result of more stable formations such as structural changes (as seen with LTP), or they might be continuously rebuilt throughout one's life. In a previous chapter we discussed several examples of cortical strengthening secondary to learning and practicing, for example, monkeys spinning a wheel (see Figure 7.13) and humans playing a musical instrument (see Figure 7.14). These studies show that the cortex changes with learning.

Synaptogenesis

One mechanism that could explain learning-associated changes in the cortical structure is

some type of synaptic growth. Indeed, there is considerable evidence showing that learning increases branching and synapse formation. We have already discussed that rats living in an enriched environment show greater branching and spine formation on their hippocampal neurons (see Point of Interest box page 29).

Spines are the small protrusions on the shaft of the dendrite. They are believed to represent the formation of new synapses thereby increasing communication between neighboring neurons. It has long been suggested that new spines are involved in memory formation. Leuner et al. tested this theory by teaching rats to blink in anticipation of a puff of air to the eye. Twenty-four hours later, they found that the conditioned rats showed a 27% increase in spine formation on the pyramidal cells from the hippocampus. The reader can perceive the structural difference in the examples in Figure 15.4. Additionally, these changes were blocked with a NMDA antagonist. Therefore, new memories correlate with new spines.

Neurogenesis

Another mechanism that could explain the development of stable memories which can last a human lifespan is the formation of new neurons. We now know that new neurons are regularly developed throughout adulthood. We have seen that rats exposed to an enriched environment, for example, also showed greater neurogenesis (see Figure 7.4). Are the new neurons produced to hold memories of the enriched environment?

Recently, Leuner et al., again teaching rats to anticipate a puff of air, looked at learning and neurogenesis. They found that those animals that showed a better performance with the task also

A Learning   **B** Control   **C** Group data

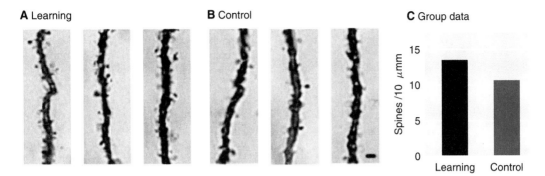

FIGURE 15.4 ● Rats taught to blink when a sound preceded a puff of air to their eyes showed greater spine density 24 hours later. (From Leuner B, Falduto J, Shors TJ. Associative memory formation increases the observation of dendritic spines in the hippocampus. *J Neurosci.* 2003;23[2]:659–665.)

had more new neurons surviving several days after the instruction. In other words, the greater the mastery of the skill, the greater the number of newly developing neurons that survived.

Perhaps the most compelling data regarding learning and neurogenesis comes from Nottemohm and his work with songbirds (see Figure 13.9). We hope the readers have stored in their long-term memory from Chapter 13 that Nottemohm established that male canaries have a sexually dimorphic brain region called the *high vocal center* (HVC), which is directly involved in song production. Further, that the HVC fluctuates in size during the year with seasonal changes in the reproductive hormones.

The relevance of the HVC for this chapter has to do with learning new songs and the changes in the HVC. The male canary changes his song repertoire over the course of 12 months by adding new notes and discarding others. Additionally, the number of new neurons added to the HVC fluctuates throughout the year. Of particular interest, the addition of new song notes and new neurons correlate (see Figure 15.5). Although not proven, it appears that the memory of the songs come and go with the development and loss of neurons in the HVC.

Reconsolidation

Until recently, the prevailing belief about memories were that once consolidated they were resistant to change. That is, convulsions, protein synthesis inhibitors, or head trauma cannot erase long-term memories. However, Nader et al. produced a study suggesting that long-term memories can return to a labile state, vulnerable to disruption, before being consolidated again. This phenomenon is called *reconsolidation*. The essential feature of reconsolidation is that the memory must be reactivated for this process to occur.

To understand reconsolidation it is important to understand the details of the study. First, rats are taught to associate a sound with an adverse stimulation, like a foot shock. When the rats hear the sound again, they "freeze"—a sign of fear in rodents. The researchers can quantify the percent of time the animals spend "frozen". Then the rats are exposed to the sound without the foot shock, but this time they receive the protein synthesis inhibitor anisomycin injected directly into their amygdala. Amazingly, when tested again, they do not "freeze". In other words, they show no fear. They appear to have forgotten what they learned. By analogy it is as though the long-term memory was ice, which melts to water when reactivated,

STRESS AND MEMORY

Although not necessarily accurate, singularly traumatic experiences are known to produce long-lasting, intense memories. Chronic stress, on the other hand, corrupts the memory-storage process. Humans given stress levels of cortisol demonstrate impaired declarative memory within days. As we discussed in Chapter 6, Hormones and the Brain, the likely mechanism is excess glucocorticoids causing atrophy of hippocampal dendrites, shrinking the hippocampus, and decreasing hippocampal neurogenesis.

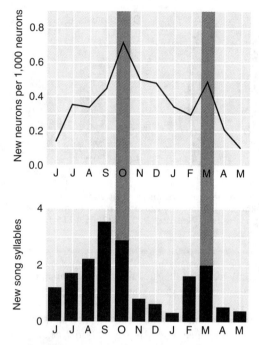

FIGURE 15.5 ● The development of new neurons correlates with the development of new song syllables. (Adapted from Kirn J, O'Loughlin B, Kasparian S, et al. Cell death and neuronal recruitment in the high vocal center of adult male canaries are temporally related to changes in song. *Proc Natl Acad Sci U S A.* 1994;91[17]:7844–7848.)

and then freezes again in the reconsolidation process—but now in a different shape.

While there is still much to be learned about reconsolidation, it provides a possible explanation for some of the healing power of psychotherapy. Do patients reactivate their memories in the course of telling their stories? However, because the patient is now in a safe environment, the memory can be reconsolidated without as much negative affect. Hopefully, this is true and can be further understood in the future as a way to improve the effectiveness of psychotherapy.

ORGANIZATION OF DECLARATIVE MEMORY

One of the great mysteries of neuroscience involves finding the location of long-term declarative memories. Where are they stored in the brain? How are they formed and why do they decay? Unfortunately, there are only basic explanations for these intriguing questions.

Hippocampus

The hippocampus (see Figure 2.5) is crucial for consolidation of long-term memories. The importance of the hippocampus became painfully obvious with the famous case of H.M. H.M. had struggled with minor seizures since the age of 10 and major seizures since the age of 16. Despite aggressive anticonvulsant medications, the seizures increased in frequency and ultimately the patient was unable to work. In 1953, at the age of 27, H.M. underwent a large bilateral resection of the medial temporal lobes in an effort to remove the nidus of the seizures. Figure 15.6 shows the areas of the brain removed.

The surgery successfully quieted the seizures, but unfortunately left H.M. with profound antegrade amnesia. Although his personality remained the same and his IQ even improved a bit from 104 to 112, he displayed severe and pervasive memory impairments. Specifically, he showed a normal immediate memory, but could not consolidate those memories into enduring traces. For example, when a person exited and within a few minutes re-entered his room, H.M. was unaware

---

FAULTY EYEWITNESS IDENTIFICATION AND RECONSOLIDATION

DNA technology has opened a window on some major errors in the criminal justice system. Hundreds of inmates have been released from jails and prisons when the DNA evidence shows that they could not have committed the crime. Eyewitness identification errors account for the largest single cause of wrongful incarcerations. Even more amazing, some eyewitnesses refuse to accept the DNA evidence. They persist in believing their identification.

Although there are many reasons a memory can be wrong, reconsolidation may explain the persistence in maintaining an inaccurate identification. It is possible that the victim, when confronted with the line-up, reactivates the memory of the crime. At that moment the memory returned to a labile state, which was then reconsolidated, but now with the face of the wrong culprit.

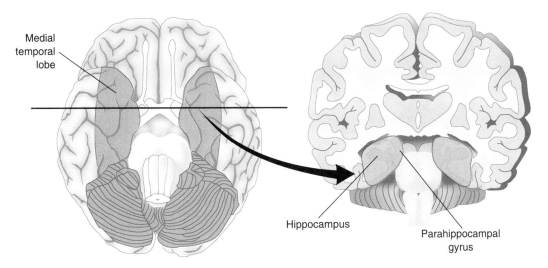

Medial temporal lobe

Hippocampus

Parahippocampal gyrus

FIGURE 15.6 ● Two views of H.M.'s brain identifying the areas that were removed in surgery, which left him with antegrade amnesia. (Adapted from Bear MF, Connors BW, Paradiso MA, eds. *Neuroscience: exploring the brain*, 3rd ed. Baltimore: Lippincott Williams & Wilkins; 2007.)

of that person's earlier visit. However, his remote memories remained intact. In fact, he would frequently speak of events before the surgery, in part because he was not developing new memories. To use a computer metaphor, it is as though H.M. has a "read only" hard drive for memory storage. He can retrieve old memories but cannot write new ones.

This unfortunate outcome for H.M. highlighted the essential role of the medial temporal lobe in forming long-term memories. Subsequent studies with animals and humans have established the hippocampus and the parahippocampal gyrus as crucial for encoding and consolidating memories of events and objects in time and space. For example, numerous studies have shown that lesions of a rat's hippocampus impair its ability to remember the location of the hidden platform in a water maze.

Further studies with H.M. established that the amnesia was not as widespread as initially perceived. For example, H.M. was asked to participate in a mirror-tracing task. While viewing his hand in a mirror, H.M. was asked to trace a star while keeping the pencil between the lines. H.M. improved at this task in ten trials on the first day (see Figure 15.7). He did even better on the second and third days. Remarkably, when asked about the task, he stated he had never seen the test before. This highlights what we addressed at the beginning of the chapter: there are different types of memory. H.M.'s explicit memory is disrupted, but his implicit memory remains intact. Consequently,

this type of memory must be stored through different mechanisms—ones that are independent of the hippocampus.

H.M. is still alive. More recent studies of his memory suggest that his declarative memory deficit is not as absolute as previously thought. For example, he was able to draw a reasonably accurate floor plan of his house although he had moved there 5 years after his operation. Likewise, when he looks in a mirror he is not startled by his appearance. This suggests that some declarative memories are being stored. Whether this is due to some residual hippocampal tissue or through other mechanisms is not known.

MEMORY AND PLEASURE

We discussed in Chapter 9, Pleasure, that memories associated with getting high could induce cravings in drug addicts. Conversely, it is well documented that pleasure enhances learning. Indeed, dopamine neurons from the ventral tegmental area directly innervate the medial temporal lobe. Recent brain imaging studies have shown simultaneous activation of the ventral tegmental area and medial temporal lobe when subjects are remembering rewarding experiences.

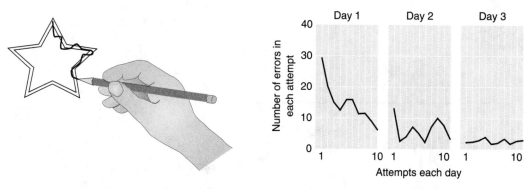

FIGURE 15.7 ● The mirror-tracing task asks subjects to trace between two stars while watching their hand in a mirror. The patient H.M. showed improvement at this task although he had no recollection of having taken the test before. (Adapted from Kandel ER, Schwartz JH, Jessell TM, eds. *Principles of neural science*, 4th ed. New York: McGraw-Hill; 2000.)

Neocortex

Sensory information comes into the brain and is processed in specific regions of the neocortex. The parahippocampal gyrus receives afferent projections from these cortical areas. The hippocampus has efferent projections back to these cortical regions, which appear to serve as storage sites for long-term memories. Figure 15.8 is a schematic representation of this process.

Damage to the hippocampus impairs the formation of new memories, but what affects remote memories? Bayley et al. examined eight patients with damage to their medial temporal lobes. All patients had problems storing new memories. Then they studied their ability to recall remote autobiographic memories. Only the three patients who also had significant additional damage to the neocortex showed impairment with remote memories. However, the exact location of long-term memories remains a mystery. It appears that remote memories are stored throughout the cortex rather than in one specific location. Anatomic studies with monkeys have established hippocampal projections to the cortical regions shown in Figure 15.9. These studies suggest that declarative memories are stored in the dorsolateral prefrontal cortex, cingulate gyrus, parietal lobe, and temporal lobe.

System Consolidation

When your computer saves a file to the hard drive, that data is placed in a specific location where it remains unchanged until it is modified. When we put items in our closets, they stay in the same location until we return for them. Storage in the brain, on the other hand, is more dynamic. There is evidence that memories undergo continuing remodeling even weeks and months after they are formed. This process is called *system consolidation*.

Looking at which part of the brain is activated during retrieval of recent and remote memories

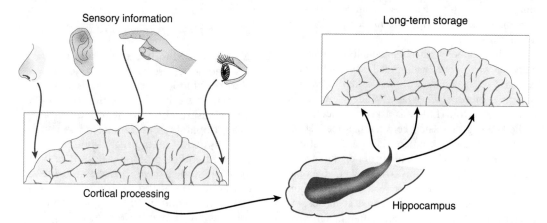

FIGURE 15.8 ● Experiences enter the brain through the senses and are initially processed in the cortex. This information then goes to the hippocampus before being stored in the cortex.

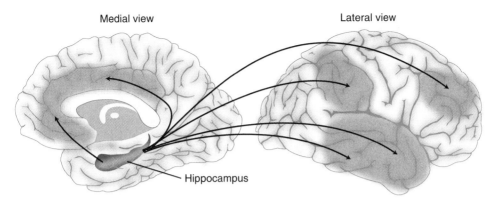

Medial view   Lateral view

Hippocampus

FIGURE 15.9 ● Efferent projections from the hippocampus go to the cortical areas shaded in gray. It is thought that long-term declarative memories are physically contained within these regions. The exact mechanism remains a mystery. (Adapted from Van Hoesen GW. The parahippocampal gyrus: New observations regarding its cortical connections in the monkey. *Trends Neurosci.* 1982;5:345–350.)

provides a good understanding of system consolidation. Researchers in France taught mice to navigate a maze. Placing the mice back in the maze at either 5 days or 25 days reactivated those memories. Cerebral metabolic activity was then measured in a functional scanner. At 5 days the mice had greater activity in their hippocampus. Those tested after 25 days had less activity in the hippocampus and greater activity in the cortical regions such as the cingulate gyrus and frontal cortex. This shows that memories are initially dependent on hippocampus. Then, by some process of consolidation that occurs over days, the memories become independent of the hippocampus and reside in a distributed pattern in the cortex.

The same researchers also looked at the remodeling of memories within layers of the cortex. As before, they taught the mice to negotiate a maze and then retested their memory at either 1 day or 30 days. This time they sacrificed the mice and measured Fos (a marker of gene activation) in the parietal cortex. They found that total Fos activity was the same at days 1 and 30. However, the location of activity within the layers of the parietal cortex changed from days 1 to 30. Figure 15.10 shows the change in Fos activity by layer. Note how the recent memory activates neurons in layers V and VI. Memory after 30 days, in comparison, shows greater activity in layers II and III.

These studies show that memories in the brain are not simply created and stored in a fixed and static receptacle awaiting recall. Memories appear to undergo remodeling as they become independent of the hippocampus and possibly as they are relocated in the layers of the cortex. And all this is done "off line," without conscious recall of the memory, possibly during sleep.

FORGETTING

From the standpoint of a mental health practitioner, problems with forgetting may be more relevant in day-to-day clinical practice than problems with forming new memories. Sometimes patients forget too much, as with Alzheimer's disease or, at the other extreme, cannot forget horrific traumatic memories they wish would disappear. While the cellular and molecular mechanisms of learning and memory are becoming clearer, the mechanisms of forgetting remain poorly understood.

The importance of forgetting can be understood from a standpoint of storage. Our brains are simply

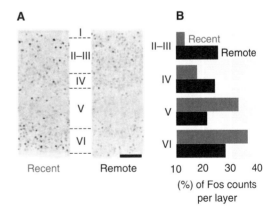

FIGURE 15.10 ● **A:** Micrographs from parietal lobes of mice tested at day 1 (recent) and day 30 (remote). **B:** Percentage of Fos counts per layer. (Micrograph from Maviel T, Durkin TP, Menzaghi F, et al. Sites of neocortical reorganization critical for remote spatial memory. *Science.* 2004;305[5680]:96–99. Reprinted with permission from AAAS.)

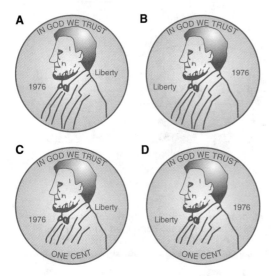

FIGURE 15.11 ● Because the brain retains so few details about objects, it is hard to identify which penny is an actual representation of the 1-cent coin. Few viewers will recognize that none of the drawings are a good match because Lincoln is facing the wrong direction.

not large enough to retain all the details of our lives. To further minimize what is retained it is likely the brain only stores broad outlines of the information. An example of this can be shown with Figure 15.11. Although the reader has seen pennies thousands of times over the past years, it is still hard to correctly identify the accurate drawing of the penny. This example highlights one reason we fail to remember: detailed memories were never stored in the first place. Likewise, any interference at the time of consolidation will impair future recall. However, this is different from forgetting what was once learned.

Numerous experiments have documented a continuous decline for remote memories with the passage of time. The "forgetting curve" in Figure 15.1 shows a hypothetical drop in the ability to recall unrehearsed information with the passage of time. Memories simply grow weaker as we age. How this occurs is poorly understood.

One possible mechanism assumes a passive decay over time. If the connections holding the memory are not used, they become weaker with time. Alternatively, the memory could be overwritten with new information and distorted or lost. Figuratively, it is as though an unused path through the woods is lost as the forest grows over it.

Actively forgetting is another possible mechanism that the brain could use. In this case it would be more like going through one's closet and throwing away items not worn in the past

year or two. Recent research suggests that active forgetting does occur in the brain.

The reader will recall that protein kinases phosphorylate transcription factors such as CREB to promote gene expression (see Figure 5.5). As is typical in the Yin and Yang mechanisms of the body, different proteins *dephosphorylate* CREB and turn off gene expression. The proteins that dephosphorylate are called *protein phosphatases*, and one of them, called *protein phosphatases 1* (PP1), has been implicated in forgetting. First, the research group established that inhibiting PP1 enhanced learning efficacy.

In a second experiment in a water maze, the researchers tested memory for the location of the hidden platform. Mice with PP1 inhibition remembered equally well at 8 weeks as they did on day 1. However, the control mice showed a decay in memory of the platform location as early as 2 weeks and seemed to have completely forgotten by 8 weeks. These results suggest that forgetting is an active function perpetrated by the brain to clean out memories not being utilized.

Electroconvulsive Therapy

One of the great controversies in psychiatry involves electroconvulsive therapy (ECT) and memory loss. Some patient groups have consistently complained that ECT erases long-term memories (retrograde amnesia). Some advocates of ECT have argued that only memories around the time of the treatment are truly lost while long-term memories are preserved. This is a difficult issue to test.

Squire et al. conducted a study over 30 years ago that provides some clarification. They asked patients to recall the names of television programs on the air during a single year between 1957 and 1972. Different versions of the test were administered before ECT and again after ECT. The results are shown in Figure 15.12A. Note the loss of more recent long-term memories with ECT while older memories are unaffected (and equally poor). These results support our discussion of system consolidation in humans continuing for years. That is, memories less than 2 years old continue to be vulnerable to disruption.

This same research group sought to extend the findings in this study to determine the length of disruption for recent long-term memories. They followed up the study of the patient's memory for television programs broadcast only in the 1 to 3 year time frame before ECT and several times after ECT. The results are shown in Figure 15.12B. Note that the patients show impaired memory immediately after ECT and even 1 week later.

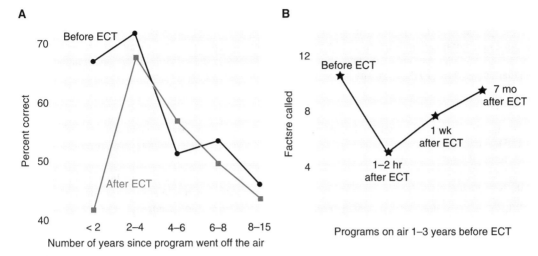

FIGURE 15.12 ● **A:** Patient's memory for television programs in the preceding years, before and after ECT. **B:** Longitudinal assessment of memory only for programs broadcast 1–3 years preceding ECT. ECT, electroconvulsive therapy. (Adapted from Squire LR, Slater PC, Chace PM. Retrograde amnesia: Temporal gradient in very long-term memory following electroconvulsive therapy. *Science*. 1975;187[4171]:77–79 and Squire LR, Slater PC, Miller PL. Retrograde amnesia and bilateral electroconvulsive therapy. *Arch Gen Psychiatry*. 1981;38[1]:89–95.)

MIND OF A MNEMONIST

Some people have extraordinary memories. One such person was studied at length in Russia for over 30 years during the time of Stalin. This man, called S. by the psychologist Aleksandr Luria, had an unbelievable capacity to accurately recall long lists of words, syllables, or numbers. For example, when shown the nonsense formula in Figure, S. studied it briefly and then after a few minutes reproduced it without error. Even more remarkable, when spontaneously and without warning asked to recall the formula 15 years later, he did so flawlessly.

$$N \cdot \sqrt{d^2 \times \frac{85}{vx}} \cdot \sqrt[3]{\frac{276^2 \cdot 86x}{n^2v \cdot ?\,264}}\ n^2b$$

$$= sv\frac{1624}{32^2} \cdot r^2s$$

A nonsense mathematical formula created to test S.'s memory. (Adapted from Luria AR. *The mind of a mnemonist*. New York: Basic Books; 1968.)

S. had an unusual ability to generate vivid enduring images in his mind of what he experienced. When it time for him to recall the items, he simply reproduced the images in his mind and read them as one would read symbols on a page. While the stable quality of these images allowed S. to earn a living as a performing mnemonist, it also cluttered his mind. He had trouble forgetting. S. was actually encumbered by past visual images that were activated by similar topics in conversation and reading. The associated images led to mental wanderings taking his mind far from the task in front of him. His gift for details interfered with his grasp of the "big picture."

Was there something different about S.'s brain? Unfortunately, S. lived before the time of brain imaging technology, so any differences in his brain's size or functions that might explain his extraordinary memory remain unknown. He also lived before the revolution in genetics. Might he have had an unusual variant of a protein synthesis gene that allowed for better immediate memory formation?

However, by 7 months their memory seems to have returned to baseline.

Perhaps the important point is that long-term memories are not impervious to erasure. We know that memories can be induced with electrical stimulation as with LTP. It seems logical that memories can also be disrupted with electrical activity. ECT is the most effective treatment for depression and has been life saving for many individuals. However, our memories are who we are. We need to be careful when using treatments that can alter life memories.

QUESTIONS

1. Learning to tie shoes is what kind of memory?
   a. Declarative.
   b. Implicit.
   c. Explicit.
   d. Antegrade.

2. Which of the following does not fit with the others?
   a. Short-term memory.
   b. DNA → RNA.
   c. Gene expression.
   d. Protein synthesis.

3. Anisomycin
   a. Enhances extinction.
   b. Accelerates memory formation.
   c. Limits neurogenesis.
   d. Inhibits protein synthesis.

4. All of the following are true about reconsolidation, except
   a. It was an unexpected finding.
   b. It suggests long-term memories are malleable.
   c. Is demonstrated with the use of D-cycloserine.
   d. Helps explain errors in eyewitness identification.

5. The patient H.M. is impaired with which of the following?
   a. Ability to build new long-term memories.
   b. Retrieve long-term memories.
   c. Develop new procedural memories.
   d. Understand explicit instructions.

6. Evidence of system consolidation includes
   a. More mature memories are more dependent on the hippocampus.
   b. Mature memories are more prevalent in the prefrontal cortex.
   c. Cortical layers II and III have less remote memories.
   d. Older memories are more active in the neocortex.

7. All of the following are true about forgetting long-term memories, except
   a. Memories decay with time.
   b. Protein phosphatases have been implicated in forgetting.
   c. Forgetting can be enhanced with anisomycin.
   d. Interference during consolidation increases forgetting.

8. ECT has all of the following effects on memory, except
   a. Inhibits consolidation.
   b. Induces forgetting of remote long-term memories.
   c. Erases recent long-term memories.
   d. Some memories are completely lost.

See Answers section at end of book.

Intelligence

INTELLIGENCE

The topic of intelligence can generate strong feelings. Specifically, the idea that there is one monolithic kind of intelligence that is reflected by a single number plotted on a bell shaped curve is hard to accept. Can one number determine a person's life? Other variables such as interpersonal skill, emotional resilience, creativity, and motivation are factors independent of intelligence, which are critical for success in a career in specific and life in general. Likewise, a person can show great aptitude in one area of life, yet struggle in another. Having said that, it is important to acknowledge there is considerable evidence of a general mental ability called *intelligence*, which has a predictive value.

It has been shown that all credible tests of mental ability rank individuals in about the same way; that is, people who do well on one type of test tend to do well on the others and *vice versa*. Such tests (e.g., the Wechsler Intelligence Scale, which gives an IQ score) are believed to measure some global element of intellectual ability. This global element is called "g" or fluid intelligence. G is conceptualized as reasoning and novel problem-solving ability. Others have described it as the ability to deal with complexity. There is no pure measure of g. An IQ score is an approximation of g.

Some argue that g is only useful to predict academic success or success in situations that resemble school. Arguing against this, others point to data showing the predictive correlates between IQ and employment, marriage, incarceration, and income. From our standpoint, we are interested in the associations between g and the neural substrate of the brain.

Genetics

Before we delve into the neuroscience of intelligence, it is worth discussing some compelling studies on the heritability of cognitive skills. The Colorado Adoption Project that started in 1975 followed up 200 adopted children from childhood through adolescence. They compared the cognitive ability of the children with their adoptive parents and their biologic parents. A control group of children raised by their biologic parents was included for comparison.

Figure 16.1 shows the correlations for verbal and spatial abilities over time between the children and the parents. Note how the adopted children have almost zero correlation between them and their adopted parents. Their cognitive skills more closely match their biologic parents. Another finding of interest is that the correlations improve with age. We become more like our biologic parents as we age—at least with regard to intelligence.

Brain Size

A consistent finding in neuroscience has been the association between brain size and intelligence; that is, all other things being equal, bigger brains really are better. Nottebohm in his work with songbirds found a noteworthy example. The reader will remember that male songbirds have an enlarged high vocal center (HVC), which plays an essential role in his song production. Nottebohm meticulously recorded the diversity of song syllables that each bird produced and then compared

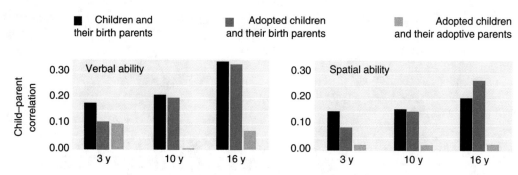

FIGURE 16.1 ● The correlation between children and their biologic parents increases with age for verbal and spatial abilities. The shared environment between adopted children and their parents had little effect on verbal or spatial intelligence scores. (Adapted from Plomin R, DeFries JC. The genetics of cognitive abilities and disabilities. *Sci Am.* 1998;278[5]:62–69.)

this with the size of his HVC. The results are plotted in Figure 16.2, and show a robust correlation.

An extensive song repertoire is not the same as reasoning and problem solving. It is probably closer to having a large fund of knowledge (sometimes called *crystalline intelligence*). However, for our purposes it shows an association between brain size and a learned task.

With humans, there is a long history of studies comparing brain size and intelligence. In the early days they would simply compare head circumference (hat size) with rough estimates of intelligence. However, there is more to intelligence than just brain size, otherwise whales and elephants would have ruled the world. That important

variable is the relative size of the brain to the size of the body.

Modern imaging studies allow the *in vivo* measurement of brain volume. McDaniel conducted a meta-analysis of imaging studies comparing brain volume and intelligence. He identified 37 high-quality studies with a total of 1,530 people. The correlation between brain volume and intelligence across the studies was 0.33. In other words, differences in brain volume explain some of the differences in IQ, but there is also a lot more that remains unexplained.

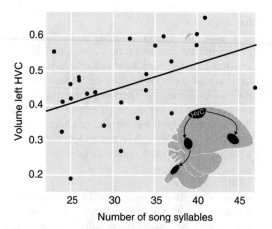

FIGURE 16.2 ● Adult male canaries with a large repertoire of song syllables also tend to have a large high vocal center (HVC) while those with small repertoire have a small HVC. (Adapted from Nottebohm F. The road we travelled: Discovery, choreography, and significance of brain replaceable neurons. *Ann N Y Acad Sci.* 2004;1016:628–658.)

INTELLIGENCE & ANXIETY

A recent prospective study reported an intriguing association between IQ at the age of 6 and post-traumatic stress disorder (PTSD) symptoms after trauma at the age of 17. Those children with an IQ of 115 or greater were only one fifth as likely to develop PTSD as similarly traumatized children with an IQ of 100 or less. These results suggest that greater intelligence is in some way protective against the development of secondary anxiety.

Frontoparietal Network

The study of patients with brain lesions has been a staple in neuroscience since the days of Broca. Unfortunately, the analysis of intelligence in patients with frontal lobe lesions has been confusing. Such patients can have significant deficits with planning and problem solving, yet retain a normal IQ. Duncan showed this was an artifact of the type of test used to measure IQ. Specifically, the Wechsler Adult Intelligence Scale (WAIS) tests some aspects of intelligence that emphasize knowledge. This may reflect g at the time of learning rather than at the time of testing.

Duncan reasoned that intelligence tests that give a better estimate of current g (novel problem solving) would reflect the deficits in patients with frontal lobe injuries. An example of a patient and control are shown here.

	WAIS IQ	Novel Problem-Solving IQ
Frontal lobe–damaged patient	130	108
Healthy control	128	131

The WAIS IQs are equal, but the patient with frontal lobe impairment struggles with novel problems. These results, along with the results of larger studies like them, suggest that frontal lobe functions may play a large role in intelligence.

Functional imaging studies, while subjects perform complex tasks, reveal regional activity that may correlate with intelligence. Researchers in Korea examined the activity in the brain during simple g and complex g tasks. Figure 16.3A shows examples of simple and complex tasks that subjects performed while in the functional scanner. The difference in activity between the tasks reveals a frontoparietal network enlisted to solve the difficult problem (Figure 16.3B). Greater efficiency and speed within this network may reflect differences in intelligence.

Cortical Development

Measurements of intelligence remain relatively stable over a person's lifespan. Yet, we know that the brain is a dynamic organ with more remodeling capability than we could have imagined just a decade ago. Likewise, there is a shrinking of the gray matter during adolescence as individuals mature. It is unclear how these fluctuations relate to intelligence.

Giedd et al. at National Institute of Mental Health (NIMH) recently completed a longitudinal study of cortical thickness and intellectual ability from childhood through adolescence for more than 300 children. The most significant finding was that it was not the absolute thickness of the gray matter that correlated best with intelligence, but rather the rate of change. This was most prominent in the prefrontal cortex (PFC). Figure 16.4 shows the cortical thickness for one point on the right

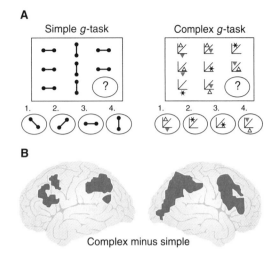

FIGURE 16.3 ● Subjects were shown simple and complex patterns of symbols and asked to fill in the empty space with the choices provided (A). Subtracting the activity when performing the simple tasks from the activity during the complex tasks reveals a frontoparietal network (B). (Adapted from Lee KH, Choi YY, Gray JR, et al. Neural correlates of superior intelligence: Stronger recruitment of posterior parietal cortex. *Neuroimage.* 2006;29[2]:578–586.)

superior frontal gyrus for subjects with superior intelligence and average intelligence. Note how those with superior intelligence have less gray matter as children, which peak later, and then show a more rapid thinning compared with the average children.

These findings are not what were expected. Smart children do not simply have more gray matter. Rather, it is the dynamic properties (perhaps even efficient pruning of unneeded connections) of the cortical maturation that are somehow superior in intelligent children. The significance of this finding remains unclear.

Performance Enhancement

There is considerable interest in medications that could enhance cognitive performance. Pharmacologic interventions to increase problem-solving skills would be valuable tools in the treatment of such disorders as traumatic brain injury, Alzheimer's disease, and schizophrenia. However, if they worked not only to reverse disease-related deficits but also to enhance healthy brains, there would be a large demand from people without disorders who seek to enhance performance. The prospect of "lifestyle" medications for intelligence is worrisome, especially in a meritocracy such as ours where profession and income are largely

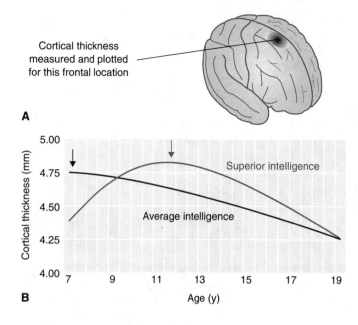

Cortical thickness measured and plotted for this frontal location

A

B

FIGURE 16.4 ● Measurements at the indicated point of the right superior frontal gyrus (**A**). Comparison of the cortical thickness at the point in (**A**) through adolescence for those with superior intelligence compared with those with average intelligence (**B**). (Adapted from Shaw P, Greenstein D, Lerch J, et al. Intellectual ability and cortical development in children and adolescents. *Nature.* 2006;440[7084]:676–679.)

dependent on school performance and intelligence as measured in school tests.

Although there are no budding treatments in the development pipeline, there are actually several products currently available. The best-known agents are the stimulants such as the amphetamines and methylphenidate. Studies have repeatedly shown that these agents will improve cognitive skills in healthy subjects. For example, Figure 16.5 shows how methylphenidate decreased reaction times and errors of omission in healthy subjects in a dose-dependent manner.

Surveys of college students have documented the abuse and misuse of the stimulant medications. Hall et al. found 17% of the male students and 11% of the female students at a midwestern university reported illicit use of prescription stimulant medications. In general, students at more competitive universities and those with lower grades are at greater risk for misuse of the stimulants.

DISORDER: ATTENTION-DEFICIT/HYPERACTIVITY DISORDER

It is not uncommon in clinical practice for a parent to try out their child's stimulant and experience a favorable response. The parent will conclude that they also have attention-deficit/hyperactivity disorder (ADHD). Often such parents will present with a request for a prescription for themselves. However, improved productivity while taking methylphenidate or amphetamine is a normal response and does not constitute the presence of a disorder.

Other pharmacologic agents are also known to enhance cognitive skills. The new medication

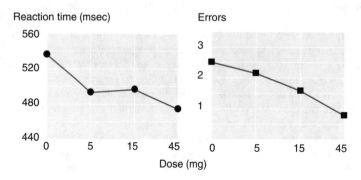

FIGURE 16.5 ● Healthy men (average age 22) displayed a dose-dependent improvement with methylphenidate, as measured on a continuous performance test. (Adapted from Cooper NJ, Keage H, Hermens D, et al. The dose-dependent effect of methylphenidate on performance, cognition and psychophysiology. *J Integr Neurosci.* 2005;4[1]:123–144.)

modafinil marketed for narcolepsy and excessive fatigue has been shown to improve cognitive performance in healthy subjects. Readily available agents such as caffeine and nicotine have also been shown to improve performance. In general, the trend is that the agents that improve alertness also improve cognitive performance. Nature's own performance-enhancing condition (hypomania) is well known to increase productivity (see Figure 16.12). A possible explanation is that the accelerated activity in the brain induced with stimulants, caffeine, or hypomania, results in faster connections. All other things being equal, faster brains may be "smarter".

DEFICITS

It is beyond the scope of this text to review all known cognitive deficits. However two topics are worth discussing: mental retardation (MR) and dyslexia. Both have distinct abnormalities that give us greater understanding of the brain.

Mental Retardation
Dendritic Pathology
MR is a non-progressive developmental disorder affecting global cognitive function. By definition MR is characterized by an IQ of 70 or below (two standard deviations below the norm of 100). In the United States, this comprises approximately 1% to 2% of the population. There are numerous causes of MR, including genetic aberrations, toxin exposure *in utero*, and malnutrition.

Severe forms of MR often have readily apparent structural abnormalities, for example, microcephaly. However, most subjects with MR show little, if any, obvious changes in brain anatomy. Their brains look roughly normal when examined with magnetic resonance imaging (MRI). In the 1970s, researchers began postmortem examination of the brains of retarded children and discovered extensive dendritic spine abnormalities (see Figure 16.6). Subsequent studies have found aberrant spine morphology and/or reduced dendritic branching as a consistent finding in MR in a variety of syndromes.

The importance of spine architecture for learning and memory has been discussed in several chapters in this book (e.g., see Figures 7.11, 9.13, 13.6, and 1.4). It is reasonable to assert that deficits in spine morphology impair the network connectivity essential for information processing. Likewise, there is only a short step to imagine that problems with information processing play a large role in the cognitive deficits of MR.

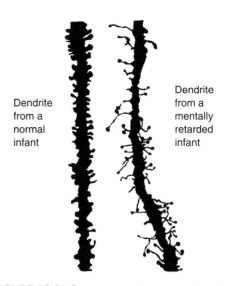

Dendrite from a normal infant

Dendrite from a mentally retarded infant

FIGURE 16.6 ● Dendrites from a healthy child and one with mental retardation (MR), highlighting the abnormal spine morphology in the child with MR. (Adapted from Purpura DP. Dendritic spine "dysgenesis" and mental retardation. *Science.* 1974;186[4169]:1126–1128.)

Deprivation
Deprivation in early infancy is a well-known cause of cognitive impairment. Studies on animals have established the lasting impact of early environmental impoverishment. Studies on humans have usually relied on case reports. The fall of the totalitarian government ruled by Nicolae Ceausescu in Romania in 1989 gave the world a group of unfortunate children who could be systematically studied and followed up.

Under the Ceausescu regime, some children were raised in institutions under conditions of severe deprivation. When Romania was opened to the world by the new government, the shocking condition of these children was revealed. Most were severely malnourished, with significant developmental delays. European and American families responded by adopting many of these children.

It is assumed that most of these children were put into the institutions as very young babies. Consequently, the age at which they were adopted approximates the length of time they were raised in a deprived environment. Likewise, it is known that these children moved into enriched environments after adoption.

The cognitive skills of 131 of these adoptees have been studied and compared with 50 UK adoptees who were adopted before 6 months of age. IQ tests have been administered to all these children throughout their childhood. Significant improvements were seen at the assessments of 4-year-old and 6-year-old Romanian children. Many children displayed an encouraging "catch-up" with the UK adoptees. Recently, the examination results of the 11-year-old Romanian adoptees were reported and are shown in Figure 16.7.

The figure shows the profound and lasting effects of early institutional deprivation. Of particular interest is the dose–response relationship between IQ and the number of years spent in an impoverished environment. Children removed from deprivation before 6 months of age had almost no lasting impairment. However, those children who stayed in the institutions for more than 6 months had 20-point reductions compared with the UK adoptees. These results reiterate the work by Hubel and Wiesel regarding critical periods of development (see Figures 7.9 and 7.11).

Dyslexia

Unlike MR, dyslexia is a localized impairment. Classified as a learning disorder, dyslexia presents as an unexpected difficulty in reading in a person with otherwise normal intelligence and motivation. Dyslexia may be the most common neurobehavioral disorder in children. Estimates of the prevalence range from 5% to 17.5%.

While speech develops naturally, reading is an acquired skill. Children must learn that letters on a page represent the sounds of spoken language. Children with dyslexia have trouble decoding the letters into the sounds of words. Comprehension can be normal once the word is recognized, but sounding out the word is laborious. Reading is effortful and slow for such children. Additionally, the impairment does not spontaneously remit.

The Shaywitzs have been studying dyslexia for almost 20 years at Yale. In a large study they examined 144 children (70 with dyslexia) in a functional MRI (fMRI). The children read real words and pseudowords while being scanned. Figure 16.8 shows the difference in activity in the brains of the normal readers compared with those with dyslexia. Note the increased activity for normal readers at two regions in the left hemisphere: a frontal region and a temporal/occipital region. These regions are thought to be critical for analyzing written words.

In a remarkable application of their findings, Shaywitz et al. conducted a treatment study to see if the dormant regions in the dyslexic children could be awakened. Thirty-seven children, who were second or third graders, with dyslexia received 50 minutes of daily tutoring in their schools for 1 year. They focused on phonics: associating letters and combinations of letters with sounds. Children in the treatment group showed

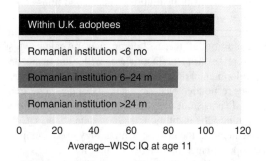

FIGURE 16.7 ● A dose–response effect is shown for different amounts of institutional deprivation on IQ at 11 years of age. WISC, Wechsler Intelligence Scale for Children. (Adapted from Beckett C, Maughan B, Rutter M, et al. Do the effects of early severe deprivation on cognition persist into early adolescence? Findings from the English and Romanian adoptees study. *Child Dev.* 2006;77[3]:696–711.)

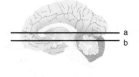

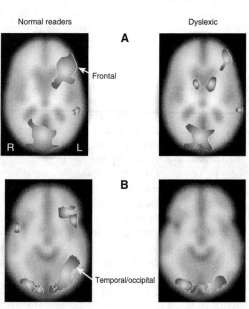

FIGURE 16.8 ● Children with dyslexia and healthy readers were scanned while reading. Normal readers showed greater activation of the frontal region as well as the temporal/occipital region. (Adapted from Shaywitz SE, Shaywitz BA. Dyslexia (specific reading disability). *Biol Psychiatry.* 2005;57[11]:1301–1309.)

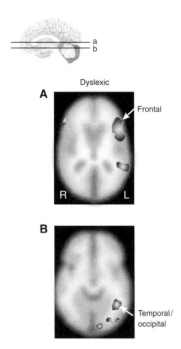

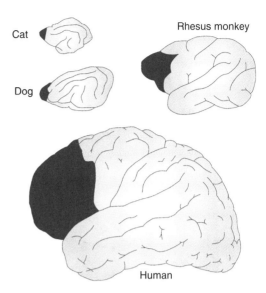

FIGURE 16.10 ● The prefrontal cortex (PFC) is proportionally larger in humans compared with other mammals.

FIGURE 16.9 ● Dyslexic children who received a phonics-based reading intervention over 1 school year showed increased activation in the regions of the brain associated with fluent reading. (Adapted from Shaywitz SE, Shaywitz BA. Dyslexia (specific reading disability). *Biol Psychiatry*. 2005;57[11]:1301–1309.)

improved reading accuracy, fluency, and comprehension after 1 year.

Of particular interest were the results of the repeated fMRIs 1 year after the study ended (2 years after the start of the study). The baseline scans subtracted from the followup scans revealed regions activated in the intervening years. The newly activated regions (see Figure 16.9) correspond to the same regions active in fluent readers: frontal and temporal/occipital.

CREATIVITY

Creativity is conceptualized as the capacity to generate novel approaches to a problem. Some call it the ability to perceive what remains hidden from the view of others. However, being creative is not just producing something different. Any fool can make a mess that has never been created before and call it art. The talent comes in creating new works that are meaningful and useful.

The ability to be creative is one of the outstanding traits of human beings. A unique feature of humans within the animal kingdom is the relative size of the PFC. Figure 16.10 shows the remarkable increase in size of the PFC for

humans compared with three other mammals. Recent MRI studies on humans and other primates compared the relative volumes of white and gray matter in the PFC. The largest difference was found with the PFC white matter (see Figure 16.11). The authors suggested that this difference may be a measure of "connectional elaboration." They postulate that the superior cognitive skills in humans could be a result of more connections, not just more neurons. With regard to the topic of this section, we can imagine that more connections increase the potential for new and creative solutions to problems.

The PFC clearly plays a significant role in the creative process. PFC has been identified as mediating behaviors such as planning, working memory, attention, and information processing. It seems likely that the PFC contains the mechanisms to create something new—to envision the world differently. Indeed, creative individuals have greater PFC blood flow, compared with less creative subjects, during a test designed to bring out new and novel solutions. The motivation to start and finish a project may also depend on the PFC.

Another interesting aspect of creativity is the association with mental illness. Individuals such as artist Vincent Van Gogh, writer Ernest Hemingway, and Nobel laureate John Nash are good case examples of highly imaginative people who also struggled with mental illness. The composer Robert Schumann provides one of the most compelling examples of mental illness and the creation

A   Rhesus monkey   Human

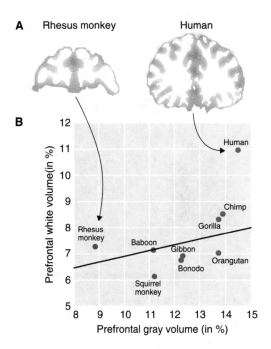

B

FIGURE 16.11 ● Gray and white matter comparisons in the prefrontal cortex (PFC) for rhesus monkeys and humans (**A**). The proportion of white matter in the PFC (compared with total white matter) is larger for humans than other primates (**B**). (Adapted from Schoenemann PT, Sheehan MJ, Glotzer LD. Prefrontal white matter volume is disproportionately larger in humans than in other primates. *Nat Neurosci.* 2005;8[2]:242–252.)

of art (see Figure 16.12). Schumann attempted suicide twice and eventually died in an asylum. He had also two known active periods during which he had symptoms of hypomania. Graphing his musical works by the years he created that correlates them shows a remarkable fluctuation in productivity with mood.

Larger studies confirm a correlation between creativity and mental illness. A combination of two older studies from the time when people were more likely to have used the Minnesota Multiphasic Personality Inventory (MMPI) found that scores for writers and highly creative writers fell between normal and psychosis (see Figure 16.13). It is important to note that the highly creative writers were not necessarily mentally ill, just sharing some of the traits of the seriously mentally ill.

Recent studies using the current method of systematic structured interviews based on Diagnostic and Statistical Manual (DSM) criteria have replicated these findings. Thus, successful artists such as writers or visual artists have a high prevalence of mental disorders. The most common disorders

are depression and bipolar disorder. It is worth noting that whereas creative artists have a high prevalence of mood disorders, it is not the same for creative individuals in other fields such as science and engineering. Too much creative thinking may not be compatible with certain disciplines within the hard-core sciences.

The similarity between creativity and mental illness may be related to decreased filtering of thoughts and sensations. A good example of unfiltered thoughts occurs when we dream during sleep. In this uninhibited state we experience a wild variety of thoughts that are—if nothing else—unique and creative. Some think dreaming is similar to psychosis. The important point is that when the inhibitions are off (as with sleep), the mind is open to new associations. Yet, few of the new ideas are useful.

Latent inhibition describes one cognitive mechanism known to filter extraneous sensations during the awake state. *Latent inhibition* is defined as an animal's unconscious capacity to screen out and ignore stimuli that are irrelevant. Specific tests can measure an individual's capacity to ignore irrelevant stimuli. Its significance in our discussions is that individuals who have reduced latent inhibition have been shown to be more creative. Additionally, this same trait is associated with increased propensity toward psychosis. In other words, a little less inhibition may promote more creative thinking, but too much may be problematic.

A study with Harvard undergraduate students found an intriguing association between latent inhibition, IQ, and creativity. The authors categorized the students by IQ and capacity for latent inhibition. They also determined each student's creative achievement. Students scored high on creative achievement if they had published a book, recorded a musical composition, patented an invention, or won a prize for a scientific discovery. The results of this analysis are shown in Figure 16.14.

The authors concluded that highly creative individuals have a high IQ and are less likely to filter out extraneous stimuli. Such individuals have access to more information, but also have the brainpower to handle the additional information and are consequently more likely to make original connections. However, the authors speculated that too much unfiltered sensory information in lower IQ individuals may be a factor for psychotic thinking.

The changing creative expression in an artist with evolving frontotemporal dementia provides a final example of the importance of the frontal lobes in creativity. The patient was a high school art teacher who had been painting since she

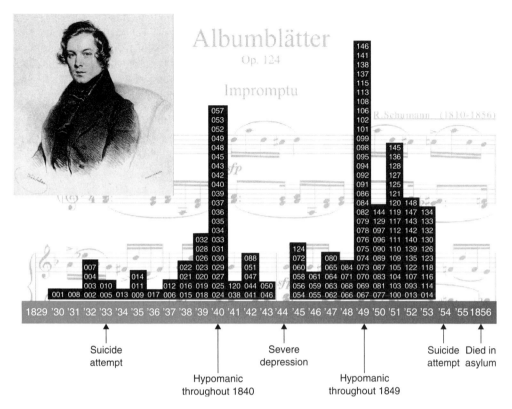

FIGURE 16.12 ● Robert Schumann's works graphed by opus number and year of completion provide a visual display of the creative potential of hypomania and the devastating effects of depression. Robert Schumann, Wien 1839, lithographie by Joseph Kriehuber. (Adapted from Jamison KR. Manic-depressive illness and creativity. *Sci Am*. 1995;272[2]:627.)

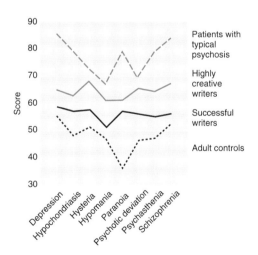

FIGURE 16.13 ● The Minnesota Multiphasic Personality Inventory (MMPI) allows the plotting of symptom severity across a spectrum—the upper graph being more severe. Highly creative writers and successful writers fall between typical psychotic patients and healthy controls. (Adapted from Simonton DK. Are genius and madness related? Contemporary answers to an ancient question. *Psychiatric Times*. 2005;22[7]:23–23.)

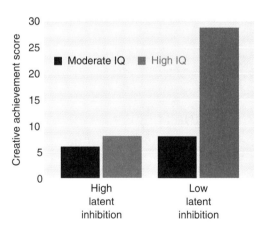

FIGURE 16.14 ● Undergraduate students with high IQ and low latent inhibition (the ability to filter out irrelevant stimuli) showed greater creative achievement. (Adapted from Carson SH, Peterson JB, Higgins DM. Decreased latent inhibition is associated with increased creative achievement in high-functioning individuals. *J Pers Soc Psychol*. 2003;85[3]:499–506.)

was a child. In 1986, at the age of 43, she began developing cognitive problems. Grading papers, preparing for class, and remembering students' names became increasingly difficult. In 1995 she took early retirement. By 2000 she required caregiver support for her activities of daily living. An MRI showed moderate bifrontal atrophy along with mild left temporal atrophy. Her final painting was in 2001.

While she was losing cognitive skills and becoming socially awkward, she was also becoming increasingly uninhibited in her artistic expression. Her paintings, which had been previously more traditional, were now impressionistic, abstract, and emotional. Clearly, the inhibitions within the PFC were removed as the disease progressed and the patient became more expressive in her art. However, when the dementia progressed too far, she was no longer able to paint. Once again, we see a spectrum in which a moderate amount of inhibition increases creative expression while too much leads to frank impairment.

QUESTIONS

1. All of the following apply to g, except
   a. Fund of knowledge.
   b. Novel problem solving.
   c. Fluid intelligence.
   d. Ability to handle complexity.

2. All of the following are true about the male canary's HVC, except
   a. The size is influenced by testosterone.
   b. Greater volume equals greater repertoire of songs.
   c. The size is an indirect measure of g.
   d. The size fluctuates with the seasons.

3. Indications that the PFC is a major site of intelligence include all of the following, except
   a. Active during problem solving.
   b. Lesions produce problem-solving deficits.
   c. Larger relative size in more intelligent animals.
   d. Larger proportion of gray matter in humans compared with other primates.

4. Impaired spine formation on dendrites is seen with all of the following, except
   a. Opioid abuse.
   b. Memory formation.
   c. MR.
   d. Impoverished environment.

5. All of the following are true about dyslexia, except
   a. Impaired ability to decode words.
   b. Right hemisphere problem.
   c. Inactive temporal/occipital region during reading.
   d. Increased frontal activity with proper treatment.

6. Most creative individuals in the sciences have the following, except
   a. Active PFC.
   b. Low latent inhibition.
   c. Mental illness.
   d. Above average IQ.

See Answers section at end of book.

Attention

INTRODUCTION

The last aspect of cognition that we will review is the ability to attend to external or internal stimuli. Like memory, attention is one of the oldest and most studied areas of cognitive science. One hundred years ago researchers used stopwatches and psychological tests to measure attention. More recently, ablation studies or the placement of microelectrodes into the brains of monkeys advanced the understanding of attention. Now brain imaging studies can observe, in real time, the shifting focus of an awake human solving a puzzle. One hundred years of research have given us a better understanding of the power of the brain to focus on relevant stimuli, although some aspects of the neurobiology of attention remain totally unknown.

Attention in a broad sense describes the mechanism that weighs the importance of various stimuli and selects the one that will receive the brain's focus. The brain has limited capacity for attention. Numerous psychological tests have demonstrated the brain's finite capacity to attend as more and more stimuli are added. A relevant example from modern life involves driving while talking on a cell phone. A recent study found that drivers using a cell phone had a fourfold increase in the chance of a serious accident. Handsfree phones were equally problematic. Attending to a conversation detracts the driver from attending to events on the road.

The capacity to concentrate and maintain one's attention is inversely related to the ability to ignore other stimuli. Responding to other stimuli—whether internal or external—changes the brain's focus. The brain cannot attend if it is wandering from one thought to another. The capacity to ignore extraneous stimuli is integral to successful adaptation.

The border collie in Figure 17.1 shows an example of selective attention. The dog is not only focused on the frisbee, but is also actively ignoring other objects of potential interest around him. In this state he will ignore female dogs, squirrels, children, even food. He will not sniff the scent of other dogs or leave his own mark on the shrubbery. He appears to focus solely on the flying sphere.

Athletes provide another example of the intimate relationship between attending and ignoring. The quarterback who has dropped into the pocket and is able to ignore all the noise and violence around him while he searches for an open receiver is an extraordinary example of attending and ignoring. Likewise, when the artist or the absent-minded professor gets lost in work, he/she is ignoring most sensory inputs coming into the brain. Fortunately, treatments that improve attention also improve the capacity to screen out the unessential.

How does the brain decide what is important and what can be ignored? The answer is that we do not know. We will review the regions with important roles in attention, but the ultimate integration remains a mystery.

Measuring Attention

Continuous performance tests (CPTs) give an objective estimate of an individual's attention and impulsivity. Subjects watch a computer screen and

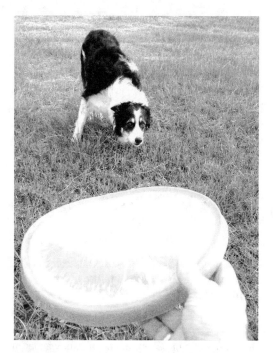

FIGURE 17.1 ● A border collie ignores everything else around him while focusing on the frisbee.

hit a button or click a mouse whenever a specified sequence of symbols or letters appears (see Figure 17.2A). Such tests reflect the subject's capacity to attend as well as the ability to restrain impulsive answers. Results are compared with normative data for individuals in one's age group.

Attention changes across the lifespan. Figure 17.2B shows the percent errors on one CPT (Test of Variables of Attention) for 1,590 individuals from the ages of 4 to 80+. Note how adults have the best attention. These findings correlate with the maturing of the brain (see Figure 7.7), a process that continues into adulthood.

ADHD AND ADULTHOOD

Attention-deficit hyperactivity disorder (ADHD) was once considered a childhood disorder. More recently, it has become popular for adults to get treatment for this condition. However, a recent meta-analysis of followup studies found that most children with ADHD fail to meet the full criteria for the disorder as adults—only 10% to 15%.

WORKING MEMORY
Prefrontal Cortex

Working memory describes what is actively being considered at any moment. If the brain contained a tiny person in a control room orchestrating the body's responses, working memory would be what he sees on the monitors in front of him. It is temporary, limited in capacity, and must be continually refreshed. Traditionally, working memory has been associated with the prefrontal cortex (PFC). It most certainly resides there, but may also include connections with the parietal lobes, as we saw with intelligence (see Figure 16.3).

Trauma to the PFC impairs working memory. Phineas Gage is the most famous case that shows the effects of frontal brain damage on working memory. He was the young railroad worker who had a tamping iron explode through his frontal cortex (see Figure 11.4). This resulted in a dramatic change in his personality. He went from being

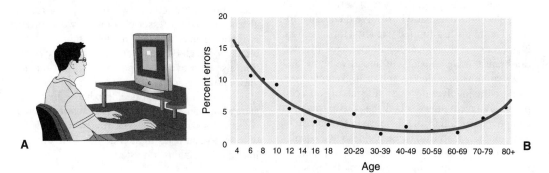

FIGURE 17.2 ● **A:** A continuous performance test provides an objective measure of attention and concentration. **B:** Percent errors as measured by the Test of Variables of Attention (TOVA) are age dependent. (Adapted from Greenberg LM, Crosby RD. *A summary of developmental normative data on the T.O.V.A. ages 4 to 80+.* Unpublished manuscript available through The TOVA company; 1992.)

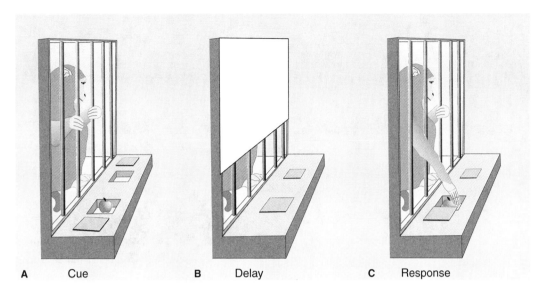

A Cue   **B** Delay   **C** Response

FIGURE 17.3 ● The delayed-response task. **A:** The screen is raised and the monkey observes a piece of fruit placed in one of the wells. **B:** The screen is lowered and the wells are covered. **C:** After a specific period of time the screen is raised and the monkey has one chance to remember the correct location of the fruit. (Adapted from Purves D, Augustine GJ, Fitzpatrick D, et al. *Neuroscience*, 3rd ed. Sunderland, MA: Sinauer; 2004.)

responsible and organized to impulsive and inattentive. The inability to hold a sustained thought in his working memory meant he was unable to focus on a task for any meaningful length of time.

Researchers developed a way to test working memory in monkeys, called the *delayed-response task*. In this task, a monkey is shown a piece of fruit being placed in one of two randomly chosen receptacles (see Figure 17.3). This is called the *cue*. A screen is then pulled down obscuring the monkey's view and lids are placed over both receptacles. When the screen is lifted, the monkey gets one chance to remove the correct lid and receive his reward. The significance of this test is that the monkey must hold the visual image of the location of the fruit in his working memory during the delay period. Healthy monkeys learn this task quickly. Monkeys with frontal lobe lesions perform poorly.

In the 1970s researchers began putting microelectrodes into individual neurons in the PFC of monkeys while they participated in the delayed-response task (see Figure 17.4A). They found that neurons reacted differently during the task. Some neurons were active only during the cue and response periods whereas other neurons became active during the delay period (Figure 17.4B). These *delay neurons* appear to be anatomic correlates of the working memory.

The delay neurons start firing with the presentation of the cue and stop with the response. These neurons seem to literally hold the memory of the task. When the monkeys incorrectly responded, the delay neurons were usually inactive. If the monkeys were distracted during the delay period, the delay neurons would typically settle down and the monkeys would make incorrect responses or not respond at all.

After the studies, the researchers sacrificed the monkeys and identified the location of the microelectrodes. The results from several of the monkeys are condensed from one section of their right PFC and shown in Figure 17.4C. The cue neurons and delay neurons are shown in different colors. Note how the delay neurons are more common than the cue neurons and cluster together. It is likely the delay neurons do not work independently but are part of a network that holds the image in working memory.

Catecholamines

Working memory is modulated by the catecholamines, dopamine (DA) and norepinephrine (NE). Pharmacologic interventions that increase DA and NE in the PFC enhance working memory and improve attention. Alternatively, agents that block DA receptors, such as haloperidol, have been shown to degrade performance on delay-response tasks.

Phillips et al. recently examined the relationship between accuracy on a delay-response task and DA release in the PFC. They placed microdialysis

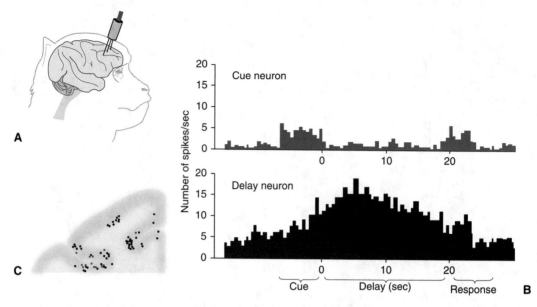

FIGURE 17.4 ● **A:** Microelectrodes placed into individual neurons in the prefrontal cortex (PFC) and monitored during the delay-response task. **B:** Neuronal activity in cue neurons (brown) and delay neurons (black) during the delay-response task. **C:** The location of the cue and delay neurons in the right PFC. (Adapted from Fuster JM. Unit activity in prefrontal cortex during delayed-response performance: Neuronal correlates of transient memory. *J Neurophysiol.* 1973;36[1]:61–78.)

probes in the PFC of rats (see Figure 9.4A), which allowed continual analysis of extracellular DA concentrations while the rat performed the task. The rats were tested using an eight-arm radial maze (see Figure 17.5A). In the *training* phase, rats were given 5 minutes to explore a radial-arm maze that had four randomly chosen arms baited with food. During the *delay*, the rats were confined at the center of the maze in the dark from 30 minutes to 6 hours. In the *test* phase, food was placed on the opposite arms from the training phase and the rats were given 5 minutes to locate the rewards. Errors

were scored as entries into unbaited arms. Extracellular DA was analyzed at baseline and during the testing phase.

The results show a remarkable inverse correlation between extracellular DA in the PFC during the testing phase and errors (Figure 17.5B). When the delay was only 30 minutes, the efflux of DA into the PFC increased over the baseline by 75% and the rat made only few error journeys into unbaited arms. However, as the delay was increased the DA efflux decreased and the errors mounted.

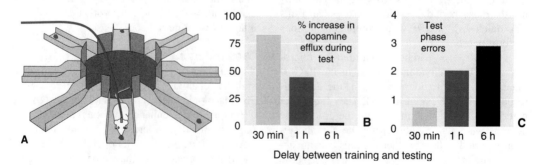

FIGURE 17.5 ● **A:** Radial-arm maze with four arms baited. **B:** Percent increase in extracellular dopamine (DA) at the testing phase. **C:** Errors at the testing phase. (Adapted from Phillips AG, Ahn S, Floresco SB. Magnitude of dopamine release in medial prefrontal cortex predicts accuracy of memory on a delayed response task. *J Neurosci.* 2004;24[2]:547–553.)

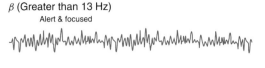

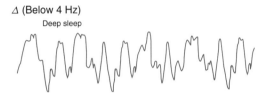

FIGURE 17.6 ● The four common electrocardiographic rhythms. The goal of neurofeedback is to help the user learn to generate more of the attentive rhythms and less of the calm rhythms.

EXECUTIVE FUNCTION VERSUS WORKING MEMORY

The terms executive function and working memory are often used synonymously in the literature. Some researchers prefer one term while others prefer the other, yet they describe different functions in the brain. Executive function includes working memory as well as other higher-level cognitive skills such as organizing priorities and planning initiation strategies. Although executive function and working memory describe different functions in the brain, they share the same underlying mechanisms. Both reside in the PFC, are impaired with frontal lobe damage, and fluctuate with catecholamine modulation.

Biofeedback

Neurofeedback (also called *electro EEG biofeedback*) is a treatment option that allows patients to exercise their brain to improve attention and concentration. The EEG frequencies are divided into four basic categories (see Figure 17.6). β Waves are the frequency pattern produced when a person is alert and concentrating. The goal of neurofeedback is to spend more time in β rhythm and less in α and θ rhythm.

Neurofeedback utilizes a computer that interprets the EEG frequencies from the user and provides them with feedback through a symbol on the computer screen. The user learns to move the image across the screen by generating the correct β rhythms. It is the mental equivalent of lifting weights or jogging.

Although there have not been good, randomized controlled trials, results in the literature are about 75% positive. Recently a group in Montreal completed a small controlled trial with functional imaging before and after biofeedback treatment in children with ADHD. Treatment consisted of 40 sessions of neurofeedback, each lasting an hour, over 15 weeks. The neurofeedback group not only improved their scores on measures of attention, but also increased the activation of the anterior cingulate cortex (see Figure 17.7). The brain, like the skeletal muscles and cardiovascular system, seems to respond to exercise and training.

REWARD AND IMPULSE CONTROL

Sustained attention to a particular task requires an individual to ignore other appealing stimuli. Controlling the impulse to take the immediate, smaller reward and waiting for the larger, delayed reward is essential for completing any project.

INATTENTION EPIDEMIC

The diagnosis and treatment of inattention has exploded during the last decade. Some believe this is because patients with true disorders are finally being recognized. Others postulate that the epidemic is a result of loosening the criteria for what is considered as a disorder. Still others wonder if the epidemic is a result of our fast-paced, complex life style. Too much information coming too quickly means that we fail to learn the skill of patience.

Neuropsychological testing

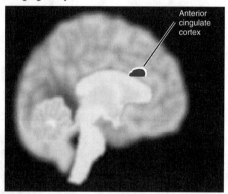

Test	Before	After
Digit Span	9.8	11.6[a]
Continuous Performance Test	77.5	85[b]
Conners Parent Rating Scale Inattention	71.6	58.9[c]
Conners Parent Rating Scale Hyperactivity	79.4	64.3[a]

A

[a] p <0.05   [b] p <0.005   [c] p <0.001

Imaging study

Anterior cingulate cortex

B

FIGURE 17.7 ● **A:** Neuropsychological testing improved after 40 sessions of neurofeedback. **B:** The anterior cingulate cortex showed greater activity after the neurofeedback treatment. (Adapted from Levesque J, Beauregard M, Mensour B. Effect of neurofeedback training on the neural substrates of selective attention in children with attention-deficit/hyperactivity disorder: A functional magnetic resonance imaging study. *Neurosci Lett.* 2006;394[3]:216–221.)

People who cannot control these impulses are at a disadvantage. In an amazingly simple study, a group at Stanford examined the ability of children to wait for the larger reward and then followed up their outcome as adolescents.

In the study, 4-year-old children were sequestered in a room with an assistant who placed a marshmallow on a table. The children were told that the assistant had to run an errand and would be stepping out of the room. They were also told they could eat the one marshmallow, but if they could wait until the assistant returned, they could have two marshmallows. The assistant left the room for approximately 15 minutes and the childrens' response was observed. Some children ate the marshmallow right away whereas others showed varying degrees of restraint.

The social and academic performance of these children was reassessed in their adolescence. The children who were better at inhibiting the impulse to immediately eat the one marshmallow were more resilient, confident, and dependable as adolescents. Additionally, they were more successful students and even scored higher on the SAT. The SAT scores for the more impulsive children are contrasted with those who showed more self-control. The total scores of the two groups are approximately 100 points different.

	Impulsive eaters	Patient waiters
Verbal	524	610
Math	528	652

Clearly, the ability to suppress the desire to grab the immediate reward was associated with or was part of behaviors that have a profound impact on one's life. People who can delay gratification appear to achieve more in the long run.

Nucleus Accumbens and Dopamine

The ability to delay gratification is controlled, in part, by DA activity in the nucleus accumbens (NAc). We also talked earlier about how being able to fully attend to a task can even be joyful. Pleasurable activities increase the release of DA in the NAc (see Figure 9.6). People are less likely to respond to other stimuli if they are engaged in activities they enjoy. Stimulant medications also increase the DA released at the NAc and increase impulse control. People report that stimulants enable them to block out irrelevant stimuli with great ease.

Clearly, other areas of the brain influence the NAc. For example, the orbitofrontal cortex, the hippocampus, and the amygdala are three regions with important projections to the NAc (see Figure 9.3). However, the NAc is uniquely wired to focus attention on the more favorable rewards.

Other evidence of the role of the NAc in impulsive behavior comes from lesion studies on rats. Rats can learn to choose a larger, delayed reward over a smaller, immediate reward. Lesions of the NAc will reverse this behavior. The rats with damaged NAcs become more impulsive and choose the immediate reward more frequently.

Impulsivity and Youth

Why are adolescents so impulsive and prone to taking risks? One possible explanation is that the frontal cortex has not yet matured—an issue discussed in Chapter 11, Anger and Aggression,

BOREDOM

It is no great revelation to say that people have a hard time staying focused on boring tasks. The stimulant medications may improve attention (at least in part) by increasing the level of interest perceived by the brain. Volkow et al. gave methylphenidate or placebo to normal young men and imaged their brains while they solved math problems. When taking methylphenidate, the men found math less boring and more exciting (see figure).

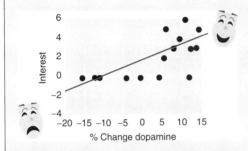

Changes in extracellular dopamine (DA) at the striatum correlated with interest in normal adults solving math problems. (Adapted from Volkow ND, Wang GJ, Fowler JS, et al. Evidence that methylphenidate enhances the saliency of a mathematical task by increasing dopamine in the human brain. *Am J Psychiatry*. 2004;161[7]:1173–1180.)

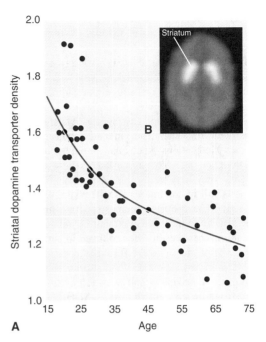

FIGURE 17.8 ● **A:** The density of the dopamine (DA) transporter at the striatum as a function of age. **B:** Distribution of DA transporter in the human brain. (Adapted from Mozley PD, Acton PD, Barraclough ED, et al. Effects of age on dopamine transporters in healthy humans. *J Nucl Med*. 1999;40[11]:1812–1817.)

in the context of explaining impulsive aggression. Another explanation points to the NAc and dopaminergic tone.

The DA reuptake pump (called the *dopamine transporter*) has been used as a measure of dopaminergic tone. New technology allows the imaging of the DA transporter density. Studies have examined the DA transporter density at the striatum (the region that contains the NAc). Figure 17.8 shows the decline in the DA transporter with age. Note the more precipitous drop in early adulthood.

Other researchers have shown that drug-naïve patients with ADHD have, on average, a slightly higher density in DA transporter at equivalent ages. For example, a 30-year-old patient with ADHD has the DA transporter density of a normal 22-year-old. Therefore, it appears that high DA transporter density (seen with younger individuals and patients with ADHD) correlates with more impulsive behavior while lower density correlates with better impulse control.

Drug Addiction

The cravings that drug addicts experience at times for their drug of choice might be the most extreme example of wanting immediate gratification. When a drug addict gets this kind of urge, there are few concerns about long-term consequences. Every clinician knows about horror stories of addicts who have squandered the family savings just to get high. What is the role of the NAc in addictive behavior?

We know that chronic cocaine use down-regulates the DA receptors at the NAc (see Figure 9.11). Likewise, we have shown that amphetamines and opioids alter the morphology of dendritic spine on neurons in the NAc (see Figure 9.13). These results and the behavior of the addicts suggest that drug abuse damages the operation of the NAc, rendering it less functional. Such an effect might be the pharmacologic equivalent of lesioning the NAc—an effect that enhances impulsive behavior.

ATTENTION-DEFICIT/ HYPERACTIVITY DISORDER

Genetics

ADHD travels in families. It is one of the most heritable psychiatric disorders we know. Pooled analyses of twin studies suggest the heritable rate may be as high as 76%.

Another consistent finding for ADHD is the treatment response from the stimulant medications. Medications such as amphetamine and methylphenidate have remarkable short-term efficacy. They may be the oldest psychiatric medications still in continuous use. The stimulants are effective because they increase extracellular DA and NE in the frontal cortex, and DA alone in the striatum. These results are produced in part by the blockade of the DA and NE reuptake transporters. It is tempting to speculate that abnormalities of the DA and NE receptors and transports will explain the strong genetic inheritance of ADHD.

Numerous studies have been conducted with ADHD, searching for abnormalities with the genes that code for the catecholamine receptors and transporters. Unfortunately, the results are not as compelling as one might hope. A recent comprehensive analysis of available genetic studies in ADHD found that 36% were positive, 17% showed a trend, and 47% were negative. Despite conflicting evidence, there are modest indications for anomalous genes for the D4 and D5 receptors as well as the DA, NE, and 5-hydroxytryptamine (5-HT) transporters in patients with ADHD.

The lack of consistent findings implicating abnormalities in catecholamine receptors and transporters may be the result of the following several factors.

1. ADHD is a complex disorder involving multiple genes, each with moderate effect.
2. ADHD is best viewed as a continuous trait rather than an all-or-none disorder.
3. Parental behaviors (which can be inherited from different genes), such as smoking or discipline style, can affect symptom expression.
4. Stimulants will improve performance for almost all individuals, not just those with disorders. This is not true for antidepressants, mood stabilizers, or antipsychotics, which offer little benefit for those without disorders.

It seems likely that this highly heritable disorder will have other neural impairments to explain the problem.

Brain Size

As discussed earlier, working memory and impulse control are important features of attention and concentration and are usually impaired in patients with ADHD. As would be expected, dysfunction in the PFC and striatum are the most common abnormal brain findings reported for ADHD.

However, the most comprehensive neuroscientific studies on children with ADHD come from Judith Rapoport's laboratory at National Institute of Mental Health (NIMH). They have conducted several large prospective case–control magnetic resonance imaging (MRI) studies of the brains of children with ADHD. One study produced multiple MRI scans of 150 children with ADHD and 139 age- and sex-matched controls. Sixty percent of the participants had at least two scans.

The most interesting finding was that children with ADHD had smaller total brain volumes by approximately 5% compared with controls. The difference held true for all four cerebral lobes (including white matter and gray matter), as well as the cerebellum. The trajectory of the total brain volumes did not change as the children aged, nor was it affected by the use of stimulant medication.

MINIMAL BRAIN DYSFUNCTION

In the past, ADHD was called *minimal brain dysfunction*, a term now considered derogatory. The findings from Rapoport's laboratory suggest that those older clinicians, without the benefits of modern imaging studies, had a subtle understanding of the pathophysiology of ADHD.

Gray Matter Thickness

In a followup study Rapoport's group examined another 300 subjects, half of whom had ADHD. This time, with better technology, they measured regional gray matter thickness. The most unique feature of this second study was that they followed up the clinical outcome as well as the structural changes in the brain of the children over time. They were able to compare the children who grew out of the disorder with those that did not.

The results showed that children with ADHD had global thinning of all the gray matter compared to the controls, although it was most prominent in the PFC. Additionally, both groups showed the usual pruning of the total gray matter as they grew through adolescence (see Figure 17.9).

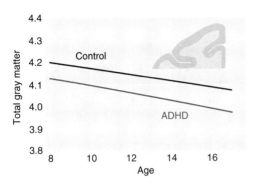

FIGURE 17.9 ● Total gray matter thickness for children with attention-deficit/hyperactivity disorder (ADHD) compared with controls. (Adapted from Shaw P, Lerch J, Greenstein D, et al. Longitudinal mapping of cortical thickness and clinical outcome in children and adolescents with attention-deficit/hyperactivity disorder. *Arch Gen Psychiatry*. 2006;63[5]:540–549.)

However, two regions were unique when correlated with clinical outcome.

1. Children who remained impaired at followup had thinner gray matter in the medial PFC at the beginning of the study.
2. Children who grew out of the disorder showed a normalization of the gray matter thickness in the right parietal cortex.

These results imply that the normalization of the parietal cortex may be a compensatory activation of the posterior attentional network. Indeed, recent research suggests that the parietal cortex may play a greater role in attention than previously considered. A recent imaging study conducted while the subjects attempted to detect and respond to the presence of an infrequent stimuli (a variation on a continuous performance test)

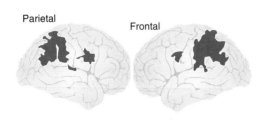

FIGURE 17.10 ● Regions of significantly greater activation in healthy subjects relative to the attention-deficit/hyperactivity disorder (ADHD) group during a target detection task. (Adapted from Tamm L, Menon V, Reiss AL. Parietal attentional system aberrations during target detection in adolescents with attention-deficit/hyperactivity disorder: Event-related fMRI evidence. *Am J Psychiatry*. 2006;163[6]:1033–1043.)

showed greater activation of the bilateral parietal lobes in the controls compared to patients with ADHD (see Figure 17.10).

NEGLECT SYNDROME

There is other evidence that the parietal lobes are important for good attention. Parietal lesions can cause a neglect syndrome in which patients ignore objects, people, and even parts of their body to one side of the center of gaze. The very existence of parts of the body on the ignored side can be denied. Figure shows an example of a patient after a right parietal stroke attempting to copy some drawings. Note how he fails to copy details from the left side of the drawings. It has been proposed that the parietal cortex is involved in attending to objects at different positions in extracellular space.

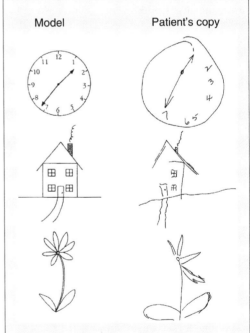

A patient after a right parietal stroke attempts to copy the drawings on the left. (From Springer SP, Deutsch G. *Left brain, right brain*. New York: Worth Publishers; 1998.)

Timing and Cerebellum

Some researchers suggest that deficits in time perception are an integral feature of ADHD. Children with ADHD are known to have problems with

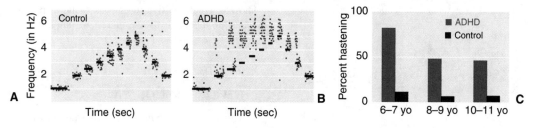

FIGURE 17.11 ● The stimulus to replicate is represented by the black lines in A: and B:. The responses by an unaffected child and one with ADHD are shown with brown dots. C: The percentage of children who hasten their responses by tapping too quickly. (Adapted from Ben-Pazi H, Shalev RS, Gross-Tsur V, et al. Age and medication effects on rhythmic response in ADHD: Possible oscillatory mechanisms? *Neuropsychologia.* 2006;44:412–416.)

temporal information processing and the timing of motor tasks. Clinical tests such as estimates of time duration or the reproduction of timed sequences are frequently impaired in children with ADHD. The finger tapping studies by Ben-Pazi provides a specific example of this problem. Children were asked to replicate the same frequency of the presented stimuli by tapping the space bar on a computer. Children with ADHD were less capable of replicating the stimuli and tended to tap faster than the stimulus presentation—getting ahead of themselves.

Figure 17.11A and B shows a comparison between a healthy control and one with ADHD. Note how the healthy control accurately replicates the same frequency of the stimuli whereas the child with ADHD was responding at a faster frequency. The propensity to hasten the response is greater for children with ADHD (Figure 17.11C). The authors speculate that the rhythmic tapping problems reflect an abnormal oscillatory mechanism for those with ADHD.

These rhythmic motor abnormalities may represent a larger timing problem for patients with ADHD. In other words, the problem is greater than just replicating the tapping of a metronome. The problems with timing may contribute to the impairments seen with higher cognitive skills required to plan and complete a project. Inconsistencies in performance, responding too fast or too slow, and procrastination are behaviors that may be impaired due to temporal processing deficits. For example, patients with ADHD typically overestimate the time left to finish a project. In short, patients with ADHD may have trouble with project planning and completion due to problems getting into a good rhythm and maintaining a consistent pace.

The cerebellum, traditionally conceptualized as controlling motor coordination, has been identified as a possible culprit in the etiology of ADHD. Studies such as those from Rapoport's laboratory have documented smaller cerebellum volumes in patients with ADHD (see Figure 17.12). Likewise, stimulant medications are known to activate the cerebellum. Finally, the cerebellum is believed to play an important role in timing responses. Taken together, these findings suggest that patients with ADHD may have impaired timing mechanisms, which may be due to cerebellar dysfunction.

In summary, it is clear that the PFC and striatum play large roles in the pathophysiology of ADHD. More recent studies suggest that the parietal cortex and cerebellar may also contribute to the problems patients experience.

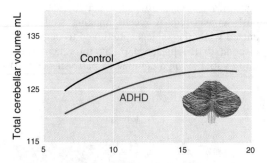

FIGURE 17.12 ● Children with attention-deficit/hyperactivity disorder (ADHD) have smaller total cerebellar volume compared with unaffected controls. (Adapted from Castellanos FX, Tannock R. Neuroscience of attention-deficit/hyperactivity disorder: The search for endophenotypes. *Nat Rev Neurosci.* 2002;3[8]:617–628.)

QUESTIONS

1. All of the following are true about CPTs, except
   a. They give an estimate of a subject's ability to attend.
   b. Scores change with age.
   c. Treatment will affect the scores.
   d. Elderly subjects perform worst.

2. A delayed-response task measures
   a. The subject's capacity to delay gratification.
   b. Impulsivity.
   c. Working memory.
   d. Relative DA activity at the NAc.

3. The goal of neurofeedback is for the subject to improve their attention by spending more time in which rhythm?
   a. α.
   b. β.
   c. θ.
   d. Δ.

4. Stimulant medications improve attention and concentration through the following mechanisms, except
   a. Increase NE efflux in the striatum.
   b. Increase NE efflux in the PFC.
   c. Increase activity in the cerebellum.
   d. Increase interest in new activities.

5. Activity at the NAc (or striatum) helps explain all of the following, except
   a. Drug addiction.
   b. Impulsivity
   c. Working memory.
   d. Adolescent behavior.

6. Children who fail to grow out of ADHD show all of the following, except
   a. Thinner total gray matter.
   b. Compensatory thickening of the parietal gray matter.
   c. Smaller total cerebellum volume.
   d. Less prefrontal gray matter.

7. Which structure is associated with which finding in ADHD?

1. PFC	A. Compensatory gray matter thickening
2. Cerebellum	B. Temporal processing
3. NAc	C. Working memory
4. Parietal cortex	D. Delay of gratification

See Answers section at end of book.

SECTION III

Disorders

Depression

INTRODUCTION

We will wrap up this review of neuroscience by looking closer at the pathophysiology of four common psychiatric disorders. The first will be the depressive disorders. Although we will often use the term *depression*, the reader should keep in mind that there are probably a multitude of discrete diseases that all end up with the syndrome we now call depression. For example, psychotic depression, atypical depression, bipolar depression, and pathologic grief may be variants of the same phenomena or they could be different conditions with different mechanisms of action. We have no objective measures to distinguish between the depressive disorders at this time. In the 1920s, we would have talked about pneumonia as one disease, as they all produced coughs and fever, although we now know that there are many different causes of pneumonia (e.g., tuberculosis, pneumococcus, H. flu, etc.).

Depression is a common condition recognized by Hippocrates (melancholia). Yet, in spite of all our technologic advances since the time of the ancient Greeks, we know surprisingly little about the pathophysiology of the disorder. We know even less about bipolar disorder.

Monoamine Hypothesis

The accidental discovery in the 1950s that the tricyclic and monoamine oxidase inhibitor medications could relieve depression transformed the treatment of the disorder. Numerous spin-off medications have been developed since the 1950s. Most are safer and better tolerated than the earlier medications, but none are more effective. In addition, they all work through the same mechanism: the monoamines. This has driven the common conceptualization of depression as a disorder of serotonin and/or norepinephrine (NE).

Again, we see that treatment response generates pathophysiology theories. Clinicians call this the *monoamine hypothesis*, and the lay public calls it a *chemical imbalance*. Unfortunately, neither is an accurate description of the biologic mechanisms of depression. At least two factors argue against the monoamine hypothesis as being the only cause of depression:

1. Medications take 6 to 10 weeks to reach full effectiveness, although the neurotransmitter activity at the synapse is altered within a few doses.
2. Studies of neurotransmitter levels in the plasma, cerebrospinal fluid (CSF), and brain tissue have failed to find deficiencies in patients who are depressed compared with healthy controls.

Clearly, the depressions are more complex than the simple replacement of an insufficient neurotransmitter.

The Depressed Brain

If a biopsy were to be done in patients with depression, it is not clear from where the tissue should be removed. However, structural imaging, functional imaging, and postmortem studies have established five regions that are consistently dysfunctional in most patients with depression. The five regions

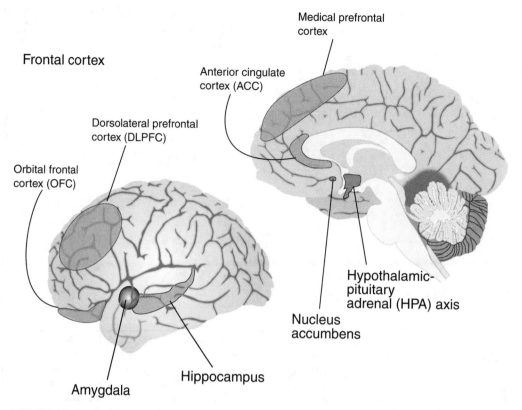

Frontal cortex

Medical prefrontal cortex

Anterior cingulate cortex (ACC)

Dorsolateral prefrontal cortex (DLPFC)

Orbital frontal cortex (OFC)

Hypothalamic-pituitary adrenal (HPA) axis

Nucleus accumbens

Hippocampus

Amygdala

FIGURE 18.1 ● The five major regions of dysfunction in depressed brains.

are shown in Figure 18.1. Note the extensive prefrontal involvement.

It is tempting to match depressive symptoms from the Diagnostic and Statistical Manual of Mental Disorders (DSM) criteria with specific regions in the brain. For example, anhedonia can be attributed to dysfunction of the nucleus accumbens or cognitive deficits to the anterior cingulate cortex. However, while a few symptoms seem to match up with a brain region, most do not. Most symptoms are likely the product of simultaneous dysfunction in several regions.

Alternatively, it is possible to envision depression as the result of overactivity in some regions and underactivity in other. For example, the hippocampus and nucleus accumbens are considered underactive in depressed patients whereas the hypothalamic-pituitary-adrenal (HPA) axis and amygdala are overactive. This is appealing because some of the symptoms of depression appear to be caused by loss of function (low motivation, lack of hope, low appetite) whereas others appear to be caused by hyperactivity (insomnia, anxiety, suicidal thoughts). However, the situation in the frontal cortex is more complex.

Frontal Cortex

The activity level in the frontal cortex in depressed patients is generally hypoactive when measured in resting positron emission tomography (PET) scans. However, the specific region affected varies from one study to the next. Likewise, functional magnetic resonance imaging (fMRIs) gives a varying picture of activity in the depressed frontal cortex. There is no consensus.

Furthermore, one would expect that successful treatment would have an activating effect on the frontal cortex, but that is not the case. Figure 18.2 shows the paradoxical effect that electroconvulsive therapy (ECT) has on the frontal cortex. Remarkably, a successful course of ECT unequivocally turns DOWN the frontal cortex. Perhaps even more confusing, antidepressants and transcranial magnetic stimulation (TMS) have been shown to activate the frontal cortex whereas cognitive-behavioral therapy decreases the activity.

How can these successful treatments have such disparate effects on the frontal cortex? The answer is not known. We think one explanation is that depression results from dysfunction of the frontal cortex and that successful treatment restores

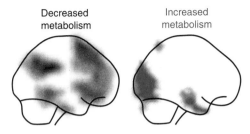

Decreased
metabolism

Increased
metabolism

FIGURE 18.2 ● Sagittal views of positron emission tomography (PET) scans on an average group of patients after a successful course of electroconvulsive therapy (ECT). (Adapted from Nobler MS, Oquendo MA, Kegeles LS, et al. Decreased regional brain metabolism after ect. *Am J Psychiatry.* 2001;158[2]:305–308.)

harmony to the region. A sports analogy may be helpful. A team that is disorganized will not be successful. Interventions that help the players to work together can improve the team's performance. However, some interventions enhance defensive skills whereas others enhance offense. In either case a team that works in harmony (whether on defense or offense) is more likely to win. Likewise with the brain, a frontal cortex that is organized and working together (whether more active or less active) may be less depressed.

THE HYPOTHALAMIC-PITUITARY-ADRENAL AXIS

Since the 1950s it has been recognized that depressed patients have excessive activity of the HPA axis. Figure 18.3 shows the increased plasma cortisol levels over 24 hours in patients with depression compared with controls. The hypercortisolemia is stimulated by increased expression

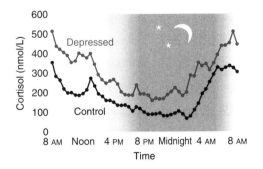

FIGURE 18.3 ● Diurnal mean plasma cortisol in depressed patients and healthy controls. (Adapted from Deuschle M, Schweiger U, Weber B, et al. Diurnal activity and pulsatility of the hypothalamic-pituitary-adrenal system in male depressed patients and healthy controls. *J Clin Endocrinol Metab.* 1997;82[1]:234–238.)

of corticotropin-releasing hormone (CRH) and reduced feedback inhibition of the HPA axis (see Figure 6.9). As discussed in Chapter 6, Hormones and the Brain, one theory of depression postulates that chronic, unremitting stress leads to the inability of the brain to turn down the HPA axis.

Postmortem studies of depressed patients have shown increased neurons in the paraventricular nucleus of the hypothalamus. The increased neurons are believed to be driving the increased activity in the HPA axis. It is unclear why these patients have more neurons in the hypothalamus. It could be genetic or a reaction to chronic stress.

DEPRESSION LABORATORY TEST

The activation of the HPA axis is so consistent in depression that there were early efforts to use it as a laboratory test to diagnose depression. Unfortunately, the sensitivity and specificity of increased adrenocorticotropic hormone (ACTH) for depression are not to the level where it is clinically useful. Other medical conditions also result in elevations of ACTH and there is even a subset of depressed patients who have low ACTH!

The dexamethasone-suppression test (DST) was piloted in the early 1980s in an alternative attempt to develop a laboratory test for depression. Patients are given dexamethasone at 11 P.M. and cortisol levels are drawn the next morning. Dexamethasone binds to the glucocorticoid receptors, which in turn inhibits the secretion of ACTH and subsequently cortisol. Healthy subjects will suppress the release of cortisol. Depressed patients will fail to suppress the cortisol and show a bump in their cortisol level the next morning. Unfortunately, the test has not been sensitive or specific enough—only 25% to 40%. It fails to detect most patients who are truly depressed, and some general medical conditions also fail to suppress cortisol.

Subsequently, with the availability of CRH, a new test has been developed using both dexamethasone and CRH (dex/CRH). Although the dex/CRH test is more accurate (the sensitivity increases to 80%), the clinical utility of this cumbersome test as a diagnostic tool remains doubtful.

Saline   BDNF

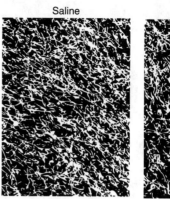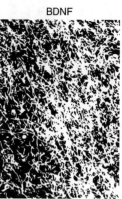

FIGURE 18.4 ● Brain-derived neurotrophic factor (BDNF) infused directly into the rat frontal cortex results in a supranormal branching of 5-hydroxytryptamine axons. (Adapted from Mamounas LA, Blue ME, Siuciak JA, et al. Brain-derived neurotrophic factor promotes the survival and sprouting of serotonergic axons in rat brain. *J Neurosci.* 1995;15[12]:7929–7939.)

Some patients with excess cortisol—either taken orally or generated internally—have reduced hippocampal volume. A recent meta-analysis of magnetic resonance imaging (MRI) studies has confirmed that hippocampal volume is reduced in patients with depression. It is believed that the excess cortisol produced by depressed patients is toxic to the hippocampus and causes the volume loss.

Effective treatments for depression (antidepressants, ECT, and lithium) are known to restore normal HPA function in most patients. It is postulated that this effect is due to increased glucocorticoid receptor production stimulated by the treatments, which has the effect of making the hypothalamus more receptive to negative feedback from cortisol. Finally, effective treatment of depression is believed to preserve and possibly restore hippocampal function (more on this later). A healthy hippocampus provides more inhibitory feedback on the HPA axis, as shown in Figure 6.9.

Consequently, depression appears to result in the breakdown of the normal relationship between the hippocampus and HPA axis. Increased cortisol from the adrenal gland causes hippocampal damage, which results in decreased inhibitory feedback on the HPA axis—which in turn causes increased cortisol release, and so forth.

Restoring normal functioning of the HPA axis as a treatment option has generated considerable interest. Several groups have tested CRH receptor blockers as novel treatments for depression. Although the early small studies were favorable, the results were not consistent and were associated with a risk of hepatotoxicity. Research in this area has stalled.

NEUROGENESIS AND BRAIN-DERIVED NEUROTROPHIC FACTOR

As discussed in Chapter 7, Adult Development and Plasticity, the brain is more dynamic than

previously thought. The brain contains undeveloped stem cells that can migrate and mature into neurons or glial cells (see Neurogenesis in Chapter 7, Adult Development and Plasticity). There is compelling evidence that this process is disrupted in depression and corrected with successful treatment.

Volume Loss

Structural imaging studies and postmortem analysis of depressed patients have documented subtle volumetric loss. The findings of a smaller hippocampus (mentioned above) are the best known, but other findings include decreased prefrontal cortex (PFC), cingulate gyrus, and cerebellum. Additionally, microscopic examinations have shown decreased cortical thickness as well as diminished neural size. One possible explanation is that HPA axis activation is neurotoxic to the brain. Another possibility involves a disruption of normal nerve growth.

The prospect that depression is related to problems with nerve growth factors opens a new way to conceptualize the pathophysiology of the disorder. A failure of neurogenesis and growth factor proteins, such as brain-derived neurotrophic factor (BDNF), may cause subtle shrinkage of the brain in depression.

BDNF is one of a family of neurotrophins that regulate the differentiation and survival of neurons (see Figure 7.8). Most likely there are a multitude of growth factor proteins maintaining and stimulating nerve growth, but BDNF is the most widely studied at this point. Figure 18.4 shows a dramatic example of the effects of BDNF on serotonergic neurons in the rat cortex. Saline or BDNF was infused directly into the rat frontal cortex for 21 days. Then the animals were sacrificed and the cortex at the site of the infusion was stained for 5-hydroxytryptamine (5-HT) neurons. Note the remarkable arborization of the 5-HT axons in the cortex of the rat exposed to BDNF.

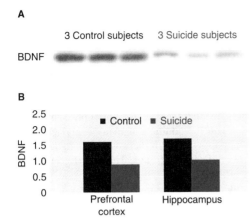

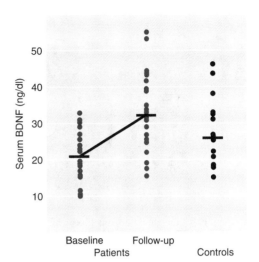

FIGURE 18.5 ● **A:** Western blots showing the immunolabeling of brain-derived neurotrophic factor (BDNF) in the prefrontal cortex in three control subjects and three suicide subjects. **B:** Averaged BDNF in the prefrontal cortex and hippocampus for both groups. (Adapted from Dwivedi Y, Rizavi HS, Conley RR, et al. Altered gene expression of brain-derived neurotrophic factor and receptor tyrosine kinase B in postmortem brain of suicide subjects. *Arch Gen Psychiatry.* 2003;60[8]:804–815.)

FIGURE 18.6 ● Serum brain-derived neurotrophic factor (BDNF) levels in depressed patients before and 8 weeks after antidepressant treatment compared with healthy controls. (Adapted from Gonul AS, Akdeniz F, Taneli F, et al. Effect of treatment on serum brain-derived neurotrophic factor levels in depressed patients. *Eur Arch Psychiatry Clin Neurosci.* 2005;255[6]:381–386.)

Growth factor proteins such as BDNF provide ongoing maintenance of neurons in the brain. Disruption of these nerve growth factors results in the reduction in the size of neurons, as well as some cell loss. Such reductions and loss may produce psychiatric symptoms.

It is difficult to assess the quantity and quality of BDNF in living humans, so the evidence connecting BDNF and depression is indirect. A postmortem analysis of suicide subjects found a marked decrease in BDNF in their PFC and hippocampus compared with controls (see Figure 18.5).

Psychiatric Treatment and Brain-Derived Neurotrophic Factor

Of great interest to psychiatrists are the increases in BDNF and neurogenesis seen with treatments that relieve depression. In rats, the following interventions have been shown to increase BDNF:

1. Antidepressants
2. Lithium
3. Stimulation treatments: ECT, TMS, and VNS
4. Estrogen
5. Exercise

This is a remarkable discovery. It is the first time that one mechanism of action has been found that could explain how all these disparate modes of treatments relieve depression. Presumably, psychotherapy would also increase BDNF, but no one

has yet developed a credible animal model that could be tested.

With humans, there is less data on studies following depression treatment and BDNF levels. Recently, a group in Turkey examined serum BDNF levels in depressed patients before and after the initiation of antidepressant treatment. The results were compared with healthy control subjects. Although serum BDNF levels are not as accurate as direct central measurements, the results are still impressive (see Figure 18.6). The BDNF levels in the depressed patients before treatment were significantly less than the levels in the healthy subjects. After 8 weeks of antidepressant treatment, the serum BDNF levels increased significantly and no longer differed from those of the controls.

Neurogenesis

Numerous studies have shown that increased BDNF leads to increased neurogenesis. Therefore, interventions that increase BDNF should also increase the development of new nerve cells. A unique study with rats has demonstrated that fluoxetine stimulates neurogenesis in about the same amount of time as it takes for humans to respond to the treatment. The rats given fluoxetine did not generate new neurons at a rate any different from placebo after 5 days, but did separate from placebo by 28 days (see Figure 18.7). Of particular

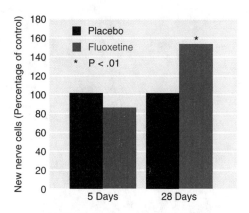

FIGURE 18.7 ● New neurons (neurogenesis) at 5 days and 28 days on rats given placebo and fluoxetine. (Adapted from Santarelli L, Saxe M, Gross C, et al. Requirement of hippocampal neurogenesis for the behavioral effects of antidepressants. *Science.* 2003;301[5634]:805–809.)

interest, it also took 28 days for the rats to change their behavior—demonstrate a greater willingness to move into open, lighted areas to eat.

Scarring the DNA

Nestler et al. at the University of Texas Southwestern Medical Center have taken these ideas one step further. They have looked at the effect of animal models of depression on the DNA that codes for BDNF. First, they stressed mice by placing them in the presence of a different aggressor mouse for 10 consecutive days. The exposed mice—called *defeated mice*—were later socially avoidant with unfamiliar mice. Such a reaction is similar to that of humans with depression and post-traumatic stress disorder (PTSD). The messenger RNA (mRNA) that encodes for BDNF was analyzed in the defeated mice and comparable controls. As expected, it was greatly reduced in the defeated mice.

The defeated mice were given imipramine, fluoxetine, or placebo for 30 days. The antidepressants not only reversed the avoidant behavior, but also returned the BDNF mRNA to almost normal levels. On the basis of these results the researchers speculated that depression (or in this case, social defeat) must affect the DNA. What they have found may change the way we view depression.

We discussed in Chapter 14, Social Attachment, how DNA must unravel in order for the mRNA to be transcribed (see Figure 14.7). Likewise, we discussed the profound effect that a mother rat's behavior has on gene expression (see Figure 14.8). The results from Nestler's laboratory suggest that depression too may be a disorder of gene expression—or what they call *gene silencing*.

The DNA in the region that codes for BDNF was examined in the defeated mice as well as healthy controls. Figure 18.8 shows the results. In the healthy controls there were a few methyl groups attached to the histones that package the DNA. In the defeated mice the methyl groups were greatly increased, which had the effect of limiting access to the DNA. The antidepressant-treated group had the addition of many acetyl groups to the histones although there was no change in the number of methyl groups. The acetyl groups have the effect of opening up the DNA and allowing BDNF mRNA to be transcribed.

Human studies examining methylation of the DNA in depressed patients have not been conducted. Although we would never biopsy the brain of a living depressed person, it would be interesting to compare methylation of the DNA in postmortem studies of depressed patients and nondepressed controls.

In summary, these studies suggest a mechanism for depression. Stress in conjunction with a genetic vulnerability decreases growth factor proteins (such as BDNF) due to "clogging" of the DNA (see Figure 18.9). This leads to thinning of the neuronal structures, which results in depressive symptoms. These structural changes make the prefrontal limbic governing system vulnerable to disruption and dysregulation. Stress, loss, or other processes cause the system to lose self-regulation. Furthermore, it appears that effective treatments such as antidepressants, lithium, ECT, and exercise (and presumably psychotherapy and good social support) will reverse the process. Presumably the treatment increases the production of growth factor proteins, such as BDNF, that result in renewed neuronal growth, more resilient self-regulating circuits, and a return to healthy mood.

Clearly, this is a simplistic description of what is a very complex and heterogenous process. Much more remains to be discovered.

Are Antidepressants Neuroprotective?

An intriguing study looking at stress, neurogenesis, and antidepressants with tree shrews suggests that antidepressants are neuroprotective. The tree shrew is actually closely related to primates and has a relatively large brain. They are nothing like a shrew.

"Stressed out" tree shrews showed reduced neurogenesis whereas the administration of an antidepressant (one that is available in Europe but not in the United States) preserved normal cell development (see Figure 18.10). Further analysis showed that the antidepressant did not suppress the elevated cortisol in the stressed tree shrews,

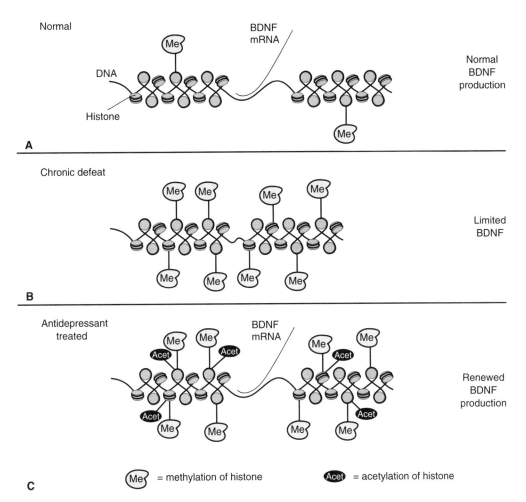

Normal

BDNF
mRNA

DNA

Me

Histone

Normal
BDNF
production

Me

A

Chronic defeat

Me   Me   Me   Me

Limited
BDNF

Me   Me   Me   Me

B

Antidepressant
treated

Me   Me   Me   Me
Acet   Acet   Acet

BDNF
mRNA

Renewed
BDNF
production

Acet   Acet
Me   Me   Me   Me

C

Me = methylation of histone   Acet = acetylation of histone

FIGURE 18.8 ● A: DNA must unravel to transcribe messenger RNA (mRNA) needed for protein translation such as brain-derived neurotrophic factor (BDNF). B: Chronic defeat (and possibly
depression) caused excessive methylation of the histones, which blocks access to the DNA. C: Antidepressant treatment renews access to the DNA by adding acetyl groups to the histones. (Adapted
from Tsankova NM, Berton O, Renthal W, et al. Sustained hippocampal chromatin regulation in a
mouse model of depression and antidepressant action. *Nat Neurosci.* 2006;9[4]:519–525.)

suggesting that the benefit was not mediated
through the HPA axis.

Sheline et al. looked at hippocampal volume in
medically healthy depressed women. They found
that hippocampal size correlated with days of

untreated depression (see Figure 18.11). This
study and the tree shrew study suggest that antidepressants might protect the brain from the
effects of depression and stress. If this is true,
one wonders if soldiers in combat would have

GLIAL CELLS

An unexpected finding in postmortem
studies of depressed patients has been
the reduced number and density of glial
cells in the PFC. Subsequent studies have
shown that electroconvulsive seizures in

rats will increase proliferation of new glial
cells but not new neurons in the PFC. Glial
cells may play a larger role in depression and its treatment than traditionally
believed.

A Normal state   **B** Depressed state   **C** Treated state

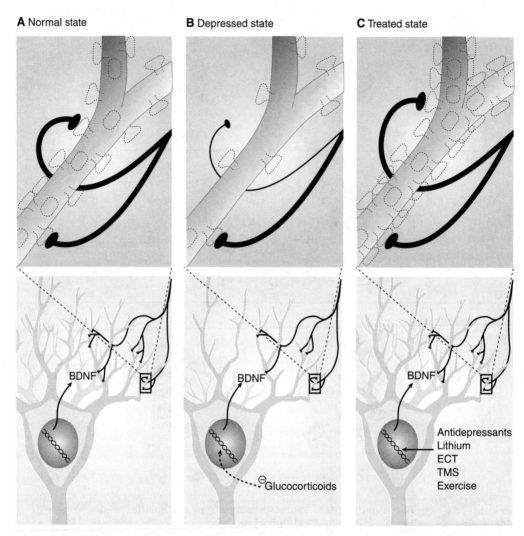

FIGURE 18.9   ●   Stress and genetics cause decreased growth factor protein production, which reduces neural substrate. Effective treatment reverses this process. BDNF, brain-derived neurotrophic factor; ECT, electroconvulsive therapy; TMS, transcranial magnetic stimulation. (Adapted from Berton O, Nestler EJ. New approaches to antidepressant drug discovery: Beyond monoamines. *Nat Rev Neurosci.* 2006;7[2]:137–151.)

less PTSD-related sequela if they were taking antidepressants during the hostilities. Clearly, more research on this important topic is needed.

BIPOLAR DISORDER

Bipolar disorder is a prevalent illness with strong genetic links and unique clinical features. Unfortunately, there is disappointingly little to report about the neuroscience of bipolar disorder. This may be due to the difficulty in distinguishing the subtle differences in bipolar patients' brains from those with unipolar depression as well as healthy controls. The essential feature of bipolar disorder—episodes of mania—is clinically very distinctive, but have no obvious structural, functional, or molecular markers yet identified in the brain.

Global Activation

One would think that manic episodes would be easy to differentiate in functional imaging studies—if the subjects could remain still enough in the scanner. In a manic episode the patient's brain appears to be revved up—going way too fast. One would imagine that the manic brain would "light up" in a functional imaging study, but that has not been the case.

The Medical University of South Carolina Functional Neuroimaging Team conducted a prospective

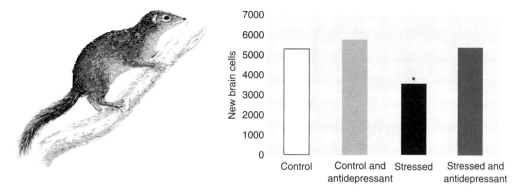

FIGURE 18.10 ● New neurons in the dentate gyrus of the hippocampus of tree shrews. The development of new cells decreased in the stressed tree shrews (black). The stressed tree shrews on the antidepressant produced new nerve cells at the same rate as the unstressed controls. (Adapted from Czeh B, Michaelis T, Watanabe T, et al. Stress-induced changes in cerebral metabolites, hippocampal volume, and cell proliferation are prevented by antidepressant treatment with tianeptine. *Proc Natl Acad Sci U S A.* 2001;98[22]:12796–12801.)

fMRI study of six rapid cycling bipolar patients in an effort to identify changes in the brain with different moods. The patients were matched with appropriate controls and asked to call the imaging center whenever in an altered mood. Numerous scans were performed at many unusual hours of the day on each patient and control. The absolute blood flow measures did change over time and were softly, but not significantly, associated with depression and mood. The results from one subject are shown in Figure 18.12. Note how the total brain activity (shown in black) roughly follows the mood changes (shown in brown). Unfortunately, larger studies attempting to show this same phenomenon have been disappointing.

Lithium and Gray Matter
Some imaging studies have found decreased size and activity in the PFC of patients with bipolar

disorder—similar to that found in patients with unipolar depression. We mentioned earlier that lithium has been shown to stimulate BDNF synthesis. A group at Wayne State University conducted a clever study matching these two concepts. They examined the gray matter volume changes in bipolar patients after initiating lithium treatment. MRI scans were conducted at baseline and after 4 weeks of lithium. A computer outlined and measured the gray matter volume in each scan (see Figure 18.13). Eight of the ten patients showed significant increases in total gray matter volume—averaging 3%.

Subsequent studies by other groups have replicated this data. Of interest, valproic acid has not been shown to have the same effect.

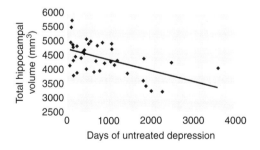

FIGURE 18.11 ● Relation between hippocampal volume and days of untreated depression in medically healthy women. (Adapted from Sheline YI, Gado MH, Kraemer HC. Untreated depression and hippocampal volume loss. *Am J Psychiatry.* 2003;160[8]:1516–1518.)

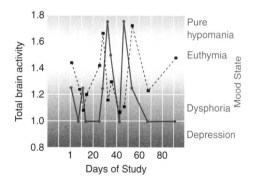

FIGURE 18.12 ● Serial functional magnetic resonance imaging (fMRI) of a rapidly cycling bipolar patient. Total brain activity in black squares. Mood states in brown circles. (Adapted from Koss S, George MS. Functional magnetic resonance imaging investigations in mood disorders. In: Soares JC, ed. *Brain imaging in affective disorders.* New York: Marcel Dekker Inc; 2003.)

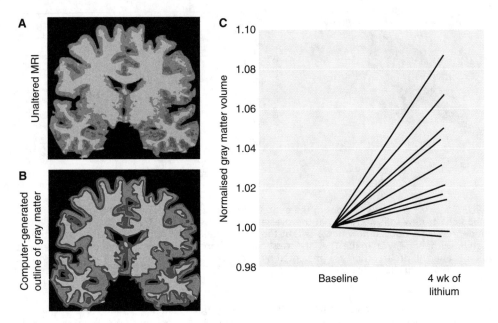

FIGURE 18.13 ● Gray matter in magnetic resonance imaging (MRI). **A:** are outlined and quantified in the computer. **B:** The change in gray matter volume is shown after 4 weeks of lithium. **C:** (Adapted from Moore GJ, Bebchuk JM, Wilds IB, et al. Lithium-induced increase in human brain grey matter. *Lancet.* 2000;356[9237]:1241–1242.)

Bipolar Summary

Although these studies are interesting, they fail to provide the neuroscientific basis for bipolar disorder that we would like to see. Haldane and Frangou reviewed the literature on imaging studies on patients with bipolar disorder. They suggest that bipolar patients share some features with unipolar depression (reduced activity in the PFC). Yet, other areas such as the amygdala are larger and more active in the bipolar patients. The authors suggest that bipolar disorder may be the result of abnormal interactions between the PFC and subcortical regions such as the amygdala—an abnormality not seen with unipolar depression. Clearly, more research is needed on this interesting topic.

BDNF UTOPIA?

One can get the impression that nerve growth factors such as BDNF are the solution to all problems. Although future psychiatric treatments may provide better ways to restore nerve growth factor deficiencies in mentally ill patients, it will not be as simple as just finding ways to get more BDNF into the brain. Too much BDNF in some regions of the brain may be detrimental. For example, Nestler et al. using the same "defeated mouse" protocol found that the defeated mice had increased BDNF in the nucleus accumbens. The researchers speculate that the development of the social phobia seen with the defeated mice may be related to too much BDNF in the brain's reward system. Additionally, "too much growth, in an uncontrolled manner" is another way to describe cancer.

QUESTIONS

1. All the following are true about the monoamine hypothesis, except
   a. It is often called a *chemical imbalance*.
   b. Explains the delay in response seen with depression treatments.
   c. Proposes deficiencies in 5-HT and norepinephrine (NE) in depressed patients.
   d. Suffers from a lack of supporting findings.

2. Postmortem studies in depressed patients have found all of the following, except
   a. Reduced neurons in the hypothalamus.
   b. Thinning of the gray matter in certain regions.
   c. Diminished neuronal size.
   d. Reduced glial cells.

3. Antidepressants may decrease depressive symptoms and improve neural survival through which of the following effects?
   a. Increased glucocorticoids and increased BDNF.
   b. Increased glucocorticoids and decreased BDNF.
   c. Decreased glucocorticoids and increased BDNF.
   d. Decreased glucocorticoids and decreased BDNF.

4. Goals for effective treatment of depression include all of the following, except
   a. Decrease HPA activity.
   b. Protect the hippocampus.
   c. Restore normal sleep architecture.
   d. Awaken the prefrontal cortex.

5. Which intervention has not been shown to increase BDNF in animal models?
   a. Cognitive behavioral therapy.
   b. Exercise.
   c. TMS.
   d. Estrogen.

6. Possible culprits in the etiology of depression include all of the following, except
   a. Cytotoxic effects of cortisol.
   b. Insufficient limbic activity.
   c. Genetic predisposition for sufficient nerve growth factors.
   d. Disorganized prefrontal activity.

7. One plausible explanation for an antidepressant's effectiveness is
   a. Removing methyl groups from scarred DNA.
   b. Restoring 5-HT and NE to their normal levels.
   c. Restoring access to the DNA.
   d. Neuroprotective effects on mRNA.

8. The pathologic mechanism of bipolar disorder is best described as
   a. Excessive prefrontal activity in manic episodes and decreased activity during depression.
   b. Too much BDNF in subcortical structures.
   c. Cortisol activation of excessive electrical activity.
   d. None of the above.

See Answers section at end of book.

Anxiety

INTRODUCTION

Anxiety is part of a mechanism developed in higher animals to handle adverse situations. The anxiety response can be conceptualized as part of the brain's alarm system firing during times of perceived danger. The characteristic responses including avoidance, hypervigilance, and increased arousal are implemented to avoid harm.

The evolutionary drive to survive has invariably enhanced a strong anxiety response. Unfortunately, in many individuals, that mechanism is overactive. The alarm fires too frequently. Such people cannot seem to turn down their internal alarm even when the coast is clear.

Diagnostic and Statistical Manual

The Diagnostic and Statistical Manual (DSM) system categorizes anxiety into a multitude of different disorders (generalized anxiety disorder [GAD], obsessive-compulsive disorder [OCD], post-traumatic stress disorder [PTSD], etc.) Although each disorder has unique clinical features, it is not clear whether they actually describe different pathologic states. The disorders have the following similar characteristics:

1. Most patients with an anxiety disorder will have features of the other disorders.
2. Many of the disorders respond to similar treatment interventions: selective serotonin reuptake inhibitors (SSRIs), benzodiazepines, exposure therapy, and so on.

3. There is little evidence to show that different disorders stem from different regions of the brain.

Many people conceptualize anxiety as though there is a basic alarm system with many features in the brain. This system is overactive to perceived threat in patients with anxiety disorder. The faulty alarm generates common symptoms in patients with anxiety disorders. The one exception is OCD, which has unique mechanisms in the brain and will be reviewed separately.

Acute Stress

The body's reaction to an acutely stressful situation is well known to all of us. The characteristic rapid heart rate, dry mouth, and sweaty palms are the body's response to increased sympathetic activity generated by a stressful situation (see Figure 2.8). Less readily apparent are the endocrine responses to acute stress.

In the late 1970s, Ursin et al. studied the endocrinologic responses of young Norwegian military recruits during parachute training. During the exercise, the recruits repeatedly jumped off a 12-meter tower and slid down a long sloping wire to learn the basic skills of parachuting. The training was designed to give the jumper a realistic sensation of the initial free fall. Measures of anxiety and performance skill as well as serum hormone levels were captured at baseline and after each jump.

Initially, anxiety was high and performance was poor. As the days and number of jumps

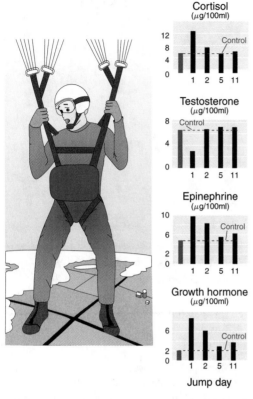

FIGURE 19.1 ● The stress of learning to parachute, on young recruits, results in changes in hormones, which return to baseline as the anxiety decreases. Parachuter. (Adapted from Rosenzweig MR, Breedlove SM, Watson NV. *Biological psychology*, 4th ed. Sunderland, MA: Sinauer; 2005.) Graphs (Adapted from Ursin H, Baade E, Levine S. *Psychobiology of stress: a study of coping men.* New York: Academic Press; 1978.)

progressed, anxiety subsided and the skills improved. The endocrinologic measures are shown in Figure 19.1. Presumably, the anxiety induces changes in the releasing hormones, which alter the pituitary hormones and ultimately the peripheral hormones (see Figure 6.4). Note how testosterone levels drop with the stress of the jumping while the other measures increase. Likewise, all return to baseline as the recruits habituate to the task.

While the average individual shows a peak in the endocrine response at the start of a difficult task, which usually subsides as the person gains mastery, this is not true for everyone. Some people have more exaggerated and persistent endocrine reactions. Kirschbaum et al. looked at salivary cortisol levels in 20 men exposed to 5 consecutive days of public speaking. For the total group, the average cortisol levels jumped on the first day and then gradually declined over the following

days. However, the men could be divided into two groups: high responders and low responders. Figure 19.2 shows the cortisol levels for these two groups.

Note how the cortisol in the low responders peaked the first day, but then quickly returned to baseline levels on the following days. These individuals appear to adjust rapidly to the stress of public speaking. The high responders, on the other hand, showed higher, more persistent peaks of cortisol. Such people appear to have a harder time turning off the stress response. Presumably, they have a stronger alarm response originating in the brain, which is driving this endocrine reaction.

NEURONAL CIRCUITRY

Multiple lines of research identify the prefrontal cortex (PFC), amygdala, hippocampus, and hypothalamic-pituitary-adrenal (HPA) axis as the regions involved with anxiety (see Figure 19.3). However, if there is one organ that represents an alarm system in the brain, it is the amygdala (see Figure 2.6).

Amygdala

In their classic studies with rhesus monkeys in the 1930s, Heinrich Klüver and Paul Bucy identified the amygdala as an important region involved with emotions. They removed large segments of the temporal lobes from wild monkeys and transformed the monkey's temperament. Aggressive and easily frightened monkeys were changed into docile, calm creatures. The entire constellation of symptoms is called the *Klüver-Bucy syndrome* and includes a host of other bizarre features, such as hypersexuality and a tendency to put objects in their mouths.

The transformation of the emotional behavior in these wild monkeys was most dramatic. The monkeys virtually became tame. They did not react fearfully to strange humans or even a snake. Of particular interest, the monkeys failed to learn from negative experience. One monkey, bitten by a snake, later approached a snake again as if nothing had happened. This is clear evidence of the survival value of anxiety.

In the intervening years it has been demonstrated that the emotional changes of the Klüver-Bucy syndrome can be elicited with the removal of just the amygdala. Other evidence points to the amygdala as an important region in the recognition and management of fear.

1. Electric stimulation of the amygdala in animals elicits fearful behavior, for example, freezing and tachycardia.
2. Humans with damaged amygdala exhibit impaired fear conditioning.

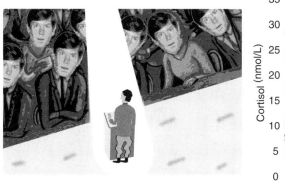
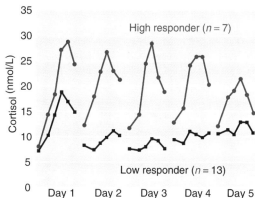

FIGURE 19.2 ● Men stressed by public speaking over 5 consecutive days showed different patterns of adrenocortical response. (Graph adapted from Kirschbaum C, Prussner JC, Stone AA, et al. Persistent high cortisol responses to repeated psychological stress in a subpopulation of healthy men. *Psychosom Med.* 1995;57[5]:468–474. Illustration adapted from Images.com.)

3. Functional imaging studies on humans show activation of the amygdala during fear learning.

Recognizing danger

Sensory information enters the brain by way of the thalamus. For example, all neurons carrying auditory and visual information synapse first in the thalamus before being sent to the appropriate cortical region for analysis. Information about danger is particularly important and needs to be recognized quickly. Work by LeDoux et al. at New York University has shown that the amygdala quickly receives some preliminary information about dangerous events even before it is processed in the cortex.

Figure 19.4 shows an example of a person coming upon a rattlesnake. This life-threatening visual information proceeds from the eyes to the thalamus. However, the thalamus sends fast but rudimentary signals to the amygdala at the same time that the full information is passed back to the visual cortex. The amygdala in turn sends responding signals to the muscles, sympathetic nervous system, and hypothalamus. The person jumps even before being consciously aware of what has been seen. LeDoux has shown with rats that the fear response is preserved even if the neural connections between the thalamus and cortex are cut. In essence, the animal startles without knowing why.

We have all had the experience of being frightened when seeing something, only to realize that it was just a rope or shadow—not a real threat. It is the fast track from the thalamus directly to the amygdala that causes the false alarm. This is considered to be "unconscious" or preconscious. We jump before we are aware. Patients with anxiety disorders can have exaggerated startle responses. They are burdened with an exaggerated, unconscious reaction to possible danger.

Anticipatory anxiety

Some people dread personal interactions in which they will be the focus of attention. Typically, they fear they will embarrass themselves. The anticipatory anxiety can ultimately restrict what they do and limit their social life and career path.

An imaging study looked at the activity in the brain of such patients who were asked to anticipate making a public speech. By subtracting the activity during anticipation from that at rest, they identified the areas of activity. Patients showed greater activity in their amygdala as well as hippocampus and insula. Figure 19.5A shows the functional

Frontal cortex

Hippocampus

Hypothalamus

Amygdala

Anterior pituitary

FIGURE 19.3 ● The important regions of the brain affecting anxiety.

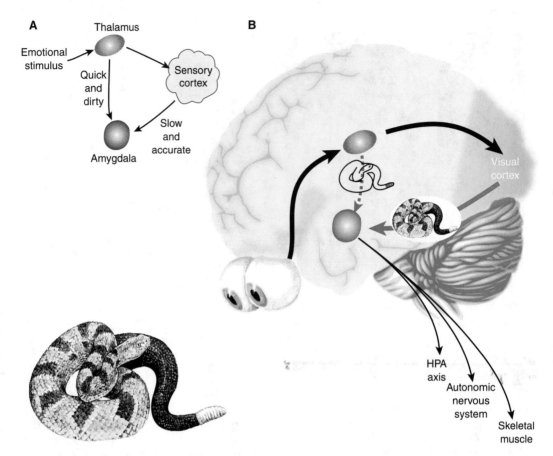

FIGURE 19.4 ● Two representations showing the two tracks that emotionally stimulating sensory information takes to the amygdala after entering the brain through the thalamus. HPA, hypothalamic-pituitary-adrenal. (Adapted from LeDoux JE. Emotion, memory and the brain. *Sci Am.* 1994;270[6]:50–57.)

magnetic resonance imaging (fMRI) slice at the level of the amygdala.

Anticipatory anxiety is not all bad. Figure 19.5B shows the hypothetical upside down U curve that many think represents the benefits and problems with anticipatory anxiety. Some anxiety is beneficial and actually improves performance; however, too much of it is overwhelming and results in a poorer outcome.

Amygdala memories

There is evidence that primitive emotionally relevant memories are stored in the amygdala. For example, in rodents:

1. Long-term potentiation (LTP) can be induced in the amygdala.
2. Protein synthesis inhibitors injected directly into the amygdala will prevent the formation of fear conditioning.

TREATMENT: AMYGDALA ACTIVITY

A small study in Sweden looked at the effects of cognitive-behavioral therapy (CBT) and the antidepressant citalopram on brain activity in patients with social phobia. Both treatments were equally effective and both reduced the amygdala activation after 9 weeks of treatment. The degree of amygdala attenuation was associated with clinical improvement 1 year later.

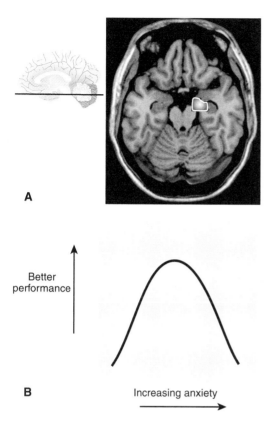

A

B Increasing anxiety

Better performance

FIGURE 19.5 ● **A:** Increased activity at the level of the amygdala when patients with anxiety anticipate making a public speech. **B:** Hypothetical upside down U curve showing benefits and problems of anticipatory anxiety. (fMRI from Lorberbaum JP, Kose S, Johnson MR, et al. Neural correlates of speech anticipatory anxiety in generalized social phobia. *Neuroreport.* 2004;15[18]:2701–2705.)

3. Chronic stress will induce increased dendritic branching in the amygdala.

These results suggest that the typical structural changes that are observed with memory formation occur in the amygdala in reaction to fearful circumstances. This may be one reason why traumatic events are so persistent. Fearful experiences form quickly, and enduring memories then reside in both the neocortex as well as the amygdala.

Prefrontal Cortex

One of the central components of anxiety is the feeling that one is not in control. Patients will complain of increased anxiety when they lose control, for example, when the door closes on an airplane, when their social support drives off, or anytime they feel trapped. Feeling in control, on the other hand, calms anxiety. The ability to reappraise a difficult situation into more favorable terms is a function of executive control. Rational reappraisal is a central feature of CBT.

The ability to cognitively master difficult circumstances and gain control likely resides in the PFC. Clearly, the PFC plays an important role in managing anxiety. However, the exact prefrontal regions involved (medial, lateral, or orbital) are ill-defined, although the medial PFC gets the most attention. The medial prefrontal cortex (mPFC), which includes the anterior cingulate gyrus, is well connected to the amygdala.

In a simple conceptualization, we can imagine that the mPFC applies the brakes to the amygdala. Several lines of evidence highlight the role of the mPFC in anxiety.

1. Lesions of the mPFC in rats reduce the ability to extinguish fears.
2. Stimulation of the mPFC inhibits a learned fear response; that is, the rat does not show anxiety.
3. The mPFC lights-up in functional imaging studies when fear is evoked in healthy subjects.
4. Subjects with anxiety disorders have reduced activity in the mPFC.

Taken together, these studies suggest that anxiety in part results from the reciprocal relation between PFC and amygdala (see Figure 19.6). This has been shown clearly in a cleaver study with traumatized combat veterans and firefighters. The subjects were shown pictures of faces expressing various emotions while in a fMRI (see Figure 19.7A). The activity in the brain when the subjects were viewing the happy face was subtracted from the brain activity when viewing the fearful face. The subjects with PTSD were compared to healthy controls.

Figure 19.7(B–D) shows the results. Note how subjects with PTSD, under the circumstances of the study, show increased activity in their amygdala and decreased activity in their prefrontal cortex. In essence, they do not have enough activity in their PFC to turn down the activity in the amygdala.

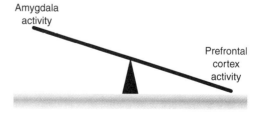

Amygdala activity

Prefrontal cortex activity

FIGURE 19.6 ● Anxiety disorders and dysregulation may be the result of too much activity in the amygdala and not enough activity in the prefrontal cortex (PFC).

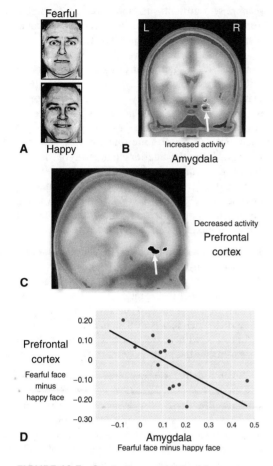

For a number of years, the reduction in volume of the hippocampus in patients with anxiety disorders has been an area of great interest. Several studies have documented smaller hippocampi in anxious patients, presumably due to the toxic effects of an activated HPA axis. However, a unique study with twins provides insight into the cause and effect of hippocampal volume.

Gilbertson et al. recruited 40 pairs of twins, in which one of each pair was exposed to combat in Vietnam and the other had stayed home. The researchers measured the hippocampal volume of each twin in an MRI. Additionally, the presence and severity of PTSD in the combat-exposed twin was

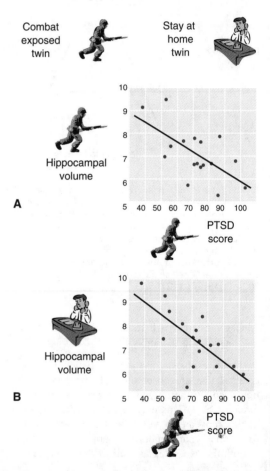

FIGURE 19.7 ● A: Traumatized subjects and controls are shown pictures of fearful faces and happy faces while in a functional magnetic resonance imaging (fMRI). The patients show increased activity in the amygdala (B) and decreased activity in the prefrontal cortex (PFC) (C) compared to the controls. Activity in the PFC and amygdala (D) have an inverse correlation for the traumatized patients. (A Adapted from Calder AJ, Lawrence AD, Young AW. Neuropsychology of fear and loathing. *Nat Rev Neurosci.* 2001;2[5]:352–363. B–D Adapted from Shin LM, Wright CI, Cannistraro PA, et al. A functional magnetic resonance imaging study of amygdala and medial prefrontal cortex responses to overtly presented fearful faces in posttraumatic stress disorder. *Arch Gen Psychiatry.* 2005;62[3]:273–281.)

Hippocampus

The hippocampus, an area involved with explicit memory acquisition (see Chapter 15, Memory), appears to interact with the amygdala during encoding of emotional memories. Although the exact role of the hippocampus in anxiety disorders remains unclear, it is an area frequently active in imaging studies during fearful situations.

FIGURE 19.8 ● A: The correlation between hippocampal volume and post-traumatic stress disorder (PTSD) score for the combat-exposed twin. B: The correlation between the stay-at-home twin's hippocampal volume and the PTSD score of his combat-exposed twin brother. (Adapted from Gilbertson MW, Shenton ME, Ciszewski A, et al. Smaller hippocampal volume predicts pathologic vulnerability to psychological trauma. *Nat Neurosci.* 2002;5[11]:1242–1247.)

assessed. As with previous reports, the twins who were diagnosed with PTSD had smaller hippocampal volumes (see Figure 19.8A). However, the most remarkable finding was that the PTSD score from the combat-exposed twin had a similar correlation with the hippocampal volume of the twin who had stayed at home (Figure 19.8B). In other words, the best prediction of a combat veterans level of PTSD and hippocampal size is not his exposure to trauma, but rather the size of his twin's hippocampus.

This finding brings to light one of the great discoveries in neuroscience. It is the interaction between nature and nurture that results in mental illness (see Figure 19.9). In other words, those at increased risk for developing PTSD are those individuals with a small hippocampus and exposure to trauma. Neither alone is sufficient.

Taken together, these findings suggest an important role for the hippocampus in the development of anxiety. These early preliminary data suggest that there is something neuroprotective about a large hippocampus that mitigates the development of PTSD, even when someone is exposed to unimaginable trauma. Possibly, a large hippocampus is better able to limit the acquisition of haunting memories or more efficient at extinguishing them once they develop.

NEUROTRANSMITTERS AND CELL BIOLOGY

γ-Aminobutyric Acid

γ-Aminobutyric acid (GABA) is the major inhibitory neurotransmitter in the brain. Activating the GABA neurons calms down the brain. Too much activation causes sluggishness and even coma. The GABA receptor has several sites that bind with other substances, which has the effect of enhancing the inhibitory activity of the GABA neurons. Figure 5.3 shows that ethanol, barbiturates, and benzodiazepines are known to bind with the GABA receptor. It is no wonder that people use and abuse these substances to calm down and reduce anxiety.

Abnormalities in the benzodiazepine GABA receptor have been implicated as a possible cause of anxiety disorders. Results of the original imaging studies and more recent genetic studies suggest that alterations in the structure or concentration of the benzodiazepine GABA receptor may predispose individuals to anxiety. However, the hypotheses have not been consistently or conclusively established.

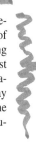

Norepinephrine

The norepinephrine (NE) neurons with cell bodies in the locus coeruleus (see Figure 4.5) are believed

---

ALCOHOLISM AND ANXIETY

There is controversy about the relation between alcoholism and anxiety. Acute alcohol intoxication reduces anxiety. Many clinicians believe that substance abusers are self-medicating their anxiety with alcohol and other calming agents. Longitudinal and genetic studies support this perception for some patients.

However, there is compelling evidence that chronic alcohol exposure induces long-term central nervous system (CNS) adaptations that cause anxiety. For example, the following have been observed.

1. Withdrawal from alcohol increases anxiety.
2. The anxiety of withdrawal decreases as abstinence persists.
3. Studies on twins have shown that anxiety disorders are common in the alcoholic twin but not the sober twin.
4. Rats exposed to chronic alcohol show alterations in GABA receptors.

5. Abstaining alcoholics showed a decreased benzodiazepine receptor distribution (Figure).

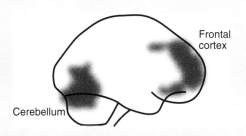

Abstaining alcoholics show decreased benzodiazepine receptor distribution in frontal cortex and cerebellum compared to controls. (Adapted from Abi-Dargham A, Krystal JH, Anjilvel S, et al. Alterations of benzodiazepine receptors in type II alcoholic subjects measured with SPECT and [123I]iomazenil. *Am J Psychiatry.* 1998;155[11]:1550–1555.)

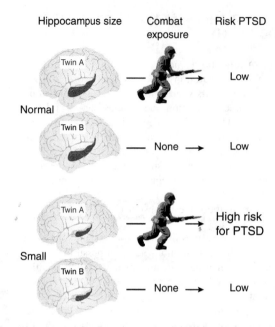

Hippocampus size   Combat exposure   Risk PTSD

Normal — Twin A — (combat) → Low

Twin B — None → Low

Small — Twin A — (combat) → High risk for PTSD

Twin B — None → Low

FIGURE 19.9 ● The risk for developing post-traumatic stress disorder (PTSD) is highest among individuals with a small hippocampus and exposure to trauma.

to be part of the stress response system and play an important role in anxiety. The following evidence supports this belief.

1. NE neurons project to the amygdala.
2. Stressed rats show increases in NE release.
3. NE stimulates the release of corticotropin releasing hormone (CRH), which in turn activates the HPA axis.
4. Peripheral NE (the sympathetic branch of the autonomic nervous system (ANS)—see Figure 2.8) produces somatic symptoms of anxiety: racing heart, sweating, dry mouth, and so on.

Brain-Derived Neurotrophic Factor

The ability of brain-derived neurotrophic factor (BDNF) to stimulate nerve cell growth has been addressed in many chapters (Chapter 7, Adult Development and Plasticity; Chapter 11, Anger and Aggression; Chapter 13, Sex and the Brain; Chapter 18, Depression). It is hypothesized that antidepressants work in part by boosting BDNF production, which in turn stimulates cell growth. However, recent work from Nestlers laboratory shows that not all BDNF is therapeutic, and some may actually play a role in the development of anxiety.

Using the same social defeat model with mice described in the previous chapter (see Scarring the DNA in Chapter 18, Depression), the researchers developed mice that displayed features of anxiety: fearful around strange mice, socially isolative, and so on. Much to the amazement of the researchers, these defeated mice showed increased BDNF in their nucleus accumbens (NAc).

The team was then able to eliminate the BDNF production in the NAc. They injected a virus that knocks out BDNF production into the neurons that supply the NAc with BDNF. These mice acted normally around strange mice and did not display any anxious behavior. Similar results were found when defeated mice were given imipramine or fluoxetine. Mice given the antidepressants or having their BDNF production knocked out failed to display anxious behavior after 10 days of social defeat.

In summary, this research implies that the development of anxiety that usually results from trauma might occur through the production of growth factor proteins in specific regions of the brain. Depression, on the other hand, might be the result of the lack of growth factor proteins in other regions. Remarkably, antidepressants seem to limit the expression of BDNF in the NAc while increasing it in other regions, such as the frontal cortex and hippocampus.

THE PARADOX OF ANTIDEPRESSANTS AND ANXIETY

If the NE system is part of the anxiety response, why does blocking NE reuptake, and consequently increasing NE at the synapse, relieve anxiety? How can more be less? For example, antidepressants such as the highly noradrenergic imipramine and the NE reuptake inhibitor reboxetine are known to reduce panic attacks. This does not make sense.

This paradox highlights that our understanding of anxiety and how the antidepressants calm the nervous system are in need of further study. Most likely, the antidepressants reduce anxiety by growth or increased strengthening of inhibitory networks.

EARLY ADVERSITY

Early adverse experiences have a significant impact on the later development of anxiety. Harry Harlow established with monkeys the profound negative impact of being raised without a mother or peer relationship. He replaced the mother of infant rhesus monkeys with an inanimate surrogate object during the first months of life. The infant monkeys displayed long-term deficits in social adaptation as well as increased anxiety-related behaviors.

We have discussed examples in which early experience changes neural structures. For example, the following have been observed.

1. Rats raised in standard wire cages have less dendritic branching than those raised in an enriched environment (see Point of Interest, page 29)

2. Licking and grooming by the rat mother effects the pups, response to stress (see Figure 14.5)
3. Children raised in Romanian orphanages have lower IQs. (see Figure 16.7)

A recent study looked at the effect of breast-feeding on anxiety in humans. Children whose parents separated or divorced when the children were between the ages of 5 and 10 years were assessed for anxiety when they turned 10. The children who were breast-fed had less anxiety and more resilience in response to the difficult circumstances. Although there are no details about the effects of breast-feeding on the brain, the results of this study seem strikingly similar to what Michael Meaney found with his high lick and groom mother rats (see Figure 14.9). Therefore, the extra attention at an early stage of life may be neuroprotective.

OBSESSIVE-COMPULSIVE DISORDER

OCD is classified as an anxiety disorder in the DSM nomenclature. However, some clinicians conceptualize OCD as a different kind of disorder. They see OCD as one extreme of a spectrum of repetitive behavioral problems: body dysmorphic disorder, certain eating disorders, gambling, and even autism. These conditions are frequently called *OC spectrum disorders*.

Regardless of the nomenclature controversy, OCD is unique among the anxiety disorders because it is driven by a different neural activity. This was first noticed in the 1930s by the behavioral sequela after von Economo's encephalitis pandemic from 1917 to 1926. Patients who had recovered from the original infection were often inflicted with OCD or parkinsonism. The basal ganglia were implicated. Symptoms of OCD are also seen with other disorders that affect the basal ganglia: Tourette's syndrome, Parkinson's disease, Sydenham's chorea, and so on.

Basal Ganglia

The basal ganglia are subcortical structures that are usually associated with movement and motor control. Disruption of the basal ganglia leads to such disorders as Huntington's disease, Parkinson's disease, and hemiballismus. However, the exact function of the basal ganglia in OCD remains unclear.

The basal ganglia are made up of interconnected nuclei—the caudate, putamen, and globus pallidus (see Figure 19.10). The caudate and putamen together are called the *striatum* and contains the NAc. Many areas of the cerebral cortex send projects to the basal ganglia that passes the signal to the thalamus, which in turn ultimately sends a signal back to the cortex. The loops that the signals take have sizable names such as corticostriatal-thalamic-cortical circuits.

Functional imaging studies of patients with OCD while they were obsessive have repeatedly shown increased activity in the orbitofrontal cortex, anterior cingulate gyrus, and basal ganglia. It is presumed that circuits between these structures are active when patients are obsessive. However, the particular circuit may depend on the particular ritual: washing, checking, or hoarding seem to activate slightly different regions. Likewise, treatment interventions, whether with psychotherapy or medications, show decreased activity in the basal ganglia for those who respond.

DOES MEDICATING ANXIETY PREVENT LEARNING?

Medication and psychotherapy alleviate anxiety through different mechanisms but with equal effectiveness. Combining the two treatment modalities is generally believed to be more efficacious than either of them alone, although this has not been conclusively established. However, some clinicians wonder whether medications limit the learning that is essential to effective psychotherapy.

There are only three large, combined psychotherapy/medication studies for the treatment of anxiety disorders that have long-term follow-up after stopping the medications.

1. Alprazolam and exposure therapy, alone and in combination, for panic disorder.
2. CBT, imipramine, or their combination for panic disorder.
3. Exposure therapy and sertraline in social phobia.

In all three trials, one outcome was the same. When the medication was stopped, the group that received a combination of medication and psychotherapy deteriorated relative to the group that received psychotherapy alone. Figure shows the result for the CBT/imipramine study for panic.

Studies have shown that extinction results from the development of new memories rather than the erasure of the old fearful memories. Does medication limit the development of new memories that are required for effective, enduring psychotherapy? These studies suggest that some therapeutic changes that usually occur in the brain with psychotherapy are impeded by the presence of the psychoactive medication.

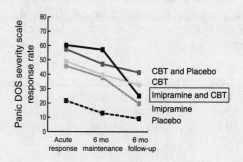

When treatment was stopped after the 6-month maintenance period, the group receiving imipramine (Imp) and cognitive-behavioral therapy (CBT) failed to sustain the benefits of psychotherapy

1. Marks IM, et al. *Brit J Psych.* 1993;162:776–787.
2. Barlow DH, et al. *JAMA.* 2000;283:2529–2536.
3. Haug TT, et al. *Brit J Psych.* 2003;182:312–318.

Psychosurgery

There is a long and troubling history of attempts to treat mental illness with neurosurgical interventions (see PREFONTAL LOBOTOMY, page 17). Consequently, many are reluctant to even consider neurosurgery as a treatment option for psychiatric diseases. However, there is good evidence that some limited procedures with treatment-resistant patients can diminish OCD symptoms.

Different techniques are preferred in various regions of the world. In the united states, the popular technique is anterior cingulotomy, which is based on the concept of interrupting the circuit between the anterior cingulate gyrus and basal ganglia. Figure 19.11 shows the location of the lesions in postsurgical MRI scans.

Follow-up studies find that approximately 30% of the anterior cingulotomy patients have a 35% or greater reduction on the Yale-Brown Obsessive-Compulsive Scale. Complications include urinary incontinence and seizures, but appear to be infrequent. A different technique used more regularly in Europe: is anterior capsulotomy. Although this procedure appears to be more effective, it is also associated with more complications, for example, cognitive and affective dysfunction. More recently, deep brain stimulation has been studied as a way to treat severe and intractable OCD in a manner that is reversible and more flexible.

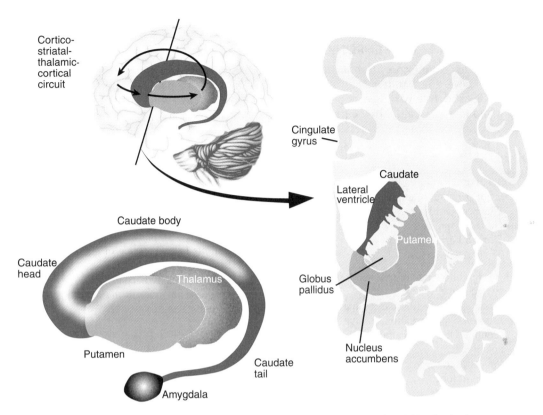

FIGURE 19.10 ● The structures of the basal ganglia and how they reside within the brain.

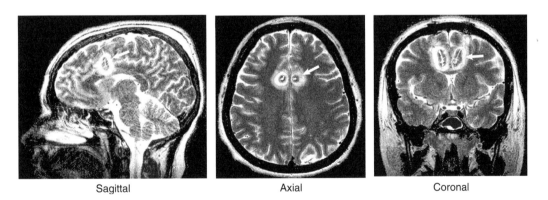

Sagittal   Axial   Coronal

FIGURE 19.11 ● Three views of anterior cingulotomy for treatment-resistant obsessive-compulsive disorder (OCD). The white *arrows* show the location of the lesions. The white rings around the lesions are secondary edema from the procedure. (Redrawn from Richter EO, Davis KD, Hamani C, et al. Cingulotomy for psychiatric disease: Microelectrode guidance, a callosal reference system for documenting lesion location, and clinical results. *Neurosurgery.* 2004;54[3]:622–628; discussion 8–30.)

CINGULOTOMY AND CHRONIC PAIN

The anterior cingulotomy has also been used for severe and unremitting pain. Figure 8.7 shows how the anterior cingulate lights-up in acute pain. The neurosurgical procedure appears to interrupt the signal and reduce pain for approximately one half to two thirds of the patients treated.

QUESTIONS

1. Which hormone initially drops owing to the stress of parachute jumping?
   a. Glucocorticoids.
   b. Gonadotrophins.
   c. Growth hormone.
   d. Mineralocorticoids.

2. All of the following are true about the Klüver-Bucy syndrome, except
   a. Made aggressive monkeys tame.
   b. Induced hypersexuality.
   c. Identified the hippocampus as important for anxiety.
   d. Was elicited through removal of most of the temporal lobe.

3. Evidence that the amygdala is important for experiencing fear
   a. Ischemic damage increases fear response.
   b. Electric stimulation reduces freezing and heart rate.
   c. Emotional trauma has no effect on the amygdala.
   d. Treatment reduces activity in the amygdala.

4. The recognition of a threatening object includes all of the following, except
   a. The brain reacts once all the signals are analyzed.
   b. Signals from the amygdala stimulate heart rate.
   c. Auditory and visual information proceed to the thalamus.
   d. Memories modulate the amygdaloid response.

5. Stimulation of the medial PFC has what effect on a rat's fear response?
   a. Inhibits the expression of anxiety.
   b. Impairs extinction.
   c. Increases the activity in the amygdala.
   d. Decreases activity in the anterior cingulate gyrus.

6. The best estimate of the volume of a combat veteran's hippocampus is
   a. The total duration of trauma he experienced.
   b. The intensity of combat trauma he experienced.
   c. The level of glucocorticoids in the morning at rest.
   d. The size of his twin's hippocampus.

7. Medications decrease anxiety in all the following ways, except
   a. Increase the GABA inhibitory signal.
   b. Increase BDNF production at the NAc.
   c. Modulation of the NE neurons.
   d. Quieting the amygdala.

8. Imaging studies show increased activity in all the following regions in OCD patients, except
   a. Orbitofrontal cortex.
   b. Anterior cingulate gyrus.
   c. Amygdala.
   d. Basal ganglia.

Schizophrenia

HISTORIC PERSPECTIVE

Over 100 years ago, Emil Kraepelin, a German psychiatrist, described the syndrome now called *schizophrenia*. Bleuler actually coined the term *schizophrenia*. Kraepelin called it *dementia praecox*. Kraepelin's major contribution to psychiatry was recognizing that schizophrenia and manic depression are different disorders. The patient with schizophrenia has a persistent deteriorating course in mental functioning whereas the patient with manic depression will experience periods of remission. Figure 20.1 shows a modern interpretation of the clinical course of schizophrenia.

Kraepelin was convinced that schizophrenia was an organic disease of the brain and spent considerable time and energy conducting postmortem studies on the brains of patients with schizophrenia. They had a good track record of identifying pathology, as one of his colleagues was the neuropathologist Alois Alzheimer. Unfortunately, Kraepelin was never able to discover a specific abnormality in the brains of schizophrenic patients. This pattern was to continue for a long time.

Numerous postmortem studies were conducted over the next 70 years comparing the brains of schizophrenic patients with healthy controls. Still no distinguishing pathology was isolated. The absence of gliosis in the tissue was of particular interest. Gliosis, sometimes called the *glial scar*, is the proliferation of astrocytes in reaction to central nervous system (CNS) injury. It is considered the hallmark of neurodegenerative disorders and is found with such conditions as Huntington's or Alzheimer's diseases as well as with trauma and ischemia.

The absence of any significant neuropathology along with the burgeoning interest in psychoanalytic theory led to psychosocial explanations for schizophrenia. Terms such as the *refrigerator mother* or the *double-bind* were developed to explain the psychological turmoil that caused schizophrenia. Some clinicians even speculated that patients voluntarily chose to be psychotic to avoid conflict in their lives.

Although the development of chlorpromazine (Thorazine) in the early 1950s dramatically changed the treatment of schizophrenia, the identification of biologic abnormalities remained elusive. In 1972, Plum summarized the frustration when he called schizophrenia the *graveyard of neuropathologists*. Schizophrenia was actually dropped from the preeminent neuropathology textbook (Greenfield's Neuropathology) for the next two editions and only added back in 1997. It was the emergence of significant findings on brain imaging studies that finally ended the debate about whether there are quantifiable (measurable) changes in the brain (more on this in the next section).

MODERN EPIDEMIC?

E. Fuller Torrey calls schizophrenia an invisible plague. He believes that schizophrenia is a modern illness that has increased so gradually that the change is not perceptible during any single person's lifetime. Additionally, the changes in diagnostic criteria that occur over the decades make

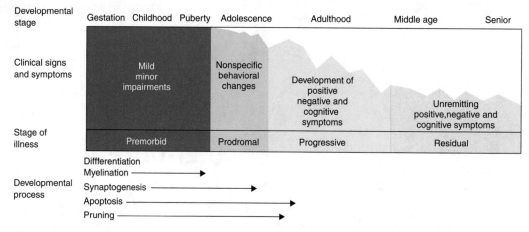

FIGURE 20.1 ● The typical clinical course of schizophrenia includes a relatively normal childhood interrupted in late adolescence or early adulthood by a dramatic deterioration from which few remit. (Adapted from Lewis DA, Lieberman JA. Catching up on schizophrenia: Natural history and neurobiology. *Neuron.* 2000;28[2]:325–334.)

comparisons between generations difficult. In spite of these difficulties, there is evidence to support Dr. Torrey's belief.

The ancient Greeks and Romans were astute observers of human behavior. Reviews of the writings from ancient times provide the following descriptions of conditions that we easily recognize:

1. Epilepsy
2. Migraine headache
3. Melancholia
4. Anxiety

5. Chronic alcoholism
6. Delirium

The ancient writers did describe psychotic symptoms including hallucinations and delusions. However, in almost every case the psychosis cleared. There are no reports that describe an initial psychotic break in late adolescence or early adulthood with a chronic unremitting course. The absence of a condition that looks like schizophrenia stands in contrast to the good clinical descriptions of other neuropsychiatric syndromes. This softly suggests

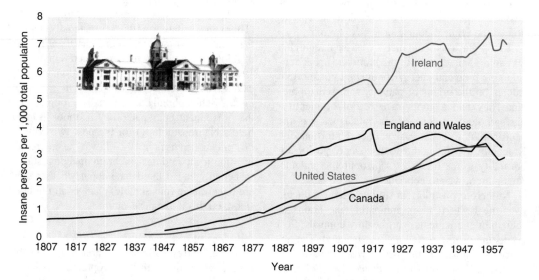

FIGURE 20.2 ● The epidemic of mental illness in the last two centuries. (Adapted from Liberman RP, Musgrave JG, Langlois J. Taunton State Hospital, Massachusetts. *Am J Psychiatry.* 2003;160[12]:2098. and Torrey EF, Miller J. *The invisible plague: the rise of mental illness from 1750 to the present.* New Brunswick, NJ: Rutgers University Press; 2001.)

POINT OF INTEREST

There is considerable evidence that people born and/or raised in urban settings are at greater risk for developing schizophrenia. For example, a Danish study compared the diagnosis of schizophrenia with where the patient resided on his/her 15th birthday. The incidence per 1,000 is as follows:

Copenhagen	6.5
Copenhagen suburbs	4.1
Provincial city	3.5
Provincial town	3.0
Rural area	2.6

What is it about urban life that increases the risk of developing schizophrenia?

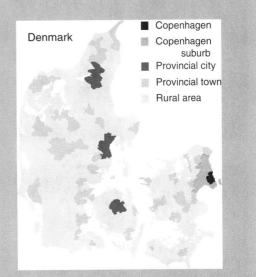

Denmark segregated by population density. (Adapted from Pedersen CB, Mortensen PB. Urbanization and traffic related exposures as risk factors for schizophrenia. *BMC Psychiatry.* 2006;6:2.)

that the illness was not present in ancient Greece or Rome.

The 19th and 20th centuries saw an explosion in the institutionalization of patients with chronic mental illness. Many of these patients had schizophrenia. Figure 20.2 shows the growth in institutionalized patients as a percentage of the total population in four countries. There are many reasons for confining the seriously mentally ill: industrial revolution, changes in social norms, lack of effective treatments, and so on. An additional explanation is the emergence of a psychiatric epidemic.

Although we may never know for sure whether schizophrenia is a modern epidemic or has been around for ages, the topic raises the issue of etiology. What causes schizophrenia? We will start with what is known about the brain of patients with schizophrenia.

GRAY MATTER

The development of brain imaging techniques provided a way to examine schizophrenic brains in live people. The first computed tomography (CT) scans in schizophrenia were published in 1976 and showed enlarged lateral ventricles in a group of patients with chronic schizophrenia. Others quickly replicated this study. However, it

was magnetic resonance imaging (MRI), with its ability to differentiate gray and white matter, that finally provided irrefutable evidence of the biologic nature of schizophrenia.

The most famous MRI studies were the original studies on twins. E. Fuller Torrey, Daniel Weinberger et al. at the National Institute of Mental Health (NIMH) recruited monozygotic twins from the united states and Canada. They originally studied 15 sets of twins who were discordant for schizophrenia: one had the illness whereas the other was unaffected. MRI was done in of all 30 participants. The most remarkable finding was that in 12 of the 15 sets of twins the affected individual was easily identified by visual inspection of corresponding coronal scans (see Figure 20.3).

The results of the twin study have been replicated and extended. The most common finding remains enlarged ventricles, but better technology has allowed more detailed analysis. Patients with schizophrenia show consistent but subtle decreases in total brain volume and total gray matter volume. These results provide an explanation for the increased ventricle size; that is, the ventricles expand to fill the void left by the loss of gray matter.

35-year-old female identical twins

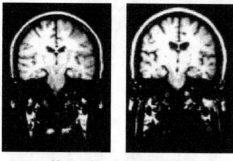

28-year-old male identical twins

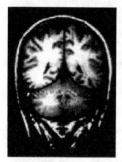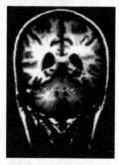

FIGURE 20.3 ● Coronal magnetic resonance imaging (MRI) of two sets of twins discordant for schizophrenia. The enlarged lateral ventricles are readily apparent in the subjects on the right. (Courtesy of Drs. E. Fuller Torrey and Daniel Weinberger.)

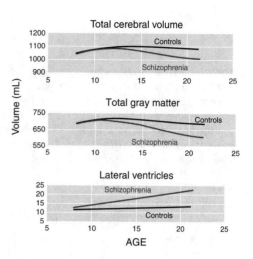

FIGURE 20.4 ● Children with schizophrenia have loss of brain volume and gray matter as well as enlargement of lateral ventricles through adolescence. (Adapted from Gogtay N, Sporn A, Rapoport J. Structural brain MRI studies in childhood-onset schizophrenia and childhood atypical psychosis. In: Lawrie S, Johnstone E, Weinberger D, eds. *Schizophrenia: from neuroimaging to neuroscience.* New York: Oxford University Press; 2004.)

Judith Rapoport's laboratory performed sequential MRI scans on children with childhood-onset schizophrenia and compared the findings with age-matched controls in an effort to follow up the changes in the brain that occur during adolescence. They found that the rate of change was greater for those children with schizophrenia. Figure 20.4 shows that the children with schizophrenia had striking loss of gray matter along with decreased brain size and increased ventricles.

Adolescence is a time of remodeling of the connections in the brain to create a more efficient organ. Processes such as pruning, apoptosis, and synaptogenesis are accepted features of the maturing brain and have been discussed in other chapters (see Figures 7.7, 16.4, and 17.9). Studies such as the one described here suggest that schizophrenia may be the result of overly exuberant remodeling of the gray matter.

Certainly, the process of gray matter reduction occurs in the same time frame as the usual onset of schizophrenic symptoms. Although no definitive evidence exists to prove this theory, some genetic studies suggest altered expression of genes that control synaptic plasticity.

Reduced Neuropil Hypothesis

As stated before, traditional microscopic examination of the gray matter of schizophrenics will not identify anything unusual. So it has been difficult to explain the gray matter loss. Investigators at Yale utilized labor-intensive three-dimensional analytic tools to estimate cellular densities. They compared neuronal density in three regions of the brain from patients with schizophrenia and from healthy controls. The regions were Brodmann's areas 9 and 46 in the prefrontal cortex (PFC) and area 17 in the visual cortex. They found increased density of neurons but not glial cells in the gray matter of schizophrenic patients (see Figure 20.5).

It appears that schizophrenic patients have the same number of neurons as healthy controls, but they are packed together in less space—called the *reduced neuropil hypothesis.* The tighter packaging of the schizophrenic neurons results from reduced cell size, less branching, and decreased spine formation. Figure 20.6 shows a drawing of this process. Figure 20.7 shows examples of actual spine formation from schizophrenic patients and controls. The key point is that it is not neuronal loss, but rather the loss of the richness of the dendritic connections that causes the reduced gray matter in schizophrenia. Presumably, this also results in deficient information processing.

Although the underlying cause of neuronal atrophy remains unknown, recent evidence suggests

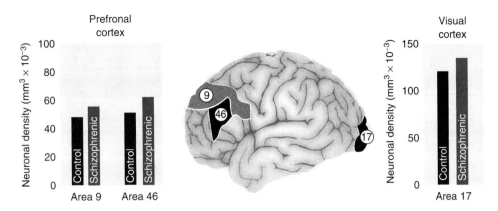

FIGURE 20.5 ● Patients with schizophrenia have increased neuronal density in all three areas of the brain tested. Glial density was no different. (Adapted from Selemon LD, Goldman-Rakic PS. The reduced neuropil hypothesis: A circuit based model of schizophrenia. *Biol Psychiatry*. 1999;45[1]:17–25.)

Health control gray matter

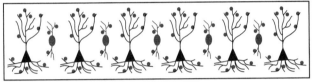

Schizophrenic gray matter

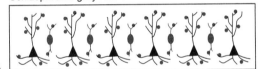

A

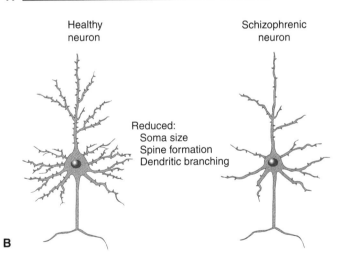

B

FIGURE 20.6 ● A: Schematic representation of the increased density but decreased size of schizophrenic gray matter. B: Suspected neuronal atrophy of schizophrenic pyramidal neurons, which results in defective connectivity. (A adapted from Selemon LD. Increased cortical neuronal density in schizophrenia. *Am J Psychiatry*. 2004;161[9]:1564.)

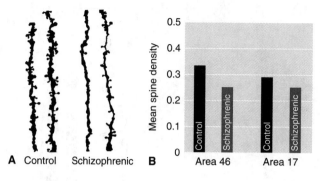

FIGURE 20.7 ● A: Drawings of actual dendrites and spines from pyramidal neurons in the dorsolateral prefrontal cortex of controls and schizophrenic patients. B: Mean spine density in frontal cortex and visual cortex from controls and schizophrenic patients. (Adapted from Glantz LA, Lewis DA. Decreased dendritic spine density on prefrontal cortical pyramidal neurons in schizophrenia. *Arch Gen Psychiatry.* 2000;57[1]:65–73.)

a role for altered neuronal apoptosis. Apoptosis is usually associated with programmed cell death (see Figure 7.8). However, sublethal apoptotic activity may result in synaptic elimination without frank cell death. Apoptosis is controlled by pro- and antiapoptotic proteins, which may be aberrant in schizophrenia.

One further point worth mentioning is that these studies highlight the extensive involvement of schizophrenia, that is it is not a disorder of just one region of the brain. Rather, schizophrenia seems to affect almost the entire cortex.

Functional Brain Imaging

Traditionally, the hallmark of schizophrenia has been the hallucinations and delusions. In actuality, the symptoms of schizophrenia are made up of the following three categories of impairment.

1. Positive symptoms: hallucinations and delusions
2. Negative symptoms: lack of motivation, apathy, and so on
3. Cognitive impairment

The cognitive dysfunction, which includes problems with attention, memory, and executive function, may be the most detrimental aspect of the illness. They have a greater negative impact on the individual than the positive symptoms. Likewise, cognitive functioning is the best predictor of long-term outcome from the disorder.

The pattern of cognitive impairment in schizophrenia implicates the frontal cortex. *Hypofrontality* is a term sometimes used to describe this problem. However, functional imaging studies have given inconsistent results. Weinberger et al. recognized that the function of the frontal lobe must be measured when it is engaged in a cognitive challenge.

To test this theory, patients and healthy controls underwent xenon, XE 133, inhalation procedure for regional cerebral blood flow measurements while they were performing the Wisconsin Card Sort test (see Figure 20.8). The control subjects showed increased activation of their frontal lobes while performing the test, but the schizophrenic patients did not. Furthermore, there was a good correlation between the change in blood flow in the frontal cortex and percent errors on the test.

In summary, these results suggest that the cognitive impairment in patients with schizophrenia comes from impaired frontal lobes. Atrophic, disconnected neuronal cells presumably cause the PFC dysfunction.

Inhibitory Neurons

The activity of the large pyramidal neurons in the gray matter is modulated by smaller local interneurons (see Figure 2.2). Most of the interneurons are γ-aminobutyric acid (GABA) neurons and hence inhibitory. There are several types of GABA neurons. Figure 20.9A shows two of them: the parvalbumin in brown and the calretinin in black. The location of their inhibitory input seems to have different effects on the pyramidal neuron.

The GABA interneurons are important in the discussion of schizophrenia because there is evidence that the parvalbumin neurons are impaired in patients with the disorder. GABA is synthesized from a number of enzymes, one of which is called *glutamic acid decarboxylase* (GAD). One form of messenger RNA (mRNA) that encodes for GAD (GAD67) has been shown repeatedly to be decreased in patients with schizophrenia. It is one of the most consistent findings in postmortem studies. Figure 20.9(B, C) shows the results of a study comparing the expression of GAD67 in patients and controls.

Of particular interest, the deficit in GAD67 expressing interneurons seems to be limited only to the parvalbumin neurons and is not found in other GABA neurons. Furthermore, the number of parvalbumin neurons is not reduced in patients with schizophrenia. So the GABA neurons that are implicated in schizophrenia are not limited in number, but have decreased expression of important genes that might impair the function of the cortex.

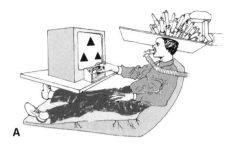

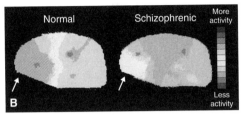

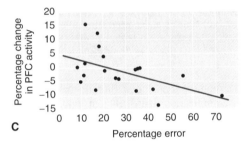

FIGURE 20.8 ● **A:** Subjects were scanned while performing the Wisconsin Card Sort task. **B:** Healthy subjects displayed increased blood flow to the prefrontal cortex (PFC) whereas those with schizophrenia did not. **C:** Percent errors on the task correlated with change in PFC blood flow. (Adapted from Weinberger DR, Berman KF, Zec RF. Physiologic dysfunction of dorsolateral prefrontal cortex in schizophrenia. I. Regional cerebral blood flow evidence. *Arch Gen Psychiatry.* 1986;43[2]:114–124.)

Working memory depends on the coordinated firing of pyramidal neurons in the PFC. The inhibitory interneurons are essential for the synchronization of the output from the pyramidal neurons. Tasks such as the delayed response task (see Figure 17.3) require inhibitory control to bridge the time between stimulus presentation and behavioral response. The cognitive impairment in patients with schizophrenia may be due to a failure to properly coordinate the pyramidal neurons.

WHITE MATTER

Schizophrenia also appears to be a disorder of disrupted connectivity. The white matter tracks that connect different regions of the cortex, as well as the cortex with the deeper brain structures,

may also play an important role in the disruption of good connections. White matter is composed of the myelinated axons that transport the signals generated by the neurons. Figure 20.10 shows a drawing of some of the long and short white matter tracks. Disruption of the integrity of the white matter tracks leads to degradation of the neuronal signal.

Imaging

MRI studies on patients and controls have found a small but nonsignificant trend toward reduced white matter in schizophrenia. Recently, a new imaging technology has been developed to assess the quality of the white matter tracks. Diffusion tensor imaging (DTI) measures the sum of vectors of water diffusion along axons. The images produced show remarkable detail of the white matter tracks (see Figure 20.11).

Many studies using DTI have found abnormalities in patients with schizophrenia compared with healthy controls. Some insight into the significance of these findings can be found from looking at the result of DTI studies in other demyelinating diseases. For example, multiple sclerosis and human immunodeficiency virus also produces changes in the DTI analysis. These results suggest that all three diseases may share some similar white matter degradation.

Myelin
Oligodendrocytes

Oligodendrocytes are one of the glial cells that support the neurons. Specifically, the oligodendrocytes provide layers of myelin that insulate the axons and enhance the speed of transmission of neural impulses (see Figure 3.13). Diseases that affect the integrity of the myelin sheath impair the function of the brain and can cause psychotic symptoms in some cases. One particular disease—metachromatic leukodystrophy—usually begins with demyelination of the frontal lobes.

The rare late-onset form of metachromatic leukodystrophy occurs in about the same time frame as schizophrenia—from adolescence to young adulthood. Reviews of such cases have noted that over half the individuals had psychotic symptoms including auditory hallucinations and bizarre delusions.

Others have looked at the oligodendrocyte population in patients with schizophrenia. Hof et al. counted the number of oligodendrocytes in the white matter of Brodmann's area 9. They found that there was a 27% decrease in the number of oligodendrocytes in the patients with schizophrenia compared with the controls (see Figure 20.12).

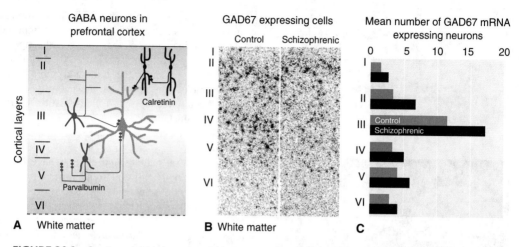

GABA neurons in
prefrontal cortex

Cortical layers

Calretinin

Parvalbumin

A   White matter

GAD67 expressing cells

Control   Schizophrenic

B   White matter

Mean number of GAD67 mRNA
expressing neurons

Control
Schizophrenic

C

FIGURE 20.9 ● **A:** γ-Aminobutyric acid interneurons have inhibitory input on the pyramidal neurons in the prefrontal cortex. **B:** GAD67 expression cells from the prefrontal cortex of a control and a patient with schizophrenia. **C:** Mean number of GAD67 messenger RNA (mRNA) expression neurons by gray matter layer. (**A** adapted from Tamminga C, Hashimoto T, Volk DW, et al. GABA neurons in the human prefrontal cortex. *Am J Psychiatry.* 2004;161[10]:1764. **B, C** adapted from Akbarian S, Kim JJ, Potkin SG, et al. Gene expression for glutamic acid decarboxylase is reduced without loss of neurons in prefrontal cortex of schizophrenics. *Arch Gen Psychiatry.* 1995;52[4]:258–266.)

Genetics

The application of microarray analysis (see Figure 1.10) has further implicated the involvement of myelin in schizophrenia. Hakak et al. applied postmortem tissue from patients with schizophrenia and controls to microarray chips to identify gene expression. In other words, they wanted to see which genes were active in which subjects.

More than 6,000 genes were compared between the schizophrenic and control subjects. Only 17 genes were significantly downregulated in the schizophrenic patients. Of these, six were myelin related. The other 11 showed no particular pattern.

The authors concluded that the results give a clear indication that deficient oligodendrocytes and myelination are involved in schizophrenia.

AUDITORY HALLUCINATIONS

In 1863, Broca described lesions of the left frontal cortex in patients with language expression deficits (see Figure 1.3). Roughly 10 years later, Wernicke described a different language deficit associated with lesions of the superior temporal

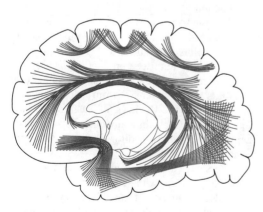

FIGURE 20.10 ● A drawing of the white matter tracks connecting various regions in the brain. (Adapted from Gray's Anatomy of the Human Body as displayed at Bartleby.com.)

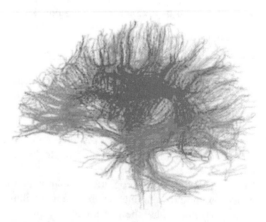

FIGURE 20.11 ● Visualization of white matter tracks in the brain using diffusion tensor imaging (DTI) technology. (Adapted from Brun A, Park HJ, Knutsson H, et al. *Coloring of DT-MRI fiber traces using laplacian eigenmaps.* Available at http://lmi.bwh.harvard.edu/papers/papers/brunEUROCAST03.html. 2003.)

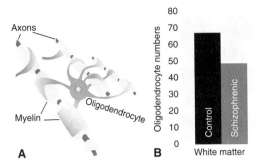

FIGURE 20.12 ● **A:** One oligodendrocyte can provide the myelin covering over many axons. **B:** Patients with schizophrenia have less oligodendrocytes in their white matter. (Graph adapted from Hof PR, Haroutunian V, Friedrich VL Jr, et al. Loss and altered spatial distribution of oligodendrocytes in the superior frontal gyrus in schizophrenia. *Biol Psychiatry.* 2003;53[12]:1075–1085.)

lobe. The region Wernicke described was a part of what is now called the *auditory cortex*. The perception of sound starts in the ear, then proceeds through the brain stem and thalamus before reaching the auditor cortex on the superior aspect of the temporal lobe (see Figure 20.13). White matter tracts called the *arcuate fasciculus* connect the auditory cortex with the frontal cortex.

Wernicke and later Kraepelin both postulated that auditory hallucinations were due to temporal lobe abnormalities. Indeed, an auditory aura preceding a seizure suggests the temporal lobe as the nidus of the electric activity. Likewise, hallucinations can result from strokes that involve the temporal lobes. So neurologic causes of auditory

hallucinations point to the temporal lobe. Until recently, it was just speculation about the neuronal correlates of auditory hallucinations with schizophrenia.

A group in Switzerland has done extensive imaging studies of schizophrenic patients when they were hallucinating. In the past, the time it took to scan a person was so long it obscured the difference between the hallucinating state and the nonhallucinating state. Now with rapid fMRI scans the differences can be detected. Patients were asked to press a button with the onset of hallucinations and keep it pressed for as long as they lasted. Images during hallucinations were compared with images when the voices were silent. Figure 20.14A shows the activity in the gray matter of the auditory cortex during hallucinations for one patient.

POINT OF INTEREST

Numerous researchers have documented a correlation between auditory hallucinations and the size of the temporal lobe; that is, a smaller temporal lobe predicts more hallucinations. This seems counterintuitive. Why does less brain tissue produce positive symptoms?

Recently, this same research grouped used DTI imaging to look at white matter tracts in schizophrenic patients with hallucinations compared with patients without hallucinations and

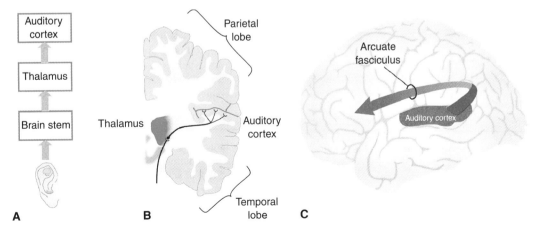

FIGURE 20.13 ● **A:** Pathways from the ear to the cortex. **B:** Auditory signals synapse in the thalamus before reaching the auditory cortex. **C:** The Arcuate fasciculus is composed of white matter tracts that connect the auditory cortex with the frontal cortex.

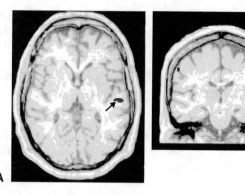
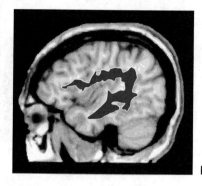

FIGURE 20.14 ● **A:** Functional magnetic resonance imaging (fMRI) showing the gray matter regions activated when they are experiencing auditory hallucinations. **B:** Diffusion tensor imaging showing the areas of altered white matter tracts for patients who hear auditory hallucinations compared to healthy controls. (**A** From Dierks T, Linden DE, Jandl M, et al. Activation of Heschls gyrus during auditory hallucinations. *Neuron.* 1999;22[3]:615–621. **B** From Hubl D, Koenig T, Strik W, et al. Pathways that make voices: White matter changes in auditory hallucinations. *Arch Gen Psychiatry.* 2004;61[7]:658–668.)

healthy controls. Remarkably, they found that patients with hallucinations have significantly more alterations of the white matter tracts of the arcuate fasciculus (Figure 20.14B).

Taken together, these studies suggest that auditory hallucinations are derived from abnormalities in the regions that register external sounds. The patient with auditory hallucinations may misidentify inner speech as coming from an external source due to lack of integrity of the system. It is reminiscent of a phone or television picking up other signals and playing more than one sound track at a time.

Another significance of these studies is that they identify abnormalities for patients with schizophrenia that include both the gray matter and white matter for one symptom. Clearly, schizophrenia is a complex disorder with broad effects on the brain.

ETIOLOGY

Schizophrenia is a complex disorder that has defied scientific explanation. As reviewed here, schizophrenia looks like a disorder of disconnectedness. There is no specific brain region affected, but rather a dysfunction of circuits within and between regions. Additionally, the onset of the full disorder suggests a neurodevelopmental disruption. It is plausible to envision that schizophrenia results from the abnormal expression of genes that govern maturational processes. However, what goes wrong and how does all this occur?

Genetics

One of the most consistent findings in schizophrenia research is the inheritable nature of the illness and related illnesses. Figure 1.1 shows the striking power of the genes with this disorder. The closer one is related to someone with schizophrenia, the more likely that person is to get the illness. However, even the monozygotic twin of a person with schizophrenia only has approximately a 50% chance of getting the illness. Furthermore, patients with schizophrenia are less likely to procreate. If this is a genetic disorder with Mendelian properties, we would expect it to decline in frequency over many generations. Clearly, there is more involved than just genes in the traditional sense.

Environment
Prenatal Complications

Adverse environmental events are known to be potential triggers for developing schizophrenia. Maternal infection is one well-known risk factor for schizophrenia. Obstetric complications are also associated with schizophrenia. A large prospective study that followed up children from birth through adulthood found that the odds of schizophrenia increased linearly with increasing number of hypoxia-associated obstetric complications.

Famine

Two large epidemiologic studies of *in utero* exposure to maternal starvation have shown an increased risk of schizophrenia among the offspring. In October 1944, a Nazi blockade of the western Netherlands precipitated a famine that did not remit until liberation in May 1945. During the blockade, daily food rations fell to <500 calories per person per day. In followup studies, the risk of developing schizophrenia in exposed children had

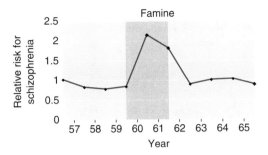

FIGURE 20.15 ● The relative rate of developing schizophrenia doubled for those born during the famine during 1960 to 1961 in one region of China.

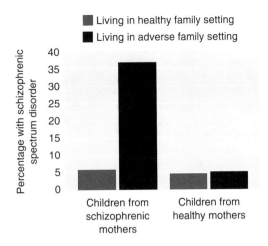

FIGURE 20.16 ● Children born to schizophrenic mothers and raised in more dysfunctional family environments were at increased risk of developing schizophrenic spectrum disorders.

doubled. Additionally, there was also a significant increase in births with neural tube defects.

The second study looked at the effects of famine caused by the Great Leap Forward in China during 1960 to 1961. Similar results were found (see Figure 20.15). In both situations the birth rate dropped during the famine. Some speculate that the lack of folate in the diet had a detrimental effect on the developing fetal brain. Folate is needed for DNA synthesis and repair. Its absence can lead to chromosomal instability.

Finnish Adoption Study

Many people conceptualize schizophrenia as resulting from some interaction between genes and the environment, but it has been hard to tease out the relation between these factors. The Finnish Adoption Study provides some interesting data to help understand this interaction. Researchers collected the names of all women who were hospitalized in Finland from 1960 to 1979 and diagnosed with schizophrenia. Then they identified the children from these women who were adopted away. They collected a similar number of adopted children as matched controls.

Detailed and blinded assessments were made of the adoptive families by experienced psychiatrists. Using specific scales, they divided families into those that were more healthy and those that were more dysfunctional. Additionally, each child was assessed for a schizophrenia spectrum disorder based on *Diagnostic and Statistical Manual of Mental Disorders-Third Edition-Revised* (DSM-III-R) criteria, for example, schizophrenia, delusional disorder, depressive disorder with psychotic features, schizotypal personality disorder, and so on.

The remarkable results of this study are shown in Figure 20.16. Only the children born to mothers with schizophrenia and raised in an adverse family household showed an increased risk of developing schizophrenic spectrum disorders. This is a clear example of a genetic–environment interaction. Children at genetic risk for schizophrenia appear to be more sensitive to problems in the environment.

Gene Expression

In several chapters of this book we have discussed the enduring effects that life events can have on the DNA (see Figures 14.9 and 18.8). Environmental events change the genes. Enhancing or silencing specific genes changes behavior. This enables animals to adapt their behavior to their particular environment. However, some events seem to silence important genes and have devastating effects on behavior. Schizophrenia may be such a condition.

Researchers are starting to look at changes in gene expression in patients with schizophrenia in efforts to better understand the disorder. To proceed with such an examination, an important protein must first be identified and then the DNA that encodes for that protein must be analyzed. One such protein is reelin, a protein expressed by GABA interneurons. Reelin has been recognized as important for neuronal migration, axonal branching, and synaptogenesis throughout brain development. Additionally, reelin and its mRNA have been found to be reduced in postmortem brains of schizophrenic patients.

We have previously discussed that the addition of methyl groups to the DNA limits the transcription of that gene. The methyl groups essentially

at the University of California in San Diego recently looked at the methylation of the reelin DNA from gray matter from postmortem brains of patients with schizophrenia. Not surprisingly, they found a distinct methylated signal in 73% of the schizophrenic samples but only in 24% of the control samples. To put it another way, the schizophrenic DNA was three times more likely to be methylated.

Not only does this give a possible mechanism to explain the failure of gene expression in patients with schizophrenia, but also fits with other environmental events that increase the risk of developing the disorder. Therefore, certain insults such as transient ischemia are known to increase DNA methylation. Additionally, folate is necessary for normal DNA methylation. This may explain why fetal hypoxia and maternal famine predispose some individuals to develop schizophrenia.

This is not to say that DNA methylation is the only mechanism to explain schizophrenia. Spontaneous mutation during spermatogenesis is another possible cause. It is known that schizophrenia is associated with increased paternal age and older fathers are more likely to have increased *de novo* germline mutations. The important point is that changes to DNA—particularly vulnerable DNA—can be a way for us to understand the genetic/environmental etiology of schizophrenia.

The take home message is this: There are likely to be multiple genetic vulnerabilities to schizophrenia, which are rarely expressed but not uncommon. Insults from the environment, such as diet, infection, ischemia, and so on, have detrimental and lasting effects on the DNA. Those individuals having both genetic vulnerability and environmental insult are the ones who develop schizophrenia.

THE DOPAMINE HYPOTHESIS

It does not seem proper to write an entire chapter on schizophrenia without mentioning dopamine. The dopamine hypothesis is an old and enduring theory purporting that overactivity of the dopamine system is part of the pathogenesis of schizophrenia. It was first proposed in 1966 on the basis of pharmacologic studies. Dopamine blocking agents provided the first effective treatment for the positive symptoms of schizophrenia. Alternatively, amphetamines, which increase dopamine at the synaptic cleft, can induce psychosis.

Although popularity of the dopamine blocking agents is at an all time high, the belief that dopamine overactivity causes schizophrenia has receded. Modulation of dopamine activity may be effective in diminishing psychotic symptoms, but there is minimal evidence to implicate the dopamine neurons in the pathogenesis of the disorder. More likely it is the disconnections among the glutamate and GABA neurons that are the culprits.

QUESTIONS

1. Neurodevelopmental causes that could explain schizophrenia include excessive amounts of all of the following, except
   a. Pruning.
   b. Synaptogenesis.
   c. Apoptosis.
   d. Myelination.

2. Evidence that schizophrenia is a biologic disorder includes all of the following, except
   a. The difference in lateral ventricles in the twin study.
   b. Gliosis in the PFC.
   c. Gray matter reduction in childhood-onset schizophrenia.
   d. Hypofrontality.

3. All of the following support the reduced neurophil hypothesis, except
   a. Oligodendrocyte dysfunction.
   b. Reduced neural cell size.
   c. Limited spine formation on the dendrites.
   d. Increased density of gray matter.

4. Evidence that GABA interneurons are impaired in schizophrenia
   a. Increased methylation of calretinin DNA.
   b. Reduced parvalbumin neurons.
   c. Reduced GAD67.
   d. Increased reelin.

5. All of the following suggest white matter impairment in schizophrenia, except
   a. Microarray analysis.
   b. DTI.

c. Oligodendrocyte cell counts.

d. Significantly reduced white matter volume.

6. Auditory hallucinations have been shown to activate which region on fMRI?
a. Superior temporal lobe.
b. Broca's area.
c. Wernicke's area.
d. Arcuate fasciculus.

7. All are plausible theories on the etiology of schizophrenia except:
a. Methylation of DNA.
b. Spontaneous mutations.
c. Dopamine hypothesis.
d. Genetic/environmental interactions.

8. Match the following:

1. Bleuler E   A. Psychoanalytic
2. E. Fuller D   theory
    Torrey   B. Distinguished
3. Kraepelin B   schizophrenia from
4. Plum F   bipolar disorder
5. Refrigerator   C. Hypofrontality
    mother A   D. Invisible epidemic
6. Wisconsin   E. Coined the term
    Card Sort C   schizophrenia
                        F. Graveyard of
                            neuropathologists

See Answers section at end of book.

Alzheimer's Disease

HISTORIC PERSPECTIVE
Human Longevity

Although historic records indicate that older people have always existed, old age was once rare. Before the 20th century, few people lived beyond 50. Now, 95% of the children born in developed countries live past that age (see Figure 21.1). Changes in health care, sanitation, and nutrition (to name a few) have had a profound impact on life expectancy. The ultimate result is that more and more people are living to ripe old ages. With more people living into their geriatric years, more aging-related central nervous system (CNS) problems are becoming prevalent.

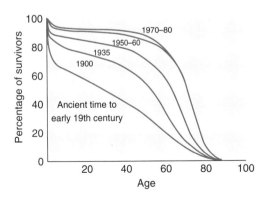

FIGURE 21.1 ● The percentage of people living beyond the age of 60 has increased dramatically in the last two centuries. (Adapted from Kandel ER, Schwartz JH, Jessell TM, eds. *Principles of neural science*, 4th ed. New York: McGraw-Hill; 2000.)

POINT OF INTEREST

The maximum human life span is approximately 125 years and has not changed in over 100,000 years. Cell culture studies suggest that each species has a biologic clock that influences its life span. For example, fibroblasts will only divide a limited number of times before dying. The number of divisions is related to life span (see Table).

Lifespan and cell division of different species

Species	Maximum life span (y)	Maximum fibroblast doubling
Galapagos tortoise	175	125
Man	125	60
Mouse	4	28

The important point is that life span and age-related illnesses such as dementia are likely to be controlled by different mechanisms.

All nerve cells are affected by aging. Sensory and motor skills decline with age. Neurodegenerative disorders such as Parkinson's disease, amyotrophic lateral sclerosis, and Huntington's disease become more prevalent as people get older. Cellular and molecular changes that accumulate over time render neurons vulnerable to damage. Most likely, the damage results from a combination of genetic vulnerability and environmental hits.

Dementia, the progressive deterioration of cognitive skills, is perhaps the most worrisome development for all of us. There are numerous causes of dementia, including cerebral vascular accidents, alcoholism, and infections. Alzheimer's disease (AD) is the most common cause of dementia. The surge in dementia cases as the baby boomers age is expected to overwhelm the health care system unless some intervention is discovered.

Alois Alzheimer

The disease we now call Alzheimer's was first discussed when Alois Alzheimer presented a case in 1906 of a woman with the early onset of dementia. Her symptoms started in middle age with a change in personality and mild memory impairment. She was institutionalized when she became paranoid and unmanageable. Alzheimer repeatedly examined the woman as he followed up her deteriorating clinical course. Four and a half years after her initial symptoms, she was bedridden in a fetal position until she died.

The autopsy revealed gross atrophy of the cortex without localized foci. With the application of the new staining methods (see Figure 1.4), Alzheimer found sclerotic plaques scattered throughout the cortex, especially in the upper layers. Additionally, he noted that many of the cortical neurons were reduced to dense bundles of neurofibrils. Alzheimer thought that his description of plaques and neurofibrillary tangles in a patient with "presenile dementia" was a new and unique condition.

In fact, Alzheimer's finding was cognitive loss associated with the following:

1. Cortical atrophy
2. Plaques outside the neurons
3. Tangles inside the neurons

These findings have become the description of the dementia that bears his name. Figure 21.2 shows a schematic representation of what Alzheimer might have seen when he looked through his microscope.

ALZHEIMER'S DISEASE

Surprisingly, what Alzheimer saw remains the focus of research now. However, the application of modern technology has greatly advanced the understanding of the pathophysiology of atrophy, plaques, and tangles.

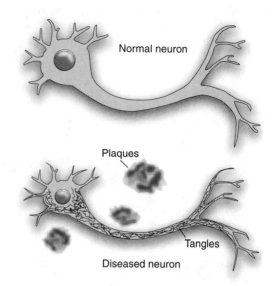

FIGURE 21.2 ● Alzheimer's disease includes the constellation of neuronal shrinkage, plaques, and neurofibrillary tangles.

Cortical Atrophy

The most striking feature of the Alzheimer's brain is the dramatic shrinkage of the cortical tissue secondary to neuronal cell death. AD is a bit like losing hair. It starts years before it is actually noticed and progresses slowly. In some people it starts sooner and proceeds faster. Almost everyone experiences some hair loss with aging.

Brain volume loss is also a "normal" feature of aging. Brain volume peaks in adolescence and then declines as much as 0.2% to 0.5% per year. Patients with AD have a more aggressive loss. Likewise, some people are genetically predisposed to early onset AD.

Examination of the AD brain at autopsy shows extensive atrophy. Figure 21.3 compares two views of normal brains with AD brains. The enlargement of the ventricles and sulci in combination with the decreased tissue are easily recognized.

Brain imaging, although not yet diagnostic for AD, can document the volume loss and contrast the changes for those with and without AD. Figure 21.4 shows the results of sequential magnetic resonance imaging (MRI) on a patient destined to develop familial AD. Note how his brain atrophy proceeds faster than in healthy elderly control. It is also of interest that the symptoms of AD did not appear until significant brain tissue was lost.

The decrease in energy metabolism secondary to the extensive neuronal damage can be seen in functional imaging studies such as positron

Normal brain   Alzheimer's brain

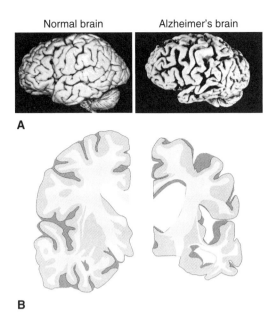

B

FIGURE 21.3 ● Gross examination (**A**) and coronal slices (**B**) show the extensive shrinkage of the brain from Alzheimer's disease. (**A** courtesy of George Grossberg and the St. Louis University Alzheimer's Brain Bank.)

emission tomography (PET). Figure 21.5 shows the marked reduction in glucose metabolism in a patient with AD compared with a healthy control. The difference is so prominent some have suggested that PET could be used to differentiate patients with AD from those normally aging. A large European study including more than 500 subjects found a 93% sensitivity and specificity for separating mild to moderate AD from normal controls. Unfortunately, they were not as effective at separating AD from other forms of dementia, and PET is even less helpful in diagnosing patients

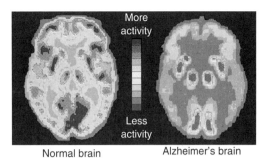

Normal brain   Alzheimer's brain

FIGURE 21.5 ● Positron emission tomography (PET) images showing glucose metabolism in a normal brain compared with an Alzheimer's disease brain. Note the reduced activity in the frontal and temporal regions of the AD brain. (Adapted from Mattson MP, Magnus T. Ageing and neuronal vulnerability. *Nat Rev Neurosci.* 2006;7[4]:278–294.)

with mild cognitive impairment and determining whether they will go on to develop AD.

Amyloid Plaques

The extracellular deposits that Alzheimer saw are called *amyloid plaques*, which is a bit of a misnomer. They are actually aggregates of fibrous protein and not amyloid at all. It was not until 1984 that the primary component of the plaques was found to be a small protein called *amyloid-β or A-β*. (To add to the confusion, the most common term used in the literature is *β-amyloid or β-amyloid*.) Specifically, it is a long 42-amino-acid chain called A-β-42 that seems to be the real culprit, although there may be others that are more noxious.

A-β is cleaved from a larger molecule called *amyloid-β precursor protein* (APP). APP is a large protein protruding through the cell wall (see Figure 21.6). It is found in cells throughout the

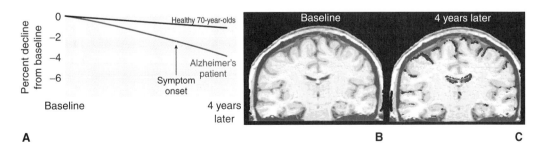

A   **B**   **C**

FIGURE 21.4 ● **A:** Sequential magnetic resonance imaging (MRI) scans show the aggressive brain atrophy in a patient with alzheimer's disease (AD) compared with healthy geriatric controls. **B:** MRI in a patient with AD at baseline and (**C**) 4 years later. Brown overlay represents tissue loss compared with baseline. (Adapted from Fox NC, Schott JM. Imaging cerebral atrophy: Normal ageing to Alzheimer's disease. *Lancet.* 2004;363[9406]:392–394.)

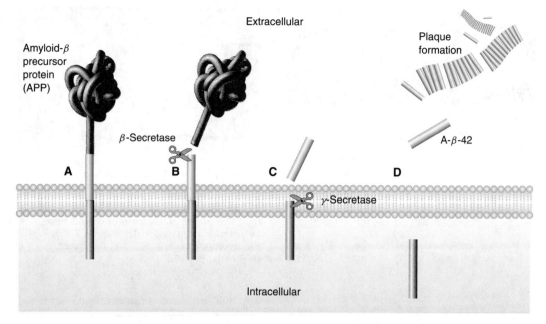

Extracellular

Amyloid-β
precursor
protein
(APP)

Plaque
formation

β-Secretase

A-β-42

A   B   C   D

γ-Secretase

Intracellular

FIGURE 21.6 ● Amyloid plaques are formed from the cleavage of amyloid precursor protein (APP) into smaller proteins that clump together. (Adapted from Wolfe MS. Shutting down Alzheimer's. *Sci Am.* 2006;294[5]:72–79.)

body, but is prominent in neurons. The functions of APP are not fully understood, but may include regulating neuronal survival, neural neurite outgrowth, and synaptic plasticity.

APP is cleaved into smaller portions by at least two enzymes called β- and γ-*secretase*. The final cleavage results in the generation of A-β-42 (and others) that coalesces into long filaments. It is the clumping of the filaments that form the amyloid plaques. Pharmacologic inhibition of the activity of the secretase enzymes has been of interest to those seeking ways to slow down the development of plaques.

Amyloid Hypothesis

Many believe that amyloid plaques are the source of the problem with AD. Two lines of reasoning suggest this is true. First, some people carry a genetic predisposition for early-onset AD usually developed before the age of 65. In all cases where they have identified the gene, the genetic abnormality causes an increased production of A-β. The toxicity of A-β is the other evidence that supports the amyloid hypothesis. A-β is toxic to neurons grown in petri dishes. Furthermore, A-β can impair the development of long-term potentiation (LTP) as well as the memory for a maze in rodents.

Recently, researchers from England have reported the results of a long-term study with marmoset monkeys. The monkeys received cerebral injections of A-β or other brain tissue that did not contain β-amyloid. Because the monkeys died, their brains were analyzed for amyloid plaques (see Figure 21.7). Monkeys that were injected with A-β were much more likely to have cerebral amyloidosis at autopsy. These results not only show the toxic effects of A-β, but also imply that the presence of A-β seeds the progression.

GENE EXPRESSION

In previous chapters we have discussed how the addition of methyl groups to the DNA structure can silence gene expression (see Figures 14.8 and 18.8). This in turn can cause psychiatric symptoms. The opposite may be happening with Alzheimer's disease; that is, the awakening of improper gene expression through demethylation. There is some indirect evidence that demethylation of the DNA sequence coding for β-secretase results in increased production of that enzyme. This could result in greater production of A-β and a faster progression of the disease.

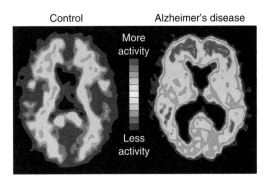

FIGURE 21.8 ● The Pittsburgh compound binds with the amyloid and lights up in a positron emission tomography (PET) scan allowing the identification of patients with Alzheimer's disease. (Adapted from Klunk WE, Engler H, Nordberg A, et al. Imaging brain amyloid in Alzheimer's disease with Pittsburgh compound-B. *Ann Neurol.* 2004;55[3]:306–319.)

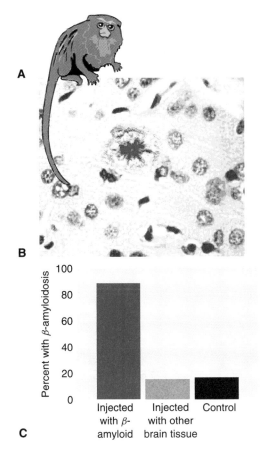

FIGURE 21.7 ● Marmoset monkeys (A) can develop cerebral amyloid plaques (B). Monkeys injected with A-β were much more likely to develop amyloidosis in the next 3 to 4 years. (Adapted from Ridley RM, Baker HF, Windle CP, et al. Very long-term studies of the seeding of beta-amyloidosis in primates. *J Neural Transm.* 2006;113:1243–1251.)

The exact mechanisms of the toxicity of A-β remain murky. Some research suggests that it is the soluble form of the protein that causes the damage. Other research suggests that it is not the A-β-42 protein, but different A-β proteins as yet unidentified. Furthermore, it is not clear why the plaques coalesce in the first place. Some evidence hints that the genetic forms of AD result from an overproduction of APP whereas the more common sporadic cases result from the failure to clear the excess A-β. Clearly, efforts to treat the disorder would benefit from better understanding of these issues.

Pittsburgh Compound

The first step in any treatment approach is an accurate diagnosis of the condition. Historically,

the gold standard for the diagnosis of AD has been at autopsy—a bit late to start treatment. As noted earlier, imaging studies are poor at differentiating AD from other forms of dementia. More recently, researchers have been looking at ways to detect the presence of amyloid deposits in subjects even before symptoms appear. One agent with such potential is Pittsburgh compound-B. This tracer binds to the amyloid and can be visualized in a PET scan. Figure 21.8 shows the results of a scan comparing a healthy control with a patient with AD. With this scan, unlike the PET scan in Figure 21.5, the subject with the disease lights up when the Pittsburgh compound attaches to the amyloid deposits.

Although only a few small studies have been reported to date, the results are encouraging. A test that can accurately identify the developing pathology of AD will be essential for any treatment interventions that seek to halt the progression of the disease.

Neurofibrillary Tangles

The final major pathology of AD is the intracellular neurofibrillary tangles. The neurofibrillary tangles come from the proteins on the microtubules of the neuron. The microtubules are the internal cytoskeleton that provides structure for the cell, and more importantly, transports essential molecules and organelles from the cell body to the synapses. Damage to the microtubules causes the peripheral aspects of the neuron to effectively starve.

The tau proteins bind to the microtubules and provide stability. The problem seems to start with the hyperphosphorylation of the tau proteins (see Figure 21.9). Too many phosphates attached to the tau proteins cause them to detach from the microtubules. It is these detached proteins that clump together and form the neurofibrillary tangles, which in turn clog the neuron's axons and dendrites and cause the cell to die. What causes the hyperphosphorylation remains unclear but seems to be initiated by β-amyloid—possibly soluble A-β that diffuses across the cell wall.

CEREBRAL SPINAL FLUID

Tau protein is increased in the cerebral spinal fluid (CSF) of patients with AD. The diagnostic accuracy of the disease may be enhanced from measurements of specific proteins in the CSF, as well as better imaging studies—in patients with signs of cognitive decline.

AD Progression

AD is a relentlessly progressive disorder. There are no remissions. The first signs are marked by subtle decline in memory. As the disease advances, changes in personality and language skills develop. Eventually even motor functions are impaired. Understanding the spread of the pathology of AD gives a greater appreciation of the changing clinical picture.

The progression of the disease can be staged by the development and progression of neurofibrillary tangles. In a landmark analysis of more than 2,500 brains in Germany over 10 years, Braak documented the insidious evolution of AD. Figure 21.10 shows the results. The initial stages start in the entorhinal cortex of the hippocampus. From there the disease spreads into the temporal and frontal cortex. The final stages involve the entire brain, with the greatest deposits remaining in the regions where it all started.

PREVENTION AND TREATMENT

The number of cases of AD is expected to quadruple in the next 40 years if nothing is done to prevent or treat the disease. Current treatments can temporarily improve cognition in those affected, but do nothing to alter the underlying pathophysiology of the condition. Those of us on the other side of our life curve hope that the scientific community will develop effective interventions in the near future. Several of the favorable prospects are discussed in the subsequent text.

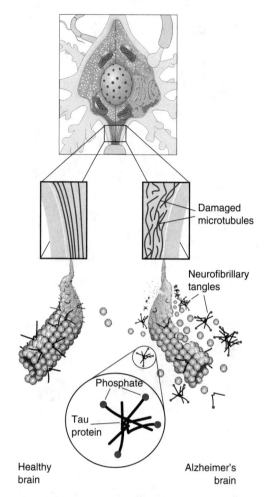

FIGURE 21.9 ● Hyperphosphorylation of the tau proteins produces neurofibrillary tangles that damages the microtubules. The result is impaired axonal transport and ultimately cell death.

Vaccine

Immunizations against childhood diseases have transformed the practice of pediatrics over the last century. The possibility of using vaccines to treat and/or prevent AD is an exciting application of this old intervention, which could likewise transform the practice of geriatric medicine. The trick is to get the immune system to attack the amyloid plaques without attacking other parts of the brain.

The basic plan is laid out in Figure 21.11. Peripheral injections of A-β-42 are ingested by antigen-presenting cells. A-β antigens are presented to T cells, which in turn activate B cells. Anti-Aβ antibodies produced by the B cells attack the amyloid plaques as well as soluble Aβ. Microglial cells then clean the plaques through phagocytosis.

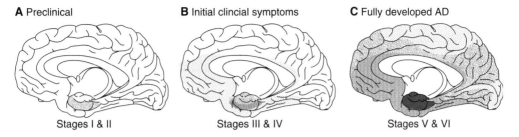

A Preclinical   **B** Initial clincial symptoms   **C** Fully developed AD

Stages I & II   Stages III & IV   Stages V & VI

FIGURE 21.10 ● The spread of neurofibrillary tangles in Alzheimer's disease. (Adapted from Braak H, Braak E. Frequency of stages of Alzheimer-related lesions in different age categories. *Neurobiol Aging.* 1997;18[4]:351–357.)

The vaccine was initially tested in mice genetically engineered to overexpress APP (APP mice). Such mice will develop amyloid plaques and memory loss by the age of 12 months. They have become the accepted animal model of AD. Immunotherapy with APP mice has produced extraordinary results (see Figure 21.12). Clearing of amyloid plaques and preservation of cognitive functions have been repeatedly documented in animal studies.

In 2001, clinical trials of a synthetic version of the β-amyloid protein for use as a vaccine were started in humans. Initial safety studies were completed without a hitch. Unfortunately, the larger phase II study had to be stopped after several months when 6% of the participants developed an excessive inflammatory response (meningoencephalitis). Further analysis has suggested that T-cell activation may have been the problem.

Followup studies on the 372 subjects who were immunized have found some encouraging results. Those individuals who did mount an antibody response to A-β showed subtle signs of improved memory and cognitive skills. Furthermore,

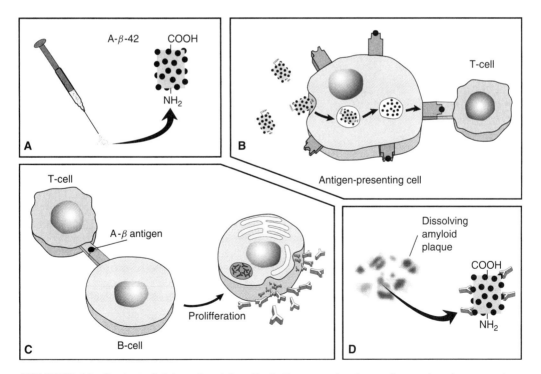

FIGURE 21.11 ● **A:** Aβ is injected peripherally. **B:** The Aβ molecules are ingested and presented to T cells by the antigen-presenting cells. **C:** T cells activate B cells, which produce anti-Aβ antibodies. **D:** The anti-Aβ antibodies attack Aβ in the amyloid plaques and are cleared by microglia. (Adapted from Schenk D, Hagen M, Seubert P. Current progress in beta-amyloid immunotherapy. *Curr Opin Immunol.* 2004;16[5]:599–606.)

postmortem studies of a few patients have documented clearing of the amyloid plaques in some regions of their brains.

The search for an effective and yet harmless treatment utilizing immunotherapy continues. Some have suggested passive immunization. Others are looking for ways to induce clearing of the plaques without overexciting the T cells. If nothing else, this research is an important reminder that successful animal studies are no guarantee of positive results in humans.

ANTIPSYCHOTICS

Alzheimer's original patient was ultimately admitted to his ward because of her uncontrollable psychotic symptoms. Currently most clinicians would quickly place such a patient on a new generation antipsychotic medication. Yet, the use of antipsychotic medications for AD is not without problems. A recent meta-analysis looked at the effect of second generation antipsychotic medications on cognitive decline in patients with AD. They found that the medications actually worsened the cognitive decline when compared with placebo (see Table).

Meta-analysis of cognitive decline in patients treated with second generation antipsychotic medications

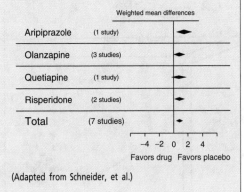

		Weighted mean differences
Aripiprazole	(1 study)	
Olanzapine	(3 studies)	
Quetiapine	(1 study)	
Risperidone	(2 studies)	
Total	(7 studies)	

-4 –2 0 2 4
Favors drug   Favors placebo

(Adapted from Schneider, et al.)

Nerve Growth Factor

The neuronal loss from AD might be prevented or at least limited with appropriate stimulation from growth factor proteins. Animal studies suggest

Hippocampus from APP genetically engineered mice

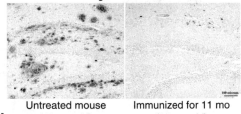

Untreated mouse   Immunized for 11 mo
A   (12 mo old)   (12 mo old)

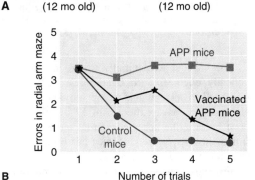

B   Number of trials

FIGURE 21.12 ● **A:** Slices of amyloid precursor protein (APP) mice hippocampi show the accumulation of amyloid plaques without and with the Aβ vaccination. **B:** Vaccinated mice display memory similar to control mice and superior to the APP mice. (**A** from Lemere CA, Maier M, Jiang L, et al. Amyloid-beta immunotherapy for the prevention and treatment of Alzheimer disease: Lessons from mice, monkeys, and humans. *Rejuvenation Res.* 2006;9[1]:77–84.), courtesy of Cynthia A. Lemere. (**B** adapted from Morgan D, Diamond DM, Gottschall PE, et al. A beta peptide vaccination prevents memory loss in an animal model of Alzheimer's disease. *Nature.* 2000;408[6815]:982–985.)

growth factor proteins may be useful for treating neurodegenerative diseases such as AD. Specifically, nerve growth factor (NGF, see Figure 1.9) has been shown to prevent cholinergic degeneration and improve memory in animals. The problem arises in choosing a method to deliver the NGF to the brain. The molecule is too large to cross the blood–brain barrier. Likewise, direct infusion into the ventricles results in excessive stimulation and intolerable side effects, for example, pain and glial cell infiltration.

An alternative method of delivery entails highjacking the DNA in autologous fibroblasts using retroviral vectors. Such fibroblasts can be induced to express NGF. In turn, they can be placed directly into the brain of the subject and deliver NGF within a few millimeters of the desired region. Because they are autologous, they do not activate an immune response.

Researchers at the University of California in San Diego completed a phase I trial with eight patients with probable AD. Fibroblasts producing NGF were injected into the subjects' cholinergic basal forebrain. Two patients had significant complications from the surgery, but with five of the remaining six, cognition stabilized or improved during the 6 to 18 months after injection. PET scans showed increased activity.

Although this treatment will not halt the development of amyloid plaques or neurofibrillary tangles, it does show that NGFs may play a role in reducing the symptoms of AD. Additionally, the study highlights that unique mechanisms can be utilized to deliver NGFs to specific regions of the brain.

Brain Reserve

Postmortem studies have found that a substantial proportion of people have the histopathology of AD, but not the cognitive failings of dementia. Prospective studies suggest the number may be as high as 40%. Some believe that this is due to *brain reserve*; that is, greater neural substrate buffers against the clinical expression of the disease. (Similar to starting with more adipose tissue during times of famine.) Indeed, prospective studies have found that individuals who have the plaques and tangles at death, but were not demented, had greater number of neurons in the frontal, parietal, and temporal cortices.

One of the most remarkable studies on this topic was the Nun Study, in which they determined the correlation between early verbal skills and later cognitive impairment. The researchers completed extensive cognitive assessments of the nuns older than 75 years in their retirement. In their early 20s, the nuns had completed an autobiographic essay when they entered the order. These essays were blindly graded for linguistic ability. The nuns with low idea density and low grammatical complexity in their autobiographies written 50 years earlier were 15 times more likely to have low cognitive scores in late life. In other words, cognitive skills in early life prevent cognitive impairment later on.

A recent study has taken this analysis one step further by including postmortem brain examination. The study included 156 individuals in whom the researchers could correlate educational background, level of cognition before death, and amyloid load in the brain at autopsy. The results are shown in Figure 21.13. The individuals with greater years of education had less cognitive impairment even with increasing amyloidosis.

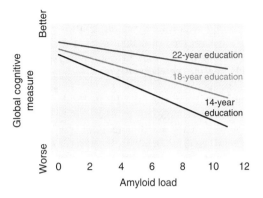

FIGURE 21.13 ● The cognitive impairment associated with amyloidosis is minimized by increasing years of education. (Adapted from Bennett DA, Schneider JA, Wilson RS, et al. Education modifies the association of amyloid but not tangles with cognitive function. *Neurology.* 2005;65[6]:953–955.)

The authors concluded that education is associated with factors that somehow reduce the effect of amyloid on cognition. They estimated that the difference between 15 years of education and 22 years is equivalent to approximately 2.6 years of amyloid progression. We think this information should provide some relief for the sort of person reading this book.

One of the mantras resulting from this line of research is "use it or lose it". The implication being that exercising the brain is neuroprotective against the pathology of AD. Clearly, the research described here shows that smarter, more educated people have greater brain resilience. What we do not know is whether these people were born with a larger reserve of neural substrate or whether a lifetime of cognitive enrichment stimulated neuronal growth, which in turn protected their brains from the effects of AD. Randomized controlled trials will be needed to answer this question.

Caloric Restriction

Caloric restriction is known to enhance longevity (see LONGEVITY, page 129). Dietary restriction may also retard the effects of AD. Studies with animals suggest that low calorie diets may protect the brain in the following ways:

1. Limiting oxidative stress
2. Reducing DNA damage
3. Increasing brain-derived neurotrophic factor (BDNF) production

A recent study shows the profound effects that calorie restriction can have on amyloid deposits in nonhuman primates. A colony of squirrel monkeys was raised on a diet reduced by 30% and compared with a freely eating control group. As the monkeys died of natural causes, their temporal cortical tissues were measured for β-amyloid, APP, and the secretase enzymes.

The monkeys on dietary restriction showed no change in the amount of APP molecule, but a remarkable reduction in A-β. The activity of β- and γ-secretase enzymes (Figure 21.6) was no different between the two groups. However, α-secretase was almost 100% more active in the diet-restricted group. α-Secretase is an enzyme that cuts the APP molecule in a manner that limits the production of β-amyloid. In other words, caloric restriction enhances the activity of an enzyme that prevents the buildup of amyloid plaques.

Although caloric restriction may be effective in altering the build up of β-amyloid, it seems unlikely to be utilized by the large number of people at risk for AD. Indeed, the industrial societies that are at most risk for AD are also the ones struggling with the obesity epidemic. However, if treatments that reduce hunger or enhance satiety can be developed (see Chapter 10, Appetite), these could be reasonable pharmacologic approaches to forestalling AD.

CABERNET SAUVIGNON

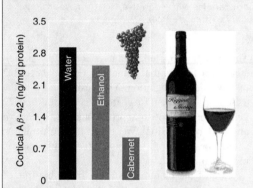

Alzheimer's modeled mice showed significant reductions in cortical β-amyloid with daily Cabernet Sauvignon. (Adapted from Wang J, Ho L, Zhao Z, et al. Moderate consumption of Carernet Sauvignon attenuates AB neuropathology in a mouse model of Alzheimer's disease. *FASEB J.* 2006;20:2313–2320.)

It is with great pleasure that we report the results of a recent study showing the cerebral benefits of moderate doses of red wine. Mice altered to overexpress APP were given daily supplements of California Cabernet Sauvignon, ethanol, or water. The wine group had not only superior memory function, but also less β-amyloid in their cortex (Figure).

We think that anyone who has finished reading every word of this book should celebrate with a little California Cabernet Sauvignon. Heck, it will give a little tweak to the nucleus accumbens, as well as promote β-amyloid clearance—all in moderation of course.

QUESTIONS

1. One hundred and twenty-five years
   a. Life expectancy.
   b. Fibroblast duration.
   c. Maximum cell divisions.
   d. Life span.

2. Alzheimer's identified all of the following, except
   a. Cortical atrophy.
   b. Amyloid plaques.
   c. β-amyloid.
   d. Neurofibrillary tangles.

3. All of the following are increased in AD, except
   a. Amyloid-β precursor protein (APP).
   b. A-β-42.
   c. Ventricular size.
   d. CSF tau protein.

4. All of the following are decreased in AD, except
   a. Cortical size.
   b. Pittsburgh Compound accumulation.
   c. Glucose metabolism.
   d. Neuronal substrate.

5. Neurofibrillary tangles are composed of
   a. Damaged microtubules.
   b. Extracellular protein tangles.
   c. Excessively phosphorylated tau.
   d. Untransportable cellular products.

6. The goal of Alzheimer's vaccine is to increase which of the following?
   a. A-β-42.
   b. T-cell activation.
   c. Memory performance.
   d. Anti-Aβ antibodies.

7. Increases with calorie restriction
   a. Amyloid-β precursor protein (APP).
   b. α-Secretase.
   c. β-Secretase.
   d. γ-Secretase.

See Answers section at end of book.

Bibliography

CHAPTER 1

1. Bear MF, Connors BW, Paradiso MA, eds. *Neuroscience: Exploring the Brain*, 3rd ed. Baltimore: Lippincott Williams & Wilkins; 2007.
2. Bouchard TJ. Twin studies of behavior: New and old findings. In: Schmitt A, Atzwanger K, Grammer K, et al. eds. *New aspects of human ethology*. New York: Plenum Publishing; 1997:121–140.
3. Finger S. *Minds behind the brain: a history of the pioneers and their discoveries*. New York: Oxford University Press; 2000.
4. Friend SH, Stoughton RB. The magic of microarrays. *Sci Am*. 2002;286:44–53.
5. Gottesman II. *Schizophrenia genesis*. New York: WH Freeman; 1991.
6. Hodgkin AL, Huxley AF. Action potentials recorded from inside a nerve fibre. *Nature*. 1939;144:710–711.
7. Illing R-B. Humbled by history. *Sci Am Mind*. 2004;14: 86–93.
8. Levi-Montalcini R. The nerve growth factor. *Ann N Y Acad Sci*. 1964;118:149–170.
9. Ramon y Cajal S *Recollections on my life. Transactions of the American Philosophical Society*, Vol. 8, Part 2. Philadelphia: The American Philosophical Society; 1937.
10. Rorden C, Karnath HO. Using human brain lesions to infer function: a relic from a past era in the fMRI age? *Nat Rev Neurosci*. 2004;5:813–819.
11. Zimmer C. *Soul made flesh: the discovery of the brain—and how it changed the world*. New York: Free Press; 2004.

CHAPTER 2

1. Bear MF, Connors BW, Paradiso MA, eds. *Neuroscience: exploring the brain*, 3rd ed. Baltimore: Lippincott Williams & Wilkins; 2007.
2. Behrstock S, Ebert A, McHugh J, et al. Human neural progenitors deliver glial cell line-derived neurotrophic factor to parkinsonian rodents and aged primates. *Gene Ther*. 2005;13(5):379–388.
3. Bower JM, Parsons LM. Rethinking the "lesser brain". *Sci Am*. 2003;289(2):50–57.
4. Fuster JM. *The prefrontal cortex: anatomy, physiology, and neuropsychology of the frontal lobe*, 3rd ed. Philadelphia: Lippincott-Raven Publishers; 1997.
5. Goldstein GW, Betz AL. The blood-brain barrier. *Sci Am*. 1986;255(3):74–83.
6. Kandel ER, Schwartz JH, Jessell TM, eds. *Principles of neural science*, 4th ed. New York: McGraw-Hill; 2000.
7. Lewis DA. Structure of the human prefrontal cortex. *Am J Psychiatry*. 2004;161(8):1366.
8. Mashour GA, Walker EE, Martuza RL. Psychosurgery: past, present, and future. *Brain Res—Brain Res Rev*. 2005;48(3):409–419.

9. Nestler EJ, Hyman SE, Malenka RC. *Molecular neuropharmacology. A foundation for clinical neuroscience*. New York: McGraw-Hill; 2001.
10. Salloway SP, Malloy PF, Duffy JD, eds. *The frontal lobes and neuropsychiatric illness*. Washington, DC: American Psychiatric Publishing, Inc; 2001.
11. Snell RS. *Clinical neuroanatomy: a illustrated review with questions and explanations*, 3rd ed. Philadelphia: Lippincott Williams & Wilkins; 2001.
12. Welch MJ, Meltzer EO, Simons FE. H1-antihistamines and the central nervous system. *Clin Allergy Immunol*. 2002;17:337–388.

CHAPTER 3

1. Bear MF, Connors BW, Paradiso MA, eds. *Neuroscience: Exploring the Brain*, 3rd ed. Baltimore: Lippincott Williams & Wilkins; 2007.
2. Fields RD. The other half of the brain. *Sci Am*. 2004; 290(4):54–61.
3. Haydon PG. GLIA: listening and talking to the synapse. *Nat Rev Neurosci*. 2001;2(3):185–193.
4. Kaufmann WE, Moser HW. Dendritic anomalies in disorders associated with mental retardation. *Cereb Cortex*. 2000;10(10):981–991.
5. Kolb B, Forgie M, Gibb R, et al. Age, experience and the changing brain. *Neurosci Biobehav Rev*. 1998;22(2): 143–159.
6. Rosenzweig MR, Breedlove SM, Watson NV. *Biological Psychology*, 4th ed. Sunderland, MA: Sinauer; 2005.
7. Tian GF, Azmi H, Takano T, et al. An astrocytic basis of epilepsy. *Nat Med*. 2005;11(9):973–981.

CHAPTER 4

1. Bear MF, Connors BW, Paradiso MA, eds. *Neuroscience: exploring the brain*, 3rd ed. Baltimore: Lippincott Williams & Wilkins; 2007.
2. Cooper JR, Bloom FE, Roth RH. *The biochemical basis of neuropharmacology*, 8th ed. New York: Oxford University Press; 2003.
3. Goff DC, Coyle JT. The emerging role of glutamate in the pathophysiology and treatment of schizophrenia. *Am J Psychiatry*. 2001;158(9):1367–1377.
4. Holmes A, Heilig M, Rupniak NM, et al. Neuropeptide systems as novel therapeutic targets for depression and anxiety disorders. *Trends Pharmacol Sci*. 2003; 24(11):580–588.
5. Iversen L. Cannabis and the brain. *Brain*. 2003;126 (Pt 6):1252–1270.
6. Nestler EJ, Hyman SE, Malenka RC. *Molecular neuropharmacology. A foundation for clinical neuroscience*. New York: McGraw-Hill; 2001.
7. Purves D, Augustine GJ, Fitzpatrick D, et al. *Neuroscience*, 3rd ed. Sunderland, MA: Sinauer; 2004.

8. Rosenzweig MR, Breedlove SM, Watson NV. *Biological psychology*, 4th ed. Sunderland, MA: Sinauer; 2005.
9. Snyder SH, Ferris CD. Novel neurotransmitters and their neuropsychiatric relevance. *Am J Psychiatry*. 2000;157(11):1738–1751.
10. Stahl SM. *Essential psychopharmacology. Neuroscientific basis of practical applications*, 2nd ed. New York: Cambridge University Press; 2000.
11. Strand FL. *Neuropeptides: regulators of physiological processes*. London: MIT Press; 1999.
12. Tsen G, Williams B, Allaire P, et al. Receptors with opposing functions are in postsynaptic microdomains under one presynaptic terminal. *Nat Neurosci*. 2000;3(2):126–132.

CHAPTER 5

1. Bear MF, Connors BW, Paradiso MA, eds. *Neuroscience: exploring the brain*, 3rd ed. Baltimore: Lippincott Williams & Wilkins; 2007.
2. Engert F, Bonhoeffer T. Dendritic spine changes associated with hippocampal long-term synaptic plasticity. *Nature*. 1999;399(6731):66–70.
3. Huang YZ, Edwards MJ, Rounis E, et al. Theta burst stimulation of the human motor cortex. *Neuron*. 2005;45:201–206.
4. Kroeze WK, Hufeisen SJ, Popadak BA, et al. H1-histamine receptor affinity predicts short-term weight gain for typical and atypical antipsychotic drugs. *Neuropsychopharmacology*. 2003;28(3):519–526.
5. LeDoux J. *The snyaptic self. How our brains become who we are*. New York: Viking; 2002.
6. Nestler EJ, Hyman SE, Malenka RC. *Molecular neuropharmacology. A foundation for clincial neuroscience*. New York: McGraw-Hill; 2001.
7. Purves D, Augustine GJ, Fitzpatrick D, et al. *Neuroscience*, 3rd ed. Sunderland, MA: Sinauer; 2004.
8. Ressler KJ, Rothbaum BO, Tannenbaum L, et al. Cognitive enhancers as adjuncts to psychotherapy: Use of D-cycloserine in phobic individuals to facilitate extinction of fear. *Arch Gen Psychiatry*. 2004;61(11):1136–1144.
9. Rogawski MA, Loscher W. The neurobiology of antiepileptic drugs. *Nat Rev Neurosci*. 2004;5(7):553–564.
10. Rosenzweig MR, Breedlove SM, Watson NV. *Biological psychology*, 4th ed. Sunderland, MA: Sinauer; 2005.
11. Strohle A, Romeo E, di Michele F, et al. Induced panic attacks shift gamma-aminobutyric acid type A receptor modulatory neuroactive steroid composition in patients with panic disorder: Preliminary results. *Arch Gen Psychiatry*. 2003;60(2):161–168.
12. Tecott LH, Smart SL. Monoamine neurotransmitters. In: Sadock BJ, Sadock VA, eds. *Kaplan and Sadock's comprehensive textbook of psychiatry*, 8th ed. Philadelphia: Lippincott Williams & Wilkins; 2005:49–60.
13. Victor M, Ropper AH. *Adams and Victor's principles of neurology*, 7th ed. New York: McGraw-Hill; 2001.

CHAPTER 6

1. Azukizawa M, Pekary AE, Hershman JM, et al. Plasma thyrotropin, thyroxine, and triiodothyronine relationships in man. *J Clin Endocrinol Metab*. 1976;43(3):533–542.
2. Bauer M, Heinz A, Whybrow PC. Thyroid hormones, serotonin and mood: Of synergy and significance in the adult brain. *Mol Psychiatry*. 2002;7(2):140–156.

3. Bauer M, London ED, Silverman DH, et al. Thyroid, brain and mood modulation in affective disorder: Insights from molecular research and functional brain imaging. *Pharmacopsychiatry*. 2003;36(Suppl 3):S215–S221.
4. Bauer M, Whybrow PC. Thyroid hormone, neural tissue and mood modulation. *World J Biol Psychiatry*. 2001;2(2):59–69.
5. Bear MF, Connors BW, Paradiso MA, eds. *Neuroscience: exploring the brain*, 3rd ed. Baltimore: Lippincott Williams & Wilkins; 2007.
6. Belanoff JK, Rothschild AJ, Cassidy F, et al. An open label trial of C-1073 (mifepristone) for psychotic major depression. [see comment]. *Biol Psychiatry*. 2002;52(5):386–392.
7. Constant EL, de Volder AG, Ivanoiu A, et al. Cerebral blood flow and glucose metabolism in hypothyroidism: A positron emission tomography study. *J Clin Endocrinol Metab*. 2001;86(8):3864–3870.
8. Fava M, Labbate LA, Abraham ME, et al. Hypothyroidism and hyperthyroidism in major depression revisited. *J Clin Psychiatry*. 1995;56(5):186–192.
9. Forrest D, Reh TA, Rusch A. Neurodevelopmental control by thyroid hormone receptors. *Curr Opin Neurobiol*. 2002;12(1):49–56.
10. Gordon JT, Kaminski DM, Rozanov CB, et al. Evidence that 3,3',5-triiodothyronine is concentrated in and delivered from the locus coeruleus to its noradrenergic targets via anterograde axonal transport. *Neuroscience*. 1999;93(3):943–954.
11. Kim JJ, Diamond DM. The stressed hippocampus, synaptic plasticity and lost memories. *Nat Rev Neurosc*. 2002;3(6):453–462.
12. Lupien SJ, de Leon M, de Santi S, et al. Cortisol levels during human aging predict hippocampal atrophy and memory deficits. *Nat Neurosci*. 1998;1(1):69–73.
13. Marangell LB, Ketter TA, George MS, et al. Inverse relationship of peripheral thyrotropin-stimulating hormone levels to brain activity in mood disorders. *Am J Psychiatry*. 1997;154(2):224–230.
14. McEwen BS. Protective and damaging effects of stress mediators. *N Engl J Med*. 1998;338(3):171–179.
15. Nestler EJ, Hyman SE, Malenka RC. *Molecular neuropharmacology. A foundation for clinical neuroscience*. New York: McGraw-Hill; 2001.
16. Raison CL, Miller AH. When not enough is too much: The role of insufficient glucocorticoid signaling in the pathophysiology of stress-related disorders. *Am J Psychiatry*. 2003;160(9):1554–1565.
17. Rosenzweig MR, Breedlove SM, Watson NV. *Biological psychology*. Sunderland, MA: Sinauer; 2005.
18. Rupprecht R, Holsboer F. Neuroactive steroids: Mechanisms of action and neuropsychopharmacological perspectives. [see comment]. *Trends Neurosci*. 1999;22(9):410–460.
19. Sapolsky RM. *Why Zebras don't get ulcers: an updated guide to stress, stress-related diseases, and coping*. New York: Barns & Noble Books; 1998.
20. Sapolsky RM. Stress and plasticity in the limbic system. *Neurochem Res*. 2003;28(11):1735–1742.
21. Snell RS. *Clinical neuroanatomy: a illustrated review with questions and explanations*. Philadelphia: Lippincott Williams & Wilkins; 2001.
22. Starkman MN, Giordani B, Gebarski SS, et al. Decrease in cortisol reverses human hippocampal atrophy following treatment of Cushing's disease. *Biol Psychiatry*. 1999;46(12):1595–1602.

23. Starkman MN, Giordani B, Gebarski SS, et al. Improvement in learning associated with increase in hippocampal formation volume. *Biol Psychiatry*. 2003; 53(3):233–238.

24. Vaidya VA, Castro ME, Pei Q, et al. Influence of thyroid hormone on 5-HT(1A) and 5-HT(2A) receptor-mediated regulation of hippocampal BDNF mRNA expression. *Neuropharmacology*. 2001;40(1):48–56.

25. Wolkowitz OM, Rothschild AJ. *Psychoneuroendocrinology: the scientific basis of clincial practice*. Washington, DC: American Psychiatric Publishing, Inc; 2003.

CHAPTER 7

1. Antonini A, Stryker MP. Rapid remodeling of axonal arbors in the visual cortex. *Science*. 1993;260(5115): 1819–1821.

2. Bear MF, Connors BW, Paradiso MA, eds. *Neuroscience: exploring the brain*, 3rd ed. Baltimore: Lippincott Williams & Wilkins; 2007.

3. Bhardway RD, Curtis MA, Spalding KL, et al. Neocortical neurogenesis in humans is restricted to development. *Proc Natl Acad Sci U S A*. 2006;103(33): 12564–12568.

4. Brown J, Cooper-Kuhn CM, Kempermann G, et al. Enriched environment and physical activity stimulate hippocampal but not olfactory bulb neurogenesis. *Eur J Neurosci*. 2003;17(10):2042–2046.

5. Elbert T, Candia V, Altenmuller E, et al. Alteration of digital representations in somatosensory cortex in focal hand dystonia. *Neuroreport*. 1998;9(16):3571–3575.

6. Gage FH. Mammalian neural stem cells. *Science*. 2000;287(5457):1433–1438.

7. Gage FH. Brain, repair yourself. *Sci Am*. 2003;289(3): 46–53.

8. Giedd JN, Blumenthal J, Jeffries NO, et al. Brain development during childhood and adolescence: A longitudinal MRI study. *Nat Neurosci*. 1999;2(10):861–863.

9. Gould E, Reeves AJ, Graziano MS, et al. Neurogenesis in the neocortex of adult primates. *Science*. 1999;286(5439):548–552.

10. Huttenlocher PR, Dabholkar AS. Regional differences in synaptogenesis in human cerebral cortex. *J Comp Neurol*. 1997;387(2):167–178.

11. Johnson JS, Newport EL. Critical period effects in second language learning: The influence of maturational state on the acquisition of English as a second language. *Cognit Psychol*. 1989;21(1):60–99.

12. Merzenich MM, Nelson RJ, Stryker MP, et al. Somatosensory cortical map changes following digit amputation in adult monkeys. *J Comp Neurol*. 1984; 224(4):591–605.

13. Mirescu C, Peters JD, Gould E. Early life experience alters response of adult neurogenesis to stress. *Nat Neurosci*. 2004;7(8):841–846.

14. Munte TF, Altenmuller E, Jancke L. The musician's brain as a model of neuroplasticity. *Nat Rev Neurosci*. 2002;3(6):473–478.

15. Nestler EJ, Hyman SE, Malenka RC. *Molecular neuropharmacology. A foundation for clinicial neuroscience*. New York: McGraw-Hill; 2001.

16. Pantev C, Engelien A, Candia V, et al. Representational cortex in musicians. Plastic alterations in response to musical practice. *Ann N Y Acad Sci*. 2001;930:300–314.

17. Purves D, Augustine GJ, Fitzpatrick D, et al. *Neuroscience*. Sunderland, MA: Sinauer; 2004.

18. Rosenzweig MR, Breedlove SM, Watson NV. *Biological psychology*. Sunderland, MA: Sinauer;2005.

19. Silver J, Miller JH. Regeneration beyond the glial scar. *Nat Rev Neurosci*. 2004;5(2):146–156.

20. Takagi Y, Takahashi J, Saiki H, et al. Dopaminergic neurons generated from monkey embryonic stem cells function in a Parkinson primate model. *J Clin Invest*. 2005;115(1):102–109.

21. Taub E, Uswatte G. Constraint-induced movement therapy: Bridging from the primate laboratory to the stroke rehabilitation laboratory. *J Rehabil Med*. 2003 (41 Suppl):34–40.

22. Wiesel TN. Postnatal development of the visual cortex and the influence of environment. *Nature*. 1982;299 (5884):583–591.

CHAPTER 8

1. Antonini A, Stryker MP. Rapid remodeling of axonal arbors in the visual cortex. *Science*. 1993;260(5115): 1819–1821.

2. Apkarian AV, Sosa Y, Sonty S, et al. Chronic back pain is associated with decreased prefrontal and thalamic gray matter density. *J Neurosci*. 2004;24(46):10410–10415.

3. Bear MF, Connors BW, Paradiso MA, eds. *Neuroscience: exploring the brain*, 3rd ed. Baltimore: Lippincott Williams & Wilkins; 2007.

4. Beecher HK. Pain in men wounded in battle. *Ann Surg*. 1946;123(1):96–195.

5. Borckardt JJ, Weinstein M, Reeves ST, et al. Postoperative left prefrontal repetitive transcranial magnetic stimulation reduces patient-controlled analgesia use. *Anesthesiology*. 2006;105(3):557–562.

6. Boucher TJ, Okuse K, Bennett DL, et al. Potent analgesic effects of GDNF in neuropathic pain states. *Science*. 2000;290(5489):124–127.

7. Cho ZH, Chung SC, Jones JP, et al. New findings of the correlation between acupoints and corresponding brain cortices using functional MRI. *Proc Natl Acad Sci U S A*. 1998;95(5):2670–2673.

8. Coghill RC, McHaffie JG, Yen YF. Neural correlates of interindividual differences in the subjective experience of pain. *Proc Natl Acad Sci U S A*. 2003;100(14):8538–8542.

9. Coghill RC, Sang CN, Maisog JM, et al. Pain intensity processing within the human brain: A bilateral, distributed mechanism. *J Neurophysiol*. 1999;82(4):1934–1943.

10. Colloca L, Beneditti F. Placebos and painkillers: Is mind as real as matter? *Nat Rev Neurosci*. 2005;6:545–552.

11. Diatchenko L, Slade GD, Nackley AG, et al. Genetic basis for individual variations in pain perception and the development of a chronic pain condition. *Hum Mol Genet*. 2005;14(1):135–143.

12. Harden RN. Chronic neuropathic pain. Mechanisms, diagnosis, and treatment. *Neurologist*. 2005;11(2):111–122.

13. Hocking B. Epidemiological aspects of "repetition strain injury" in Telecom Australia. *Med J Aust*. 1987; 147(5):218–222.

14. Hohmann AG, Suplita RL, Bolton NM, et al. An endocannabinoid mechanism for stress-induced analgesia. *Nature*. 2005;435(7045):1108–1112.

15. Hooley JM, Delgado ML. Pain insensitivity in the relatives of schizophrenia patients. *Schizophr Res*. 2001; 47(2–3):265–273.

16. Hunt SP, Mantyh PW. The molecular dynamics of pain control. *Nat Rev Neurosci*. 2001;2(2):83–91.
17. Jaffee JH, Strain EC. Opioid-related disorders. In: Sadock BJ, Sadock VA, eds. *Kaplan & Sadock's comprehensive textbook of psychiatry*, 8th ed. Philadelphia: Lippincott Williams & Wilkins; 2005:1265–1290.
18. Kandel ER, Schwartz JH, Jessell TM, eds. *Principles of neural science*, 4th ed. New York: McGraw-Hill; 2000.
19. Karai L, Brown DC, Mannes AJ, et al. Deletion of vanilloid receptor 1-expressing primary afferent neurons for pain control. *J Clin Invest*. 2004;113(9):1344–1352.
20. Mardy S, Miura Y, Endo F, et al. Congenital insensitivity to pain with anhidrosis (CIPA): Effect of TRKA (NTRK1) missense mutations on autophosphorylation of the receptor tyrosine kinase for nerve growth factor. *Hum Mol Genet*. 2001;10(3):179–188.
21. McMahon SB, Cafferty WB, Marchand F, et al. Immune and glial cell factors as pain mediators and modulators. *Exp Neurol*. 2005;192(2):444–462.
22. Melzack R, Coderre TJ, Katz J, et al. Central neuroplasticity and pathological pain. *Ann N Y Acad Sci*. 2001;933:157–174.
23. Nagasako EM, Oaklander AL, Dworkin RH, et al. Congenital insensitivity to pain: An update. *Pain*. 2003;101(3):213–219.
24. Pariente J, White P, Frackowiak RS, et al. Expectancy and belief modulate the neuronal substrates of pain treated by acupuncture. *Neuroimage*. 2005;25(4):1161–1167.
25. Petrovic P, Kalso E, Petersson KM, et al. Placebo and opioid analgesia—imaging a shared neuronal network. *Science*. 2002;295(5560):1737–1740.
26. Price DD. Psychological and neural mechanisms of the affective dimension of pain. *Science*. 2000;288(5472):1769–1772.
27. Purves D, Augustine GJ, Fitzpatrick D, et al. *Neuroscience*, 3rd ed. Sunderland, MA: Sinauer; 2004.
28. Reynolds DV. Surgery in the rat during electrical analgesia induced by focal brain stimulation. *Science*. 1969;164(878):444–445.
29. Schrader H, Obelieniene D, Bovim G, et al. Natural evolution of late whiplash syndrome outside the medicolegal context. *Lancet*. 1996;347(9010):1207–1211.
30. Staiger TO, Gaster B, Sullivan MD, et al. Systematic review of antidepressants in the treatment of chronic low back pain. *Spine*. 2003;28(22):2540–2545.
31. Tajet-Foxell B, Rose FD. Pain and pain tolerance in professional ballet dancers. *Br J Sports Med*. 1995;29(1):31–34.
32. Wager TD, Rilling JK, Smith EE, et al. Placebo-induced changes in FMRI in the anticipation and experience of pain. *Science*. 2004;303(5661):1162–1167.

CHAPTER 9

1. Adinoff B. Neurobiologic processes in drug reward and addiction. *Harv Rev Psychiatry*. 2004;12(6):305–320.
2. Adriani W, Spijker S, Deroche-Gamonet V, et al. Evidence for enhanced neurobehavioral vulnerability to nicotine during periadolescence in rats. *J Neurosci*. 2003;23(11):4712–4716.
3. Bassareo V, De Luca MA, Di Chiara G. Differential expression of motivational stimulus properties by dopamine in nucleus accumbens shell versus core and prefrontal cortex. *J Neurosci*. 2002;22(11):4709–4719.
4. Bolanos CA, Barrot M, Berton O, et al. Methylphenidate treatment during pre- and periadolescence

alters behavioral responses to emotional stimuli at adulthood. *Biol Psychiatry*. 2003;54(12):1317–1329.
5. Buhusi CV, Meck WH. Differential effects of methamphetamine and haloperidol on the control of an internal clock. *Behav Neurosci*. 2002;116(2):291–297.
6. Carlezon WA Jr, Mague SD, Andersen SL. Enduring behavioral effects of early exposure to methylphenidate in rats. *Biol Psychiatry*. 2003;54(12):1330–1337.
7. Ernst M, Nelson EE, Jazbec S, et al. Amygdala and nucleus accumbens in responses to receipt and omission of gains in adults and adolescents. *Neuroimage*. 2005;25(4):1279–1291.
8. Fone KC, Nutt DJ. Stimulants: Use and abuse in the treatment of attention deficit hyperactivity disorder. *Curr Opin Pharmacol*. 2005;5(1):87–93.
9. Garavan H, Pankiewicz J, Bloom A, et al. Cue-induced cocaine craving: Neuroanatomical specificity for drug users and drug stimuli. *Am J Psychiatry*. 2000;157(11):1789–1798.
10. Glass JM, Adams KM, Nigg JT, et al. Smoking is associated with neurocognitive deficits in alcoholism. *Drug Alcohol Depend*. 2006;82(2):119–126.
11. Goldman D, Barr CS. Restoring the addicted brain. *N Engl J Med*. 2002;347(11):843–845.
12. Kalivas PW, Volkow N, Seamans J. Unmanageable motivation in addiction: A pathology in prefrontal-accumbens glutamate transmission. *Neuron*. 2005; 45(5):647–650.
13. Kolb B, Gorny G, Li Y, et al. Amphetamine or cocaine limits the ability of later experience to promote structural plasticity in the neocortex and nucleus accumbens. *Proc Natl Acad Sci U S A*. 2003;100(18): 10523–10528.
14. Le AD, Harding S, Juzytsch W, et al. The role of corticotrophin-releasing factor in stress-induced relapse to alcohol-seeking behavior in rats. *Psychopharmacology (Berl)*. 2000;150(3):317–324.
15. Morgan D, Grant KA, Gage HD, et al. Social dominance in monkeys: Dopamine D2 receptors and cocaine self-administration. *Nat Neurosci*. 2002;5(2):169–174.
16. Nestler EJ. Molecular basis of long-term plasticity underlying addiction. *Nat Rev Neurosci*. 2001;2(2):119–128.
17. Nestler EJ, Hyman SE, Malenka RC. *Molecular neuropharmacology. A foundation for clincial neuroscience*. New York: McGraw-Hill; 2001.
18. Nestler EJ, Malenka RC. The addicted brain. *Sci Am*. 2004;290(3):78–85.
19. Olds J. Pleasure centers in the brain. *Sci Am*. 1956;195:105–112.
20. Pettit HO, Justice JB Jr. Effect of dose on cocaine self-administration behavior and dopamine levels in the nucleus accumbens. *Brain Res*. 1991;539(1):94–102.
21. Ricaurte GA, Mechan AO, Yuan J, et al. Amphetamine treatment similar to that used in the treatment of adult attention-deficit/hyperactivity disorder damages dopaminergic nerve endings in the striatum of adult nonhuman primates. *J Pharmacol Exp Ther*. 2005; 315(1):91–98.
22. Robbins TW, Everitt BJ. Drug addiction: Bad habits add up. *Nature*. 1999;398(6728):567–570.
23. Robinson TE, Gorny G, Savage VR, et al. Widespread but regionally specific effects of experimenter- versus self-administered morphine on dendritic spines in the nucleus accumbens, hippocampus, and neocortex of adult rats. *Synapse*. 2002;46(4):271–279.
24. Robinson TE, Kolb B. Persistent structural modifications in nucleus accumbens and prefrontal cortex

neurons produced by previous experience with amphetamine. *J Neurosci*. 1997;17(21):8491–8497.

25. Robinson TE, Kolb B. Structural plasticity associated with exposure to drugs of abuse. *Neuropharmacology*. 2004;47(Suppl 1):33–46.

26. Rosenbloom M, Sullivan EV, Pfefferbaum A. Using magnetic resonance imaging and diffusion tensor imaging to assess brain damage in alcoholics. *Alcohol Res Health*. 2003;27(2):146–152.

27. Schultz W. Multiple reward signals in the brain. *Nat Rev Neurosci*. 2000;1(3):199–207.

28. See RE, Fuchs RA, Ledford CC, et al. Drug addiction, relapse, and the amygdala. *Ann N Y Acad Sci*. 2003;985:294–307.

29. Tremblay L, Schultz W. Relative reward preference in primate orbitofrontal cortex. *Nature*. 1999;398(6729):704–708.

30. Volkow ND, Fowler JS. Addiction, a disease of compulsion and drive: Involvement of the orbitofrontal cortex. *Cereb Cortex*. 2000;10(3):318–325.

31. Volkow ND, Fowler JS, Wang GJ, et al. Role of dopamine in the therapeutic and reinforcing effects of methylphenidate in humans: Results from imaging studies. *Eur Neuropsychopharmacol*. 2002;12(6):557–566.

32. Volkow ND, Li TK. Drug addiction: The neurobiology of behaviour gone awry. *Nat Rev Neurosci*. 2004;5(12):963–970.

33. Wilens TE, Faraone SV, Biederman J, et al. Does stimulant therapy of attention-deficit/hyperactivity disorder beget later substance abuse? A meta-analytic review of the literature. *Pediatrics*. 2003;111(1):179–185.

34. Wilson SJ, Sayette MA, Fiez JA. Prefrontal responses to drug cues: A neurocognitive analysis. *Nat Neurosci*. 2004;7(3):211–214.

CHAPTER 10

1. Arch JR. Central regulation of energy balance: Inputs, outputs and leptin resistance. *Proc Nutr Soc*. 2005;64(1):39–46.

2. Ayyad C, Andersen T. Long-term efficacy of dietary treatment of obesity: A systematic review of studies published between 1931 and 1999. *Obes Rev*. 2000; 1(2):113–119.

3. Bear MF, Connors BW, Paradiso MA, eds. *Neuroscience: exploring the brain*, 3rd ed. Baltimore: Lippincott Williams & Wilkins; 2006.

4. Berthoud HR. Mind versus metabolism in the control of food intake and energy balance. *Physiol Behav*. 2004;81(5):781–793.

5. Butte NF, Treuth MS, Voigt RG, et al. Stimulant medications decrease energy expenditure and physical activity in children with attention-deficit/hyperactivity disorder. *J Pediatr*. 1999;135(2 Pt 1):203–207.

6. Carlson NR. *Physiology of behavior*. Boston: Pearson Education Inc.; 2004.

7. Colman E. Anorectics on trial: A half century of federal regulation of prescription appetite suppressants. *Ann Intern Med*. 2005;143(5):380–385.

8. Cone RD. Anatomy and regulation of the central melanocortin system. *Nat Neurosci*. 2005;8(5):571–578.

9. Dallman MF, Pecoraro N, Akana SF, et al. Chronic stress and obesity: A new view of "comfort food". *Proc Natl Acad Sci U S A*. 2003;100(20):11696–11701.

10. Di Marzo V, Matias I. Endocannabinoid control of food intake and energy balance. *Nat Neurosci*. 2005;8(5):585–589.

11. Havel PJ. Peripheral signals conveying metabolic information to the brain: Short-term and long-term regulation of food intake and energy homeostasis. *Exp Biol Med*. 2001;226(11):963–977.

12. Jo YH, Talmage DA, Role LW. Nicotinic receptor-mediated effects on appetite and food intake. *J Neurobiol*. 2002;53(4):618–632.

13. Kalm LM, Semba RD. They starved so that others be better fed: Remembering Ancel Keys and the Minnesota experiment. *J Nutr*. 2005;135(6):1347–1352.

14. Keesey RE, Boyle PC. Effects of quinine adulteration upon body weight of LH-lesioned and intact male rats. *J Comp Physiol Psychol*. 1973;84(1):38–46.

15. Kroeze WK, Hufeisen SJ, Popadak BA, et al. H1-histamine receptor affinity predicts short-term weight gain for typical and atypical antipsychotic drugs. *Neuropsychopharmacology*. 2003;28(3):519–526.

16. Leibel RL, Rosenbaum M, Hirsch J. Changes in energy expenditure resulting from altered body weight. *N Engl J Med*. 1995;332(10):621–628.

17. Lowell BB, Spiegelman BM. Towards a molecular understanding of adaptive thermogenesis. *Nature*. 2000; 404(6778):652–660.

18. Michelson D, Amsterdam JD, Quitkin FM, et al. Changes in weight during a 1-year trial of fluoxetine. *Am J Psychiatry*. 1999;156(8):1170–1176.

19. Rapoport JL, Buchsbaum MS, Zahn TP, et al. Dextroamphetamine: Cognitive and behavioral effects in normal prepubertal boys. *Science*. 1978;199(4328):560–563.

20. Ravussin E, Valencia ME, Esparza J, et al. Effects of a traditional lifestyle on obesity in Pima Indians. *Diabetes Care*. 1994;17(9):1067–1074.

21. de Rijke CE, Jackson PJ, Garner KM, et al. Functional analysis of the Ala67Thr polymorphism in agouti related protein associated with anorexia nervosa and leanness. *Biochem Pharmacol*. 2005;70(2):308–316.

22. Rosenzweig MR, Breedlove SM, Watson NV. *Biological psychology*. Sunderland, MA: Sinauer; 2005.

23. Roth GS. Caloric restriction and caloric restriction mimetics: Current status and promise for the future. *J Am Geriatr Soc*. 2005;53(9 Suppl):S280–S283.

24. Schwartz MW, Woods SC, Porte D Jr, et al. Central nervous system control of food intake. *Nature*. 2000;404(6778):661–671.

25. Seeley RJ, Woods SC. Monitoring of stored and available fuel by the CNS: Implications for obesity. *Nat Rev Neurosci*. 2003;4(11):901–909.

26. Strader AD, Woods SC. Gastrointestinal hormones and food intake. *Gastroenterology*. 2005;128(1):175–191.

27. Stunkard AJ, Sorensen TI, Hanis C, et al. An adoption study of human obesity. *N Engl J Med*. 1986;314(4):193–198.

28. Vaisse C, Clement K, Durand E, et al. Melanocortin-4 receptor mutations are a frequent and heterogeneous cause of morbid obesity. *J Clin Invest*. 2000;106(2):253–262.

29. Volkow ND, Wise RA. How can drug addiction help us understand obesity? *Nat Neurosci*. 2005;8(5):555–560.

CHAPTER 11

1. Bear MF, Connors BW, Paradiso MA. *Neuroscience: exploring the brain*, 3rd ed. Baltimore: Lippincott Williams & Wilkins; 2007.

2. Birbaumer N, Veit R, Lotze M, et al. Deficient fear conditioning in psychopathy: A functional magnetic resonance imaging study. *Arch Gen Psychiatry*. 2005;62(7):799–805.

3. Blair RJ. Neurobiological basis of psychopathy. *Br J Psychiatry*. 2003;182:5–7.

4. Branchi I, Francia N, Alleva E. Epigenetic control of neurobehavioural plasticity: The role of neurotrophins. *Behav Pharmacol*. 2004;15(5–6):353–362.

5. Brower MC, Price BH. Neuropsychiatry of frontal lobe dysfunction in violent and criminal behaviour: A critical review. *J Neurol Neurosurg Psychiatry*. 2001;71:720–726.

6. Coccaro EF, Kavoussi RJ. Fluoxetine and impulsive aggressive behavior in personality-disordered subjects. *Arch Gen Psychiatry*. 1997;54:1081–1088.

7. Coccaro EF, Kavoussi RJ, Hauger RL, et al. Cerebrospinal fluid vasopressin levels: Correlates with aggression and serotonin function in personality-disordered subjects. *Arch Gen Psychiatry*. 1998;55:708–714.

8. Damasio H, Grabowski T, Frank R, et al. The return of Phineas Gage: Clues about the brain from the skull of a famous patient. *Science*. 1994;264:1102–1105.

9. Ehrenkranz J, Bliss E, Sheard MH. Plasma testosterone: Correlation with aggressive behavior and social dominance in man. *Psychosom Med*. 1974;36:469–475.

10. Enserink M. Searching for the mark of Cain. *Science*. 2000;289:575–579.

11. van Erp AM, Miczek KA. Aggressive behavior, increased accumbal dopamine, and decreased cortical serotonin in rats. *J Neurosci*. 2000;20:9320–9325.

12. Fiore M, Amendola T, Triaca V, et al. Fighting in the aged male mouse increases the expression of TrkA and TrkB in the subventricular zone and in the hippocampus. *Behav Brain Res*. 2005;157(2):351–362.

13. Flynn JP. The neural basis of aggression in cats. In: Glass DC, ed. *Neurophysicology and emothion*. New York: Rockefeller University Press; 1967.

14. Gregg TR, Siegel A. Brain structures and neurotransmitters regulating aggression in cats: Implications for human aggression. *Prog Neuropsychopharmacol Biol Psychiatry*. 2001;25:91–140.

15. Hare RD. *Without conscience. The disturbing world of the psychopaths among us*. New York: Guilford Press; 1999.

16. Higley JD, Mehlman PT, Higley SB, et al. Excessive mortality in young free-ranging male nonhuman primates with low cerebrospinal fluid 5-hydroxyindoleacetic acid concentrations. *Arch Gen Psychiatry*. 1996;53(6):537–543.

17. Kiehl KA, Smith AM, Hare RD, et al. Limbic abnormalities in affective processing by criminal psychopaths as revealed by functional magnetic resonance imaging. *Biol Psychiatry*. 2001;50:677–684.

18. Lee GP, Bechara A, Adolphs R, et al. Clinical and physiological effects of stereotaxic bilateral amygdalotomy for intractable aggression. *J Neuropsychiatry Clin Neurosci*. 1998;10(4):413–420.

19. Nelson RJ. *The biology of aggression*. New York: Oxford University Press; 2006.

20. Ortiz J, Raine A. Heart rate level and antisocial behavior in children and adolescents: A meta-analysis. *J Am Acad Child Adolesc Psychiatry*. 2004;43(2):154–162.

21. de Quervain DJ, Fischbacher U, Treyer V, et al. The neural basis of altruistic punishment. *Science*. 2004;305(5688):1254–1258.

22. Raine A. Annotation: The role of prefrontal deficits, low autonomic arousal, and early health factors in the development of antisocial and aggressive behavior in children. *J Child Psychol Psychiatry*. 2002;43:417–434.

23. Raine A, Meloy JR, Bihrle S, et al. Reduced prefrontal and increased subcortical brain functioning assessed using positron emission tomography in predatory and affective murderers. *Behav Sci Law*. 1998;16(3):319–332.

24. Rosenzweig MR, Breedlove SM, Watson NV. *Biological psychology*, 4th ed. Sunderland, MA: Sinauer; 2005.

25. Sano K, Mayanagi Y. Posteromedial hypothalamotomy in the treatment of violent, aggressive behaviour. *Acta Neurochir Suppl (Wien)*. 1988;44:145–151.

26. Sheard MH, Marini JL, Bridges CI, et al. The effect of lithium on impulsive aggressive behavior in man. *Am J Psychiatry*. 1976;133:1409–1413.

27. Siegel A, Edinger H, Dotto M. Effects of electrical stimulation of the lateral aspect of the prefrontal cortex upon attack behavior in cats. *Brain Res*. 1975;93:473–484.

28. Tricker R, Casaburi R, Storer TW, et al. The effects of supraphysiological doses of testosterone on angry behavior in healthy eugonadal men–a clinical research center study. *J Clin Endocrinol Metab*. 1996;81:3754–3758.

29. Wagner GC, Beuving LJ, Hutchinson RR. The effects of gonadal hormone manipulations on aggressive target-biting in mice. *Aggress Behav*. 1980;6:1–7.

CHAPTER 12

1. Bear MF, Connors BW, Paradiso MA, eds. *Neuroscience: exploring the brain*, 3rd ed. Baltimore: Lippincott Williams & Wilkins; 2007.

2. Everson CA, Laatsch CD, Hogg N. Antioxidant defense responses to sleep loss and sleep recovery. *Am J Physiol Regul Integr Comp Physiol*. 2005;288(2):R374–R383.

3. Fosse R, Stickgold R, Hobson JA. Brain-mind states: Reciprocal variation in thoughts and hallucinations. *Psychol Sci*. 2001;12(1):30–36.

4. Frank MG, Issa NP, Stryker MP. Sleep enhances plasticity in the developing visual cortex. *Neuron*. 2001;30(1):275–287.

5. Guzman-Marin R, Suntsova N, Stewart DR, et al. Sleep deprivation reduces proliferation of cells in the dentate gyrus of the hippocampus in rats. *J Physiol*. 2003;549(Pt 2):563–571.

6. Hobson JA. *Sleep*. New York: Scientific American Library; 1989.

7. Hobson JA, Pace-Schott EF. The cognitive neuroscience of sleep: Neuronal systems, consciousness and learning. *Nat Rev Neurosci*. 2002;3(9):679–693.

8. Horne JA. *Why we sleep: the functions of sleep in humans and other mammals*. Oxford: Oxford University Press; 1988.

9. Kryger MH, Roth T, Dement WC. *Principles and practice of sleep medicine*, 4th ed. Philadelphia: Elsevier Saunders; 2005.

10. Landrigan CP, Rothschild JM, Cronin JW, et al. Effect of reducing interns' work hours on serious medical errors in intensive care units. *N Engl J Med*. 2004;351(18):1838–1848.

11. Mahowald MW, Schenck CH. Insights from studying human sleep disorders. *Nature*. 2005;437(7063):1279–1285.

12. Mansour HA, Monk TH, Nimgaonkar VL. Circadian genes and bipolar disorder. *Ann Med*. 2005;37(3):196–205.

13. Meddis R. *The sleep instinct*. London: Routledge & Kegan Paul; 1977.

14. Mujhametov LM. Sleep in marine mammals. In: Borbely AA, ed. 1984.

15. Nofzinger EA, Buysse DJ, Germain A, et al. Functional neuroimaging evidence for hyperarousal in insomnia. *Am J Psychiatry*. 2004;161(11):2126–2128.

16. Ohayon MM, Carskadon MA, Guilleminault C, et al. Meta-analysis of quantitative sleep parameters from childhood to old age in healthy individuals: Developing normative sleep values across the human lifespan. *Sleep*. 2004;27(7):1255–1273.

17. Pace-Schott EF, Hobson JA. The neurobiology of sleep: Genetics, cellular physiology and subcortical networks. *Nat Rev Neurosci*. 2002;3(8):591–605.

18. Peigneux P, Laureys S, Fuchs S, et al. Are spatial memories strengthened in the human hippocampus during slow wave sleep? *Neuron*. 2004;44(3):535–545.

19. Purves D, Augustine GJ, Fitzpatrick D, et al. *Neuroscience*, 3rd ed. Sunderland, MA: Sinauer; 2004.

20. Ralph MR, Lehman MN. Transplantation: A new tool in the analysis of the mammalian hypothalamic circadian pacemaker. *Trends Neurosci*. 1991;14(8):362–366.

21. Reiter RJ. The melatonin rhythm: Both a clock and a calendar. *Experientia*. 1993;49(8):654–664.

22. Rosenzweig MR, Breedlove SM, Watson NV. *Biological psychology*, 4th ed. Sunderland, MA: Sinauer; 2005.

23. Saper CB, Scammell TE, Lu J. Hypothalamic regulation of sleep and circadian rhythms. *Nature*. 2005;437 (7063):1257–1263.

24. Siegel JM. Why we sleep. *Sci Am*. 2003;289(5):92–97.

25. Siegel JM. Clues to the functions of mammalian sleep. *Nature*. 2005;437(7063):1264–1271.

26. Sutherland GR, McNaughton B. Memory trace reactivation in hippocampal and neocortical neuronal ensembles. *Curr Opin Neurobiol*. 2000;10(2):180–186.

27. Taheri S, Lin L, Austin D, et al. Short sleep duration is associated with reduced leptin, elevated ghrelin, and increased body mass index. *PLoS Med*. 2004;1(3):e62.

28. Van Dongen HP, Maislin G, Mullington JM, et al. The cumulative cost of additional wakefulness: Dose-response effects on neurobehavioral functions and sleep physiology from chronic sleep restriction and total sleep deprivation. *Sleep*. 2003;26(2):117–126.

29. Wehr TA, Duncan WC Jr, Sher L, et al. A circadian signal of change of season in patients with seasonal affective disorder. *Arch Gen Psychiatry*. 2001;58(12): 1108–1114.

30. Wehr TA, Turner EH, Shimada JM, et al. Treatment of rapidly cycling bipolar patient by using extended bed rest and darkness to stabilize the timing and duration of sleep. *Biol Psychiatry*. 1998;43(11):822–828.

CHAPTER 13

1. Alexander GM, Hines M. Sex differences in response to children's toys in nonhuman primates (Cercopithecus aethiops sabaeus). *Evol Hum Behav*. 2002;23:467–479.

2. Allen LS, Hines M, Shryne JE, et al. Two sexually dimorphic cell groups in the human brain. *J Neurosci*. 1989;9(2):497–506.

3. Bear MF, Connors BW, Paradiso MA, eds. *Neuroscience: exploring the brain*, 3rd ed. Baltimore: Lippincott Williams & Wilkins; 2007.

4. Breedlove SM, Arnold AP. Hormonal control of a developing neuromuscular system. II. Sensitive periods for the androgen-induced masculinization of the rat spinal nucleus of the bulbocavernosus. *J Neurosci*. 1983;3(2):424–432.

5. Cohen LS, Altshuler LL, Harlow BL, et al. Relapse of major depression during pregnancy in women who maintain or discontinue antidepressant treatment. *JAMA*. 2006;295(5):499–507.

6. Colapinto J. *As nature made him: the boy who was raised as a girl*. New York: HarperCollins; 2000.

7. Conn J, Gillam L, Conway GS. Revealing the diagnosis of androgen insensitivity syndrome in adulthood. *Br Med J*. 2005;331(7517):628–630.

8. Hines M. Sex steroids and human behavior: Prenatal androgen exposure and sex-typical play behavior in children. *Ann N Y Acad Sci*. 2003;1007:272–282.

9. Hines M, Ahmed SF, Hughes IA. Psychological outcomes and gender-related development in complete androgen insensitivity syndrome. *Arch Sex Behav*. 2003; 32(2):93–101.

10. Kinsley CH, Lambert KG. The maternal brain. *Sci Am*. 2006;294(1):72–79.

11. Laumann EO, Paik A, Rosen RC. Sexual dysfunction in the United States: Prevalence and predictors. *JAMA*. 1999;281(6):537–544.

12. LeVay S. A difference in hypothalamic structure between heterosexual and homosexual men. *Science*. 1991;253(5023):1034–1037.

13. Nelson RJ. *An introduction to behavioral endocrinology*, 3rd ed. Sunderland, MA: Sinauer; 2005.

14. Nottebohm F. The road we travelled: Discovery, choreography, and significance of brain replaceable neurons. *Ann N Y Acad Sci*. 2004;1016:628–658.

15. Pfaus JG, Shadiack A, Van Soest T, et al. Selective facilitation of sexual solicitation in the female rat by a melanocortin receptor agonist. *Proc Natl Acad Sci U S A*. 2004;101(27):10201–10204.

16. Pope HG Jr, Cohane GH, Kanayama G, et al. Testosterone gel supplementation for men with refractory depression: A randomized, placebo-controlled trial. *Am J Psychiatry*. 2003;160(1):105–111.

17. Purves D, Augustine GJ, Fitzpatrick D, et al. *Neuroscience*, 3rd ed. Sunderland, MA: Sinauer; 2004.

18. Rapp SR, Espeland MA, Shumaker SA, et al. Effect of estrogen plus progestin on global cognitive function in postmenopausal women: The Women's Health Initiative Memory Study: A randomized controlled trial. *JAMA*. 2003;289(20):2663–2672.

19. Reiner WG, Gearhart JP. Discordant sexual identity in some genetic males with cloacal exstrophy assigned to female sex at birth. *N Engl J Med*. 2004;350(4):333–341.

20. Roselli CE, Larkin K, Resko JA, et al. The volume of a sexually dimorphic nucleus in the ovine medial preoptic area/anterior hypothalamus varies with sexual partner preference. *Endocrinology*. 2004;145(2):478–483.

21. Rosenzweig MR, Breedlove SM, Watson NV. *Biological psychology*, 4th ed. Sunderland, MA: Sinauer; 2005.

22. Rust J, Golombok S, Hines M, et al. The role of brothers and sisters in the gender development of preschool children. *J Exp Child Psychol*. 2000;77(4):292–303.

23. Soares CN, Almeida OP, Joffe H, et al. Efficacy of estradiol for the treatment of depressive disorders in perimenopausal women: A double-blind, randomized, placebo-controlled trial. *Arch Gen Psychiatry*. 2001;58(6):529–534.

24. Spitzer RL. Can some gay men and lesbians change their sexual orientation? 200 participants reporting a change from homosexual to heterosexual orientation. *Arch Sex Behav*. 2003;32(5):403–417; discussion 19–72.

25. Stahl SM. *Essential psychopharmacology. Neuroscientific basis of practical applications*, 2nd ed. New York: Cambridge University Press; 2000.
26. Wallen K. Nature needs nurture: The interaction of hormonal and social influences on the development of behavioral sex differences in rhesus monkeys. *Horm Behav*. 1996;30(4):364–378.
27. Woolley CS, Weiland NG, McEwen BS, et al. Estradiol increases the sensitivity of hippocampal CA1 pyramidal cells to NMDA receptor-mediated synaptic input: Correlation with dendritic spine density. *J Neurosci*. 1997;17(5):1848–1859.
28. Yang LY, Verhovshek T, Sengelaub DR. Brain-derived neurotrophic factor and androgen interact in the maintenance of dendritic morphology in a sexually dimorphic rat spinal nucleus. *Endocrinology*. 2004;145(1):161–168.
29. Zandi PP, Carlson MC, Plassman BL, et al. Hormone replacement therapy and incidence of Alzheimer disease in older women: The Cache County Study. *JAMA*. 2002;288(17):2123–2129.
30. Zucker KJ, Bradley SJ, Oliver G, et al. Psychosexual development of women with congenital adrenal hyperplasia. *Horm Behav*. 1996;30(4):300–318.

CHAPTER 14
1. Aron A, Fisher H, Mashek DJ, et al. Reward, motivation, and emotion systems associated with early-stage intense romantic love. *J Neurophysiol*. 2005;94(1):327–337.
2. Becker JB, Breedlove SM, Crews D, et al. *Behavioral endocrinology*, 2nd ed. Cambridge: MIT Press; 2002.
3. Bosch OJ, Meddle SL, Beiderbeck DI, et al. Brain oxytocin correlates with maternal aggression: Link to anxiety. *J Neurosci*. 2005;25(29):6807–6815.
4. Bridges RS. Endocrine regulation of parental behavior in rodents. In: Krasnegor NA, Bridges RS, eds. *Mammalian parenting: biochemical, neurobiological and behavioral determinants*. New York: Oxford University Press; 1990.
5. Carr L, Iacoboni M, Dubeau MC, et al. Neural mechanisms of empathy in humans: A relay from neural systems for imitation to limbic areas. *Proc Natl Acad Sci U S A*. 2003;100(9):5497–5502.
6. Dapretto M, Davies MS, Pfeifer JH, et al. Understanding emotions in others: Mirror neuron dysfunction in children with autism spectrum disorders. *Nat Neurosci*. 2006;9(1):28–30.
7. Emanuele E, Politi P, Bianchi M, et al. Raised plasma nerve growth factor levels associated with early-stage romantic love. *Psychoneuroendocrinology*. 2006;31:288–294.
8. Engh AL, Beehner JC, Bergman TJ, et al. Behavioral and hormonal responses to predation in female chacma baboons (Papio hamadryas ursinus). *Proc R Soc Lond B Biol Sci*. 2006;273(1578):707–712.
9. Felsenfeld G, Groudine M. Controlling the double helix. *Nature*. 2003;421(6921):448–453.
10. Francis D, Diorio J, Liu D, et al. Nongenomic transmission across generations of maternal behavior and stress responses in the rat. *Science*. 1999;286(5442):1155–1158.
11. Iacoboni M. Neural mechanisms of imitation. *Curr Opin Neurobiol*. 2005;15(6):632–637.
12. Klin A, Jones W, Schultz R, et al. Visual fixation patterns during viewing of naturalistic social situations as predictors of social competence in individuals with autism. *Arch Gen Psychiatry*. 2002;59(9):809–816.

13. Klin A, Jones W, Schultz R, et al. Defining and quantifying the social phenotype in autism. *Am J Psychiatry*. 2002;159(6):895–908.
14. Li M, Davidson P, Budin R, et al. Effects of typical and atypical antipsychotic drugs on maternal behavior in postpartum female rats. *Schizophr Res*. 2004;70(1):69–80.
15. Lim MM, Wang Z, Olazabal DE, et al. Enhanced partner preference in a promiscuous species by manipulating the expression of a single gene. *Nature*. 2004;429:754–757.
16. Liu D, Diorio J, Tannenbaum B, et al. Maternal care, hippocampal glucocorticoid receptors, and hypothalamic-pituitary-adrenal responses to stress. *Science*. 1997;277(5332):1659–1662.
17. Mcgue M, Lykken DT. Genetic influence on risk of divorce. *Psychol Sci*. 1992;3(6):368–373.
18. Nelson RJ. *An introduction to behavioral endocrinology*, 3rd ed. Sunderland, MA: Sinauer; 2005.
19. Numan M, Sheehan TP. Neuroanatomical circuitry for mammalian maternal behavior. *Ann N Y Acad Sci*. 1997;807:101–125.
20. Purves D, Augustine GJ, Fitzpatrick D, et al. *Neuroscience*, 3rd ed. Sunderland, MA: Sinauer; 2004.
21. Redcay E, Courchesne E. When is the brain enlarged in autism? A meta-analysis of all brain size reports. *Biol Psychiatry*. 2005;58(1):1–9.
22. Rizzolatti G, Fogassi L, Gallese V. Neurophysiological mechanisms underlying the understanding and imitation of action. *Nat Rev Neurosci*. 2001;2(9):661–670.
23. Rosenblatt JS, Siegel HI, Mayer AD. Blood levels of progesterone, estradiol and prolactin in pregnant rats. *Adv Study Behavior*. 1979;10:225–311.
24. Rosenzweig MR, Breedlove SM, Watson NV *Biological psychology*, 4th ed. Sunderland, MA: Sinauer; 2005.
25. Schultz RT, Anderson GM. The neurobiology of autism and the pervasive developmental disorders. In: Charney DS, Nestler EJ, eds. *Neurobiology of mental illness*, 2nd ed. Oxford: Oxford University Press; 2004:954–967.
26. Taylor SE, Klein LC, Lewis BP, et al. Biobehavioral responses to stress in females: Tend-and-befriend, not fight-or-flight. *Psychol Rev*. 2000;107(3):411–429.
27. Terkel J, Rosenblatt JS. Maternal behavior induced by maternal blood plasma injected into virgin rats. *J Comp Physiol Psychol*. 1968;65(3):479–482.
28. Weaver IC, Cervoni N, Champagne FA, et al. Epigenetic programming by maternal behavior. *Nat Neurosci*. 2004;7(8):847–854.
29. Werner E, Dawson G. Validation of the phenomenon of autistic regression using home videotapes. *Arch Gen Psychiatry*. 2005;62(8):889–895.
30. Young LJ, Wang Z. The neurobiology of pair bonding. *Nat Neurosci*. 2004;7(10):1048–1054.

CHAPTER 15
1. Barad M. Fear extinction in rodents: Basic insight to clinical promise. *Curr Opin Neurobiol*. 2005;15(6):710–715.
2. Bayley PJ, Gold JJ, Hopkins RO, et al. The neuroanatomy of remote memory. *Neuron*. 2005;46(5):799–810.
3. Bear MF, Connors BW, Paradiso MA, eds. *Neuroscience: exploring the brain*, 3rd ed. Baltimore: Lippincott Williams & Wilkins; 2007.
4. Corkin S. What's new with the amnesic patient H.M.? *Nat Rev Neurosci*. 2002;3(2):153–160.

5. Frankland PW, Bontempi B. The organization of recent and remote memories. *Nat Rev Neurosci*. 2005;6(2):119–130.
6. Genoux D, Haditsch U, Knobloch M, et al. Protein phosphatase 1 is a molecular constraint on learning and memory. *Nature*. 2002;418(6901):970–975.
7. Hebb DO. *The organization of behavior*. New York: Wiley; 1949.
8. Kandel ER, Schwartz JH, Jessell TM, eds. *Principles of neural science*, 4th ed. New York: McGraw-Hill; 2000.
9. Kirn J, O'Loughlin B, Kasparian S, et al. Cell death and neuronal recruitment in the high vocal center of adult male canaries are temporally related to changes in song. *Proc Natl Acad Sci U S A*. 1994;91(17):7844–7848.
10. Lamprecht R, LeDoux J. Structural plasticity and memory. *Nat Rev Neurosci*. 2004;5(1):45–54.
11. Leuner B, Falduto J, Shors TJ. Associative memory formation increases the observation of dendritic spines in the hippocampus. *J Neurosci*. 2003;23(2):659–665.
12. Leuner B, Mendolia-Loffredo S, Kozorovitskiy Y, et al. Learning enhances the survival of new neurons beyond the time when the hippocampus is required for memory. *J Neurosci*. 2004;24(34):7477–7481.
13. Luria AR. *The mind of a mnemonist*. New York: Basic Books; 1968.
14. Maviel T, Durkin TP, Menzaghi F, et al. Sites of neocortical reorganization critical for remote spatial memory. *Science*. 2004;305(5680):96–99.
15. Meiri N, Rosenblum K. Lateral ventricle injection of the protein synthesis inhibitor anisomycin impairs long-term memory in a spatial memory task. *Brain Res*. 1998;789(1):48–55.
16. Nader K, Schafe GE, Le Doux JE. Fear memories require protein synthesis in the amygdala for reconsolidation after retrieval. *Nature*. 2000;406(6797):722–726.
17. Purves D, Augustine GJ, Fitzpatrick D, et al. *Neuroscience*, 3rd ed. Sunderland, MA: Sinauer; 2004.
18. Ressler KJ, Rothbaum BO, Tannenbaum L, et al. Cognitive enhancers as adjuncts to psychotherapy: Use of D-cycloserine in phobic individuals to facilitate extinction of fear. *Arch Gen Psychiatry*. 2004;61(11):1136–1144.
19. Rosenzweig MR, Breedlove SM, Watson NV. *Biological psychology*, 4th ed. Sunderland, MA: Sinauer; 2005.
20. Santini E, Ge H, Ren K, et al. Consolidation of fear extinction requires protein synthesis in the medial prefrontal cortex. *J Neurosci*. 2004;24(25):5704–5710.
21. Squire LR, Slater PC, Chace PM. Retrograde amnesia: Temporal gradient in very long term memory following electroconvulsive therapy. *Science*. 1975;187(4171):77–79.
22. Squire LR, Slater PC, Miller PL. Retrograde amnesia and bilateral electroconvulsive therapy. *Arch Gen Psychiatry*. 1981;38(1):89–95.
23. Van Hoesen GW. The parahippocampal gyrus: New observations regarding its cortical connections in the monkey. *Trends Neurosci*. 1982;5:345–350.

CHAPTER 16

1. Andreasen NC. *The creating brain: the neuroscience of genius*. New York: Dana Press; 2005.
2. Beckett C, Maughan B, Rutter M, et al. Do the effects of early severe deprivation on cognition persist into early adolescence? Findings from the English and Romanian adoptees study. *Child Dev*. 2006;77(3):696–711.

3. Breslau N, Lucia VC, Alvarado GF. Intelligence and other predisposing factors in exposure to trauma and posttraumatic stress disorder. *Arch Gen Psychiatry*. 2006;63(11):1238–1245.
4. Carlsson I, Wendt PE, Risberg J. On the neurobiology of creativity. Differences in frontal activity between high and low creative subjects. *Neuropsychologia*. 2000;38(6):873–885.
5. Carson SH, Peterson JB, Higgins DM. Decreased latent inhibition is associated with increased creative achievement in high-functioning individuals. *J Pers Soc Psychol*. 2003;85(3):499–506.
6. Cooper NJ, Keage H, Hermens D, et al. The dose-dependent effect of methylphenidate on performance, cognition and psychophysiology. *J Integr Neurosci*. 2005;4(1):123–144.
7. Dierssen M, Ramakers GJA. Dendritic pathology in mental retardation: From molecular genetics to neurobiology. *Genes Brain Behav*. 2006;5(Suppl 2):48–60.
8. Duncan J, Burgess P, Emslie H. Fluid intelligence after frontal lobe lesions. *Neuropsychologia*. 1995;33(3):261–268.
9. Gottfredson LS. The general intelligence factor. *Sci Am Presents: Exploring Intell*. 1998;9(4):24–29.
10. Gray JR, Thompson PM. Neurobiology of intelligence: Science and ethics. *Nat Rev Neurosci*. 2004;5(6):471–482.
11. Hall KM, Irwin MM, Bowman KA, et al. Illicit use of prescribed stimulant medication among college students. *J Am Coll Health*. 2005;53(4):167–174.
12. Jamison KR. Manic-depressive illness and creativity. *Sci Am*. 1995;272(2):62–67.
13. Lee KH, Choi YY, Gray JR, et al. Neural correlates of superior intelligence: Stronger recruitment of posterior parietal cortex. *Neuroimage*. 2006;29(2):578–586.
14. McDaniel MA. Big-brained people are smarter: A meta-analysis of the relationship between *in vivo* brain volume and intelligence. *Intelligence*. 2005;33(4):337–346.
15. Mell JC, Howard SM, Miller BL. Art and the brain: The influence of frontotemporal dementia on an accomplished artist. *Neurology*. 2003;60(10):1707–1710.
16. Nottebohm F. The road we travelled: Discovery, choreography, and significance of brain replaceable neurons. *Ann N Y Acad Sci*. 2004;1016:628–658.
17. Plomin R, DeFries JC. The genetics of cognitive abilities and disabilities. *Sci Am*. 1998;278(5):62–69.
18. Purpura DP. Dendritic spine "dysgenesis" and mental retardation. *Science*. 1974;186(4169):1126–1128.
19. Schoenemann PT, Sheehan MJ, Glotzer LD. Prefrontal white matter volume is disproportionately larger in humans than in other primates. *Nat Neurosci*. 2005;8(2):242–252.
20. Shaw P, Greenstein D, Lerch J, et al. Intellectual ability and cortical development in children and adolescents. *Nature*. 2006;440(7084):676–679.
21. Shaywitz SE, Shaywitz BA. Dyslexia (specific reading disability). *Biol Psychiatry*. 2005;57(11):1301–1309.
22. Simonton DK. Are genius and madness related? Contemporary answers to an ancient question. *Psychiatric Times*. 2005;22(7):23–23.

CHAPTER 17

1. Bear MF, Connors BW, Paradiso MA, eds. *Neuroscience: exploring the brain*, 3rd ed. Baltimore: Lippincott Williams & Wilkins; 2007.
2. Ben-Pazi H, Shalev RS, Gross-Tsur V, et al. Age and medication effects on rhythmic response in ADHD:

Possible oscillatory mechanisms? *Neuropsychologia*. 2006;44:412–416.

3. Bobb AJ, Castellanos FX, Addington AM, et al. Molecular genetic studies of ADHD: 1991 to 2004. *Am J Med Genet B Neuropsychiatr Genet*. 2005;132(1):109–125.

4. Cardinal RN, Pennicott DR, Sugathapala CL, et al. Impulsive choice induced in rats by lesions of the nucleus accumbens core. *Science*. 2001;292(5526):2499–2501.

5. Cardinal RN, Winstanley CA, Robbins TW, et al. Limbic corticostriatal systems and delayed reinforcement. *Ann N Y Acad Sci*. 2004;1021:33–50.

6. Castellanos FX, Lee PP, Sharp W, et al. Developmental trajectories of brain volume abnormalities in children and adolescents with attention-deficit/hyperactivity disorder. *JAMA*. 2002;288(14):1740–1748.

7. Castellanos FX, Tannock R. Neuroscience of attention-deficit/hyperactivity disorder: The search for endophenotypes. *Nat Rev Neurosci*. 2002;3(8):617–628.

8. Castner SA, Williams GV, Goldman-Rakic PS. Reversal of antipsychotic-induced working memory deficits by short-term dopamine D1 receptor stimulation. *Science*. 2000;287(5460):2020–2022.

9. Faraone SV, Biederman J, Mick E. The age-dependent decline of attention deficit hyperactivity disorder: A meta-analysis of follow-up studies. *Psychol Med*. 2006; 36(2):159–165.

10. Fuster JM. Unit activity in prefrontal cortex during delayed-response performance: Neuronal correlates of transient memory. *J Neurophysiol*. 1973;36(1):61–78.

11. Greenberg LM, Crosby RD. *A summary of developmental normative data on the T.O.V.A. ages 4 to 80+*. Unpublished manuscript available through The TOVA company; 1992.

12. Larisch R, Sitte W, Antke C, et al. Striatal dopamine transporter density in drug naive patients with attention-deficit/hyperactivity disorder. *Nucl Med Commun*. 2006;27(3):267–270.

13. Levesque J, Beauregard M, Mensour B. Effect of neurofeedback training on the neural substrates of selective attention in children with attention-deficit/hyperactivity disorder: A functional magnetic resonance imaging study. *Neurosci Lett*. 2006;394(3):216–221.

14. McEvoy SP, Stevenson MR, McCartt AT, et al. Role of mobile phones in motor vehicle crashes resulting in hospital attendance: A case-crossover study. *BMJ*. 2005;331(7514):428.

15. Mozley PD, Acton PD, Barraclough ED, et al. Effects of age on dopamine transporters in healthy humans. *J Nucl Med*. 1999;40(11):1812–1817.

16. Phillips AG, Ahn S, Floresco SB. Magnitude of dopamine release in medial prefrontal cortex predicts accuracy of memory on a delayed response task. *J Neurosci*. 2004;24(2):547–553.

17. Purves D, Augustine GJ, Fitzpatrick D, et al. *Neuroscience*, 3rd ed. Sunderland, MA: Sinauer; 2004.

18. Shaw P, Lerch J, Greenstein D, et al. Longitudinal mapping of cortical thickness and clinical outcome in children and adolescents with attention-deficit/hyperactivity disorder. *Arch Gen Psychiatry*. 2006;63(5):540–549.

19. Springer SP, Deutsch G. *Left brain, right brain*. New York: Worth Publishers; 1998.

20. Tamm L, Menon V, Reiss AL. Parietal attentional system aberrations during target detection in adolescents with attention deficit hyperactivity disorder: Event-related fMRI evidence. *Am J Psychiatry*. 2006;163(6): 1033–1043.

21. Toplak ME, Dockstader C, Tannock R. Temporal information processing in ADHD: Findings to date and new methods. *J Neurosci Methods*. 2006;151(1):15–29.

22. Volkow ND, Wang GJ, Fowler JS, et al. Evidence that methylphenidate enhances the saliency of a mathematical task by increasing dopamine in the human brain. *Am J Psychiatry*. 2004;161(7):1173–1180.

23. Volkow ND, Wang GJ, Fowler JS, et al. Imaging the effects of methylphenidate on brain dopamine: New model on its therapeutic actions for attention-deficit/hyperactivity disorder. *Biol Psychiatry*. 2005; 57(11):1410–1415.

CHAPTER 18

1. Berton O, McClung CA, Dileone RJ, et al. Essential role of BDNF in the mesolimbic dopamine pathway in social defeat stress. *Science*. 2006;311(5762):864–868.

2. Berton O, Nestler EJ. New approaches to antidepressant drug discovery: Beyond monoamines. *Nat Rev Neurosci*. 2006;7(2):137–151.

3. Czeh B, Michaelis T, Watanabe T, et al. Stress-induced changes in cerebral metabolites, hippocampal volume, and cell proliferation are prevented by antidepressant treatment with tianeptine. *Proc Natl Acad Sci U S A*. 2001;98(22):12796–12801.

4. Deuschle M, Schweiger U, Weber B, et al. Diurnal activity and pulsatility of the hypothalamus-pituitary-adrenal system in male depressed patients and healthy controls. *J Clin Endocrinol Metab*. 1997;82(1):234–238.

5. Drevets WC. Neuroimaging and neuropathological studies of depression: Implications for the cognitive-emotional features of mood disorders. *Curr Opin Neurobiol*. 2001;11(2):240–249.

6. Duman RS. The neurochemistry of depressive disorders: Preclinical studies. In: Charney DS, Nestler EJ, eds. *Neurobiology of mental illness*, 2nd ed. New York: Oxford University Press; 2004:421–439.

7. Dwivedi Y, Rizavi HS, Conley RR, et al. Altered gene expression of brain-derived neurotrophic factor and receptor tyrosine kinase B in postmortem brain of suicide subjects. *Arch Gen Psychiatry*. 2003;60(8):804–815.

8. Gonul AS, Akdeniz F, Taneli F, et al. Effect of treatment on serum brain-derived neurotrophic factor levels in depressed patients. *Eur Arch Psychiatry Clin Neurosci*. 2005;255(6):381–386.

9. Haldane M, Frangou S. New insights help define the pathophysiology of bipolar affective disorder: Neuroimaging and neuropathology findings. *Prog Neuropsychopharmacol Biol Psychiatry*. 2004;28(6): 943–960.

10. Haldane M, Frangou S. Functional neuroimaging studies in mood disorders. *Acta Neuropsychiatrica*. 2006; 18:88–99.

11. Holsboer F. Stress, hypercortisolism and corticosteroid receptors in depression: Implications for therapy. *J Affect Disord*. 2001;62(1–2):77–91.

12. Koss S, George MS. Functional magnetic resonance imaging investigations in mood disorders. In: Soares JC, ed. *Brain imaging in affective disorders*. New York: Marcel Dekker Inc; 2003.

13. Mamounas LA, Blue ME, Siuciak JA, et al. Brain-derived neurotrophic factor promotes the survival and sprouting of serotonergic axons in rat brain. *J Neurosci*. 1995;15(12):7929–7939.

14. Manji HK, Quiroz JA, Sporn J, et al. Enhancing neuronal plasticity and cellular resilience to develop novel, improved therapeutics for difficult-to-treat depression. *Biol Psychiatry*. 2003;53(8):707–742.

15. McQuade R, Young AH. Future therapeutic targets in mood disorders: The glucocorticoid receptor. *Br J Psychiatry*. 2000;177:390–395.

Progress in neuro-psychopharmacology & Biological psychiatry

16. Moore GJ, Bebchuk JM, Wilds IB, et al. Lithium-induced increase in human brain grey matter. *Lancet*. 2000;356(9237):1241–1242.

17. Nobler MS, Oquendo MA, Kegeles LS, et al. Decreased regional brain metabolism after ect. *Am J Psychiatry*. 2001;158(2):305–308.

18. Rajkowska G, Miguel-Hidalgo JJ, Wei J, et al. Morphometric evidence for neuronal and glial prefrontal cell pathology in major depression. *Biol Psychiatry*. 1999;45(9):1085–1098.

19. Santarelli L, Saxe M, Gross C, et al. Requirement of hippocampal neurogenesis for the behavioral effects of antidepressants. *Science*. 2003;301(5634):805–809.

20. Sheline YI, Gado MH, Kraemer HC. Untreated depression and hippocampal volume loss. *Am J Psychiatry*. 2003;160(8):1516–1518.

21. Tsankova NM, Berton O, Renthal W, et al. Sustained hippocampal chromatin regulation in a mouse model of depression and antidepressant action. *Nat Neurosci*. 2006;9(4):519–525.

22. Videbech P, Ravnkilde B. Hippocampal volume and depression: A meta-analysis of MRI studies. *Am J Psychiatry*. 2004;161(11):1957–1966.

23. Wong ML, Licinio J. Research and treatment approaches to depression. *Nat Rev Neurosci*. 2001;2(5): 343–351.

24. Zobel AW, Nickel T, Sonntag A, et al. Cortisol response in the combined dexamethasone/CRH test as predictor of relapse in patients with remitted depression. A prospective study. *J Psychiatr Res*. 2001;35(2): 83–94.

CHAPTER 19

1. Abi-Dargham A, Krystal JH, Anjilvel S, et al. Alterations of benzodiazepine receptors in type II alcoholic subjects measured with SPECT and [123I]iomazenil. *Am J Psychiatry*. 1998;155(11):1550–1555.

2. Barlow DH, Gorman JM, Shear MK, et al. Cognitive-behavioral therapy, imipramine, or their combination for panic disorder: A randomized controlled trial. *JAMA*. 2000;283(19):2529–2536.

3. Baxter LR Jr, Schwartz JM, Bergman KS, et al. Caudate glucose metabolic rate changes with both drug and behavior therapy for obsessive-compulsive disorder. *Arch Gen Psychiatry*. 1992;49(9):681–689.

4. Berton O, McClung CA, Dileone RJ, et al. Essential role of BDNF in the mesolimbic dopamine pathway in social defeat stress. *Science*. 2006;311(5762):864–868.

5. Calder AJ, Lawrence AD, Young AW. Neuropsychology of fear and loathing. *Nat Rev Neurosci*. 2001;2(5): 352–363.

6. Charney DS. Neuroanatomical circuits modulating fear and anxiety behaviors. *Acta Psychiatr Scand Suppl*. 2003(417):38–50.

7. Furmark T, Tillfors M, Marteinsdottir I, et al. Common changes in cerebral blood flow in patients with social phobia treated with citalopram or cognitive-behavioral therapy. *Arch Gen Psychiatry*. 2002;59(5):425–433.

8. Gilbertson MW, Shenton ME, Ciszewski A, et al. Smaller hippocampal volume predicts pathologic vulnerability to psychological trauma. *Nat Neurosci*. 2002; 5(11):1242–1247.

9. Gross C, Hen R. The developmental origins of anxiety. *Nat Rev Neurosci*. 2004;5(7):545–552.

10. Kirschbaum C, Prussner JC, Stone AA, et al. Persistent high cortisol responses to repeated psychological stress in a subpopulation of healthy men. *Psychosom Med*. 1995;57(5):468–474.

11. Kushner MG, Abrams K, Borchardt C. The relationship between anxiety disorders and alcohol use disorders: A review of major perspectives and findings. *Clin Psychol Rev*. 2000;20(2):149–171.

12. LeDoux JE. Emotion, memory and the brain. *Sci Am*. 1994;270(6):50–57.

13. LeDoux JE. *The synaptic self: how our brains become who we are: viking*. 2002.

14. Likhtik E, Pelletier JG, Paz R, et al. Prefrontal control of the amygdala. *J Neurosci*. 2005;25(32):7429–7437.

15. Lorberbaum JP, Kose S, Johnson MR, et al. Neural correlates of speech anticipatory anxiety in generalized social phobia. *Neuroreport*. 2004;15(18):2701–2705.

16. Maren S, Ferrario CR, Corcoran KA, et al. Protein synthesis in the amygdala, but not the auditory thalamus, is required for consolidation of Pavlovian fear conditioning in rats. *Eur J Neurosci*. 2003;18(11):3080–3088.

17. Mashour GA, Walker EE, Martuza RL. Psychosurgery: Past, present, and future. *Brain Res Brain Res Rev*. 2005;48(3):409–419.

18. Montgomery SM, Ehlin A, Sacker A. Breast feeding and resilience against psychosocial stress. *Arch Dis Child*. 2006;91(12):990–994.

19. Otto MW, Smits JAJ, Reese HE. Combined psychotherapy and pharmacotherapy for mood and anxiety disorders in adults: Review and analysis. *Clin Psychol: Sci Pract*. 2005;12(1):72–86.

20. Purves D, Augustine GJ, Fitzpatrick D, et al. *Neuroscience*, 3rd ed. Sunderland, MA: Sinauer; 2004.

21. Richter EO, Davis KD, Hamani C, et al. Cingulotomy for psychiatric disease: Microelectrode guidance, a callosal reference system for documenting lesion location, and clinical results. *Neurosurgery*. 2004;54(3):622–628; discussion 8–30.

22. Rosenzweig MR, Breedlove SM, Watson NV. *Biological psychology*, 4th ed. Sunderland, MA: Sinauer; 2005.

23. Shin LM, Wright CI, Cannistraro PA, et al. A functional magnetic resonance imaging study of amygdala and medial prefrontal cortex responses to overtly presented fearful faces in posttraumatic stress disorder. *Arch Gen Psychiatry*. 2005;62(3):273–281.

24. Stein DJ. Obsessive-compulsive disorder. *Lancet*. 2002; 360(9330):397–405.

25. Ursin H, Baade E, Levine S. *Psychobiology of stress: a study of coping men*. New York: Academic Press; 1978.

26. Vyas A, Pillai AG, Chattarji S. Recovery after chronic stress fails to reverse amygdaloid neuronal hypertrophy and enhanced anxiety-like behavior. *Neuroscience*. 2004;128(4):667–673.

27. Yen CP, Kung SS, Su YF, et al. Stereotactic bilateral anterior cingulotomy for intractable pain. *J Clin Neurosci*. 2005;12(8):886–890.

CHAPTER 20

1. Abdolmaleky HM, Cheng KH, Russo A, et al. Hypermethylation of the reelin (RELN) promoter in the brain of schizophrenic patients: A preliminary report. *Am J Med Genet B Neuropsychiatr Genet*. 2005;134(1): 60–66.

2. Adityanjee, Aderibigbe YA, Theodoridis D, et al. Dementia praecox to schizophrenia: The first 100 years. *Psychiatry Clin Neurosci*. 1999;53(4):437–448.

3. Akbarian S, Kim JJ, Potkin SG, et al. Gene expression for glutamic acid decarboxylase is reduced without loss of neurons in prefrontal cortex of schizophrenics. *Arch Gen Psychiatry*. 1995;52(4):258–266.

4. Baumeister AA, Francis JL. Historical development of the dopamine hypothesis of schizophrenia. *J Hist Neurosci*. 2002;11(3):265–277.

5. Black DN, Taber KH, Hurley RA. Metachromatic leukodystrophy: A model for the study of psychosis. *J Neuropsychiatry Clin Neurosci*. 2003;15(3):289–293.

6. Brun A, Park HJ, Knutsson H, et al. *Coloring of DT-MRI fiber traces using laplacian eigenmaps*. Available at http://lmi.bwh.harvard.edu/papers/papers/brunEUROCAST03.html. 2003.

7. Davis KL, Stewart DG, Friedman JI, et al. White matter changes in schizophrenia: Evidence for myelin-related dysfunction. *Arch Gen Psychiatry*. 2003;60(5):443–456.

8. Dierks T, Linden DE, Jandl M, et al. Activation of Heschls gyrus during auditory hallucinations. *Neuron*. 1999;22(3):615–621.

9. Evans K, McGrath J, Milns R. Searching for schizophrenia in ancient Greek and Roman literature: A systematic review. *Acta Psychiatr Scand*. 2003;107(5): 323–330.

10. Glantz LA, Gilmore JH, Lieberman JA, et al. Apoptotic mechanisms and the synaptic pathology of schizophrenia. *Schizophr Res*. 2006;81(1):47–63.

11. Glantz LA, Lewis DA. Decreased dendritic spine density on prefrontal cortical pyramidal neurons in schizophrenia. *Arch Gen Psychiatry*. 2000;57(1): 65–73.

12. Gogtay N, Sporn A, Rapoport J. Structural brain MRI studies in childhood-onset schizophrenia and childhood atypical psychosis. In: Lawrie S, Johnstone E, Weinberger D, eds. *Schizophrenia: from neuroimaging to neuroscience*. New York: Oxford University Press; 2004.

13. Hakak Y, Walker JR, Li C, et al. Genome-wide expression analysis reveals dysregulation of myelination-related genes in chronic schizophrenia. *Proc Natl Acad Sci U S A*. 2001;98(8):4746–4751.

14. Hof PR, Haroutunian V, Friedrich VL Jr, et al. Loss and altered spatial distribution of oligodendrocytes in the superior frontal gyrus in schizophrenia. *Biol Psychiatry*. 2003;53(12):1075–1085.

15. Hubl D, Koenig T, Strik W, et al. Pathways that make voices: White matter changes in auditory hallucinations. *Arch Gen Psychiatry*. 2004;61(7):658–668.

16. Hulshoff Pol HE, Schnack HG, Bertens MG, et al. Volume changes in gray matter in patients with schizophrenia. *Am J Psychiatry*. 2002;159(2):244–250.

17. Lawrie S, Johnstone E, Weinberger D. *Schizophrenia: from neuroimaging to neuroscience*. New York: Oxford University Press; 2004.

18. Lewis DA, Hashimoto T, Volk DW. Cortical inhibitory neurons and schizophrenia. *Nat Rev Neurosci*. 2005;6(4):312–324.

19. Lewis DA, Lieberman JA. Catching up on schizophrenia: Natural history and neurobiology. *Neuron*. 2000; 28(2):325–334.

20. Liberman RP, Musgrave JG, Langlois J. Taunton State Hospital, Massachusetts. *Am J Psychiatry*. 2003; 160(12):2098.

21. McClellan JM, Susser E, King MC. Maternal famine, de novo mutations, and schizophrenia. *JAMA*. 2006; 296(5):582–584.

22. Pedersen CB, Mortensen PB. Urbanization and traffic related exposures as risk factors for schizophrenia. *BMC Psychiatry*. 2006;6:2.

23. Selemon LD. Increased cortical neuronal density in schizophrenia. *Am J Psychiatry*. 2004;161(9):1564.

24. Selemon LD, Goldman-Rakic PS. The reduced neuropil hypothesis: A circuit based model of schizophrenia. *Biol Psychiatry*. 1999;45(1):17–25.

25. Sporn AL, Greenstein DK, Gogtay N, et al. Progressive brain volume loss during adolescence in childhood-onset schizophrenia. *Am J Psychiatry*. 2003;160(12): 2181–2189.

26. Suddath RL, Christison GW, Torrey EF, et al. Anatomical abnormalities in the brains of monozygotic twins discordant for schizophrenia. *N Engl J Med*. 1990; 322(12):789–794.

27. Tamminga C, Hashimoto T, Volk DW, et al. GABA neurons in the human prefrontal cortex. *Am J Psychiatry*. 2004;161(10):1764.

28. Tienari P, Wynne LC, Sorri A, et al. Genotype-environment interaction in schizophrenia-spectrum disorder. Long-term follow-up study of Finnish adoptees. *Br J Psychiatry Suppl*. 2004;184:216–222.

29. Torrey EF, Miller J. *The invisible plague: the rise of mental illness from 1750 to the present*. New Brunswick, NJ: Rutgers University Press; 2001.

30. Walker E, Kestler L, Bollini A, et al. Schizophrenia: Etiology and course. *Annu Rev Psychol*. 2004;55:401–430.

31. Weinberger DR, Berman KF, Zec RF. Physiologic dysfunction of dorsolateral prefrontal cortex in schizophrenia. I. Regional cerebral blood flow evidence. *Arch Gen Psychiatry*. 1986;43(2):114–124.

CHAPTER 21

1. Baas PW, Qiang L. Neuronal microtubules: When the MAP is the roadblock. *Trends Cell Biol*. 2005;15(4): 183–187.

2. Bennett DA, Schneider JA, Wilson RS, et al. Education modifies the association of amyloid but not tangles with cognitive function. *Neurology*. 2005;65(6):953–955.

3. Blennow K, de Leon MJ, Zetterberg H. Alzheimer's disease. *Lancet*. 2006;368(9533):387–403.

4. Braak H, Braak E. Frequency of stages of Alzheimer-related lesions in different age categories. *Neurobiol Aging*. 1997;18(4):351–357.

5. Finger S. *Origins of neuroscience: a history of explorations into brain functions*. Oxford: Oxford University Press; 1994.

6. Fox NC, Schott JM. Imaging cerebral atrophy: Normal ageing to Alzheimer's disease. *Lancet*. 2004;363(9406): 392–394.

7. Fuso A, Seminara L, Cavallaro RA, et al. S-adenosylmethionine/homocysteine cycle alterations modify DNA methylation status with consequent deregulation of PS1 and BACE and beta-amyloid production. *Mol Cell Neurosci*. 2005;28(1):195–204.

8. Hayflick L. The future of ageing. *Nature*. 2000;408 (6809):267–269.

9. Herholz K, Salmon E, Perani D, et al. Discrimination between Alzheimer dementia and controls by automated analysis of multicenter FDG PET. *Neuroimage*. 2002;17(1):302–316.

10. Kandel ER, Schwartz JH, Jessell TM, eds. *Principles of neural science*, 4th ed. New York: McGraw-Hill; 2000.

11. Klunk WE, Engler H, Nordberg A, et al. Imaging brain amyloid in Alzheimer's disease with Pittsburgh compound-B. *Ann Neurol*. 2004;55(3):306–319.

12. Lemere CA, Maier M, Jiang L, et al. Amyloid-beta immunotherapy for the prevention and treatment of Alzheimer disease: Lessons from mice, monkeys, and humans. *Rejuvenation Res*. 2006;9(1):77–84.

13. Mattson MP. Pathways towards and away from Alzheimer's disease. *Nature*. 2004;430(7000):631–639.

14. Mattson MP, Magnus T. Ageing and neuronal vulnerability. *Nat Rev Neurosci*. 2006;7(4):278–294.
15. Morgan D, Diamond DM, Gottschall PE, et al. A beta peptide vaccination prevents memory loss in an animal model of Alzheimer's disease. *Nature*. 2000;408(6815):982–985.
16. Mortimer JA. Brain reserve and the clinical expression of Alzheimer's disease. *Geriatrics*. 1997;52(Suppl 2):S50–S53.
17. Qin W, Chachich M, Lane M, et al. Calorie restriction attenuates Alzheimer's disease type brain amyloidosis in squirrel monkeys (saimiri sciureus). *J Alzheimers Dis*. 2006;10:417–422.
18. Ridley RM, Baker HF, Windle CP, et al. Very long term studies of the seeding of beta-amyloidosis in primates. *J Neural Transm*. 2006;113:1243–1251.
19. Schenk D, Hagen M, Seubert P. Current progress in beta-amyloid immunotherapy. *Curr Opin Immunol*. 2004;16(5):599–606.
20. Snowdon DA, Kemper SJ, Mortimer JA, et al. Linguistic ability in early life and cognitive function and Alzheimer's disease in late life. Findings from the Nun Study. *JAMA*. 1996;275(7):528–532.
21. Tuszynski MH, Thal L, Pay M, et al. A phase 1 clinical trial of nerve growth factor gene therapy for Alzheimer disease. *Nat Med*. 2005;11(5):551–555.
22. Wang J, Ho L, Zhao Z, et al. Moderate consumption of Carernet Sauvignon attenuates AB neuropathology in a mouse model of Alzheimer's disease. *FASEB J*. 2006;20:2313–2320.
23. Wolfe MS. Shutting down Alzheimer's. *Sci Am*. 2006;294(5):72–79.

Answers to End-of-Chapter Questions

CHAPTER 1

Part 1

1. L
2. E
3. B
4. D
5. F
6. C
7. J
8. A
9. H
10. G
11. K
12. I

Part 2

13. P
14. N
15. O
16. M
17. Q

CHAPTER 2

1. b
2. c
3. a
4. c
5. d
6. a
7. b
8. d

CHAPTER 3

1. c
2. a
3. b
4. d
5. a

6. b
7. d
8. a

CHAPTER 4

1. c
2. b
3. d
4. a
5. d
6. c
7. a
8. d

CHAPTER 5

1. c
2. b
3. c
4. a
5. d
6. b
7. d
8. d

CHAPTER 6

1. c
2. d
3. a
4. c
5. b
6. b
7. a

CHAPTER 7

1. d
2. a
3. b
4. c

5. c
6. a
7. d
8. b

CHAPTER 8

1. c
2. b
3. a
4. d
5. c
6. d
7. b
8. a

CHAPTER 9

1. c
2. a
3. d
4. b
5. a
6. c
7. d
8. a
9. b

CHAPTER 10

1. d
2. b
3. a
4. c
5. b
6. a
7. d
8. c

CHAPTER 11

1. a
2. c

3. b
4. d
5. c
6. d
7. a
8. b

CHAPTER 12

1. a
2. b
3. d
4. a
5. c
6. c
7. d
8. c

CHAPTER 13

1. d
2. a
3. c
4. b
5. d
6. c
7. a
8. b

CHAPTER 14

1. c
2. d
3. b
4. a
5. b
6. a
7. d
8. c

CHAPTER 15

1. b
2. a
3. d
4. c
5. a
6. d
7. c
8. b

CHAPTER 16

1. a
2. c
3. d
4. b
5. b
6. c

CHAPTER 17

1. d
2. c
3. b
4. a
5. c
6. b
7. 1. C
   2. B
   3. D
   4. A

CHAPTER 18

1. b
2. a
3. c
4. d
5. a

6. b
7. c
8. d

CHAPTER 19

1. b
2. c
3. d
4. a
5. a
6. d
7. b
8. c

CHAPTER 20

1. d
2. b
3. a
4. c
5. d
6. a
7. c
8. 1. E
   2. D
   3. B
   4. F
   5. A
   6. C

CHAPTER 21

1. d
2. c
3. a
4. b
5. c
6. d
7. b

Index